Community as Client:
Application of the Nursing Process

ELIZABETH T. ANDERSON, R.N., C., Dr. PH.

Professor
University of Texas
School of Nursing at Galveston
Galveston, Texas

JUDITH M. McFARLANE, R.N., C., Dr. PH.

Community Health Nursing Professor
College of Nursing
Texas Woman's University
Houston, Texas

With 8 contributors

J. B. LIPPINCOTT COMPANY   *Philadelphia*

London,   Mexico City,   New York,   St. Louis,   São Paulo,   Sydney

COMMUNITY AS CLIENT

Application of the Nursing Process

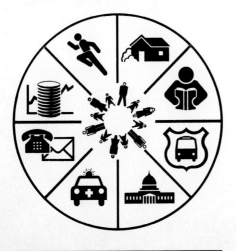

Acquisition/Sponsoring Editor: Nancy L. Mullins
Coordinating Editorial Assistant: Nancy L. McFarland
Manuscript Editor: Brenda Lee Reed
Indexer: Ellen Murray
Senior Design Coordinator: Anita Curry
Designer: Katharine Nichols
Production Manager: Kathleen P. Dunn
Production Coordinator: Fred D. Wood IV
Compositor: Tapsco, Inc.
Printer/Binder: R. R. Donnelley & Sons
Cover photographs courtesy of Community Home Health Services
Cover Design: Anne O'Donnell

1   3   5   6   4   2

Library of Congress Cataloging-in-Publication Data

Community as client.

Includes index.
1. Community health nursing.   2. Public health
nursing.   I. Anderson, Elizabeth T.   II. McFarlane,
Judith M.   [DNLM: 1. Community Health Nursing—
United States.   WY 106 C7334]
RT98.C63   1988   610.73'43   87-3518
ISBN 0-397-54564-9

Any procedure or practice described in this book should be applied
by the health-care practitioner under appropriate supervision in
accordance with professional standards of care used with regard to
the unique circumstances that apply in each practice situation. Care
has been taken to confirm the accuracy of information presented
and to describe generally accepted practices. However, the authors,
editors, and publisher cannot accept any responsibility for errors or
omissions or for consequences from application of the information
in this book and make no warranty, express or implied, with respect
to the contents of the book.

Every effort has been made to ensure drug selections and dosages are in accordance with current recommendations and practice.
Because of ongoing research, changes in government regulations
and the constant flow of information on drug therapy, reactions and
interactions, the reader is cautioned to check the package insert for
each drug for indications, dosages, and warnings and precautions,
particularly if the drug is new or infrequently used.

For *inspiriting* Community as Client, *we wish to acknowledge communities everywhere* . . .

> *public health service areas;*
> *rural villages;*
> *shelters for battered women, the homeless,*
>   *refugees, and migrants;*
> *factories;*
> *urban neighborhoods;*
> *schools* . . .

and the nurses who work in partnership with them.

Community as Client: Application of the Nursing Process
is dedicated to you.

Contributors

Kathryn J. Gardner, R.N., M.P.H.
Supervisor, Clinical Health Education
City of Houston Health Department of Health and Human Services
Houston, Texas

Chapter 13: The Teaching Role in Community Health Nursing

Janet Heinrich, R.N., Dr. PH.
Assistant Director
Congressional and Agency Relations
American Nurse's Association
Washington, DC

Chapter 3: The Political Process and Change

Linda Linville, R.N., M.S.
Director
Division of Public Health Nursing
Texas Department of Health
Austin, Texas

Chapter 14: The Management Role in Community Health Nursing

A. Russell Lokkeberg, Dr. PH.
Associate Professor and Coordinator
Health Care Administration, Texas Woman's University
Houston, Texas

Chapter 1: The Health Care System

Sally Lechlitner Lusk, Ph.D., R.N.
Associate Professor
University of Michigan
School of Nursing
Ann Arbor, Michigan

Chapter 15: The Research Role in Community Health Nursing

Robert McFarlane, Ph.D.
Consulting Ecologist
Houston, Texas

Chapter 4: Ecological Connections

Maija Selby, R.N., C., Dr. PH.
Associate Professor and Deputy Chair for Research Development
Curriculum of Public Health
School of Public Health
University of North Carolina at Chapel Hill
Chapel Hill, North Carolina

Chapter 2: Epidemiology, Demography, and Research

Nancy Stewart, R.N., M.S.N.
Assistant Director
Division of Public Health Nursing
Texas Department of Health
Austin, Texas

Chapter 14: The Management Role in Community Health Nursing

Foreword

Everyone has felt the sudden, intense delight that comes from first seeing an inspired piece of handiwork. It is this same delight that readers are apt to feel when they examine this book. The authors of this seminal work have produced a book destined to become one of the vital tools used by public/community health nurses. They have nurtured the ideas contained inside for years, clothed them with words, and brought a finished product into existence.

The nursing profession has declared public/community health nursing a specialty area of practice, differentiated from other nursing specialities by the client that it serves, which is a community, an aggregate of individuals who share a common characteristic, be it geographical, or a health or social condition. The practice is guided by the nursing process, adhering to standards of care promulgated by the profession. It diagnoses and treats human responses to actual or perceived health problems of the group that is receiving care. Data are derived by applying epidemiological methods to describe the occurrence and distribution of health problems of the group. Life and health events are defined and interpreted through the use of biostatistical, numerical data.

The roots of public/community health nursing began in the 19th century. Our revered founder of professional nursing, Florence Nightingale, influenced William Rathbone in his development of district nursing in Great Britain by establishing and defining its functions. As her ideas flowed into America they were modified. Visiting nurse associations developed independently, in different places, each providing health instruction and nursing care to the sick in their homes. This was followed a few years later by nursing services provided by official health agencies; these were focused primarily on health promotion and disease-prevention activities.

Then came Medicare and Medicaid in the 1960s. No longer was nursing practice in the community so neatly divided. Confusion developed over the role of the public/community health nurse. There was much debate and discussion, often heated, over what constituted public/community health nursing. The emphasis was primarily on individuals, families, and groups. But an idea was incubating in the School of Public Health at Houston, Texas. A project was started in 1970 that had the aim of demonstrating how to nurse a community.

For the past 16 years that idea has been refined, demonstrated, taught, and evaluated. Now for the first time the profession has at hand a text that clearly and simply explains how to nurse a community. Other books and numerous articles have discussed the concept, but none has provided a detailed guide on how to practice public/community health nursing professionally and scientifically.

Public/community health nurses have a set of instruments that serve as guides for population-focused practice. This set includes the two definitions created in 1980 by the American Nursing Association (ANA) and the Public Health Nursing/American Public Health Association (PHN/APHA); *Nursing: A Social Policy Statement* (ANA, 1980), which describes what nursing is and the process by which it is practiced; the recently revised *Standards of Community Health Nursing* (ANA, 1986); *The Guide for Community-Based Nursing Services* (ANA, 1985), which contains the Operational Definition of Public Health Nursing and a Statement of Competencies; and *Public Health/Community Health Nursing* and its companion volume, *Community-Based Nursing Services: Innovative Models* (ANA, 1986). Now *Community as Client: Application of the Nursing Process* has been added to this set, illustrating how to put it all together. No longer need the practice seem ambiguous.

The authors provide the necessary theory and conceptual framework for understanding public/community health practice; they describe the cognates upon which it is based, that is, epidemiology, demography, political processes, health organizations, and ecology. After taking the reader step-by-step through the process, examples are given to illustrate how to nurse a variety of communities. The same process is applicable to communities everywhere, whether they are in developing or developed countries.

This book will not close the subject of the practice of public/community health nursing. Rather, it invites dialogue and experimentation with the ideas presented. In the words of Thoreau, "The woods would be very silent if no birds sang except those that sing the best." Mary Gardner wrote many years ago, "Public health nursing has a heritage of open mindedness, for its development in the past has so often necessitated entrance into new and untried paths" (Public Health Nursing, p 434. New York, Macmillan, 1955).

I am honored to write this foreword. I am proud to endorse this book enthusiastically and to recommend it to each of you who are courageously practicing public/community health nursing despite the many social and economic constraints of the 1980s. The authors have performed a real service to our profession. Scotsmen, when delivering a compliment, say something or someone is "no bad." *Community as Client: Application of the Nursing Process* is "no bad."

Dorothy M. Talbot, Professor Emeritus
School of Public Health
University of North Carolina at Chapel Hill

Chapel Hill, North Carolina
May, 1986

Preface

Although the community-as-client concept represents the uniqueness of community health nursing, there is no nursing text devoted to this concept nor to its application. The community-as-client concept provides a focus for this introductory text in community health nursing. Key concepts of nursing and public health are delineated and illustrated throughout. The nursing process provides the framework for the text.

Part I: Concepts and Theories of Community Health Nursing
This section describes content areas basic to the practice of community health nursing, including: the health care system, epidemiology, demography and research, the political process, and ecological connections. The principles and processes of each concept are incorporated into the Community-as-Client Model, which is presented in Chapter 5 and used to guide Part II of the text.

Part II: Application of the Nursing Process to Community Health Nursing
The Community-as-Client Model and one sample community are used to apply each step of the nursing process to the practice of community health nursing. The student is guided through the processes of community assessment; data analysis; formulation of a community diagnosis; and the planning, implementation, and evaluation of a health plan. The emphasis is on understanding the community as a dynamic system that interacts with its environment.

Part III: Roles in Community Health Nursing
This section specifies the functions and supporting theory of the major roles —teacher, manager, and researcher—that are basic to the practice of community health nursing. Pertinent legislation that affects the delivery of each role is presented, as well as standards and criteria for practice. The concluding chapter presents issues that confront community health nursing and opportunities for practice in the areas of research, home health care, school, and occupational and international settings.

The Authors

Acknowledgments

Community as Client: Application of the Nursing Process could not have been written without the thoughts, critiques, and examples of our students. We thank each of you. Special thanks go to those whose work directly contributed to "Rosemont": Kathy Falkenhagen, Anne Stewart Helton, Mary Luckett, Carol Pyles, and Marianne Zotti.

Table of Contents

Community as Client:
Application of the Nursing Process

PART I

Concepts and Theories
of Community Health Nursing

1

The Health Care System

OBJECTIVES

The *health care system* is the environment in which a community health nurse works. It is a system made up of people, services, and facilities that strive to restore, maintain, and promote health. How the services are delivered, by whom, to whom, in what settings, and at what cost all influence the practice of community health nursing. This chapter discusses the health care system—its beginnings, its present status, and the directions in which it is evolving.

After studying this chapter you will be able to

- use information about the economic, social, and political forces affecting the health care system to practice community health nursing that is responsive to the health needs of a community

INTRODUCTION

Health care is "essential but too expensive"; hospitals are "intimidating but life-saving"; health insurance "pays most of the bills, but the premiums are unaffordable"; health care is a "right and should be made accessible to everyone." But who will pay? Why is health care so expensive? Is government regulation to blame? Is inflation? Or is the answer consumer demand for expensive diagnostic and treatment services? Health care is a major social, economic, and political issue; it is also a basic need. Legislative and popular attention revolve around the dramatic spiraling of health care costs; in twenty years, health care costs have doubled. Society is asking, "Can there be health care for all at a price that all can afford?" The business community is addressing the dilemma of costs through organizations such as preferred provider organizations, alternative delivery systems, and health maintenance organizations. These new organizations, coupled with new prospective payment systems, based on diagnostic related groups, produce a high level of uncertainty as people ask if health care can be accessible, acceptable, economical, and still maintain its quality.

Was the health care system always like this? How did the system begin? An historical perspective of health care can help us understand the present system.

HISTORICAL PERSPECTIVE: GENERATIONS OF CHANGE

Prior to 1850 health care was primarily a physician–patient relationship with treatment received in the home. With the development and acceptance of hospitals in the 1850s, health care moved out of the private home into public voluntary hospitals. The scientific method and research began to rationalize clinical care, replacing earlier reliance on unproven generalities and good intentions. Health care focused on diagnosing and treating diseases and human ailments. Each decade witnessed the control of additional diseases and an increase in life expectancy. Pneumonia and tuberculosis no longer claimed thousands of lives, women could be guaranteed safe childbirth, and the chronic conditions of diabetes and epilepsy were managed with daily medication. Vaccines, antibiotics, clean water, and safe food eliminated most of the diseases that plagued our ancestors.

In the 1950s, legislation was passed for the planning and financing of health care. Debate flourished on the notion of health care as a basic right, as something more than a privilege for people with economic means—and this debate continues today. Passage of the Hospital Construction Act in 1946 (commonly referred to as the Hill–Burton legislation) began a national plan for the equitable construction of hospitals and the provision of "charitable care" to people who could not afford to pay. Immediately thereafter, third-party health insurance companies, such as Blue Cross and Blue Shield, offered an insurance premium plan to pay for health care. Health insurance was very popular and was lobbied for by workers and adopted by business. Health insurance plans became more elaborate, offering dental, optical, home care, and a variety of extended and rehabilitation services. With each addendum to the insurance plan, premiums increased.

The 1960s witnessed federal policy and legislation to increase citizen access to health care. Government programs such as Medicare and Medicaid were started. At the same time, a technological explosion occurred based on heavy public investment in medical research. Elaborate technology was available for diagnosis and treatment, as well as for life support and life extension. As the technology developed, ethical issues began to emerge such as how to define when life begins and ends and how to select candidates for life-saving procedures such as organ transplants.

The 1970s ushered in increased government regulation and mandated community-based planning to limit hospital expansion. The goal was to contain rapidly increasing health care costs. Health systems agencies and certificates of need were two types of measures implemented to regulate health care and contain costs. All plans were basically ineffective because the costs and demand for expensive technology and care services (*i.e.,* intensive care units) continued to escalate.

The 1980s introduced legislation of deregulation and prospective payment plans. (Based on a prospective payment system and a list of DRGs hospitals were paid a set reimbursement for a given condition regardless of services rendered or days of hospitalization.) Deregulation resulted in increased competition among health providers to meet consumer demands for health. There were proposals for ADSs, and HMOs proliferated. At the same time, consumer demands for health care changed. No longer could the major diseases be treated with antibiotics and vaccines. Prevention of cancer, heart disease, and stroke required changes in lifestyle practices. Habits of smoking, alcohol use, poor diet, and lack of exercise contributed to the major diseases and killers of the 1980s. Primary prevention, early detection, and modification of lifestyle were necessary to restore or maintain health. Educated to the risk and disability of chronic disease, people wanted a healthy environment in which to live and work. Consumers demanded health-promotion programs and legislation to decrease health hazards.

ECONOMIC PERSPECTIVE: GENERATIONS OF GROWTH

Ten percent of what our nation earns (the gross national product) is spent on health care. This has increased from 5% in 1960. What is significant is that most health care is not paid for by the consumer, but by third parties.

NOTE: The term *third party* refers to an organization other than the patient (the *first party*) or the health provider (the *second party*). A third party may be a government program such as Medicare or a private health insurer such as Blue Cross.

Direct consumer payments for health care account for less than one third of all health expenditures. Third-party reimbursement ranges from 88% of all hospital care to 22% for eyeglasses. What effect do you think third-party reimbursement has on the cost of health care?

A related economic characteristic within the health care system that contributes to the problems of rising costs, unequal distribution, and lack of access by all people is the unpredictability of the need for medical care services. For example, if you decide to purchase a car, by using your knowledge of the purchase price and of your monthly expenses and income, you can save by budgeting and decide at what point you will be able to purchase the car. However, an individual, family, or community *cannot* predict their medical service needs. In any year, most people spend relatively little on health care, but some individuals experience a serious illness that is very costly. Uncertainty over illness and the required expenditures of illness stimulated the need for third-party health insurance. Insurance lowers the risk of economic disaster should unpredictable health expenses occur. Medical costs continue to rise steadily and the incentive to purchase health insurance increases. More people are purchasing more expensive health insurance each year.

Compounding the problem of cost is the fact that until recently health insurance premiums were tax-deductible for both employees and employers. Insurance reimbursement for health costs changes the usual consumer purchasing practices. People who are ill do not want to "shop" for the best buy in health care; they want restored health. In addition, once people have purchased health insurance there is a strong motivation to use the insurance even if it means incurring unnecessary costs such as staying in the hospital two additional days for one more test that could be done as an outpatient. Statements such as "the insurance company will pay for everything" are common.

Recall that the 1980s have been a decade of deregulation and encouraged competition. What effect has this had on the cost of health care services? Competition does not assure quality of care or access to care. Health services governed by competition tend to stress profits, not service. However, competition is not new to the health care system. Historically, hospitals have competed for physicians, more elaborate technology, and public recognition through research. It is the use of advertising techniques to compete for patients that is new to hospitals.

Competition for the consumer's health dollar is now influenced by employers who offer choices among various health plans, employers who provide a set dollar contribution regardless of the health plan that an employee chooses, and by limits placed upon the amount of health premiums that can be treated as a deduction for tax purposes. Health care has become big business and the change may mean that issues of access, affordability, and acceptability may be pushed aside as unimportant.

The consumer plays a major role in the escalating cost of medical care. Traditionally, advanced technology reduces labor costs, but new technology in health care has resulted in new diagnostic and treatment services that require workers with specialized skills and training. As the consumer becomes aware of diagnostic and curative treatments, the demand for such services increases, as does the cost. Coupled with this is the dramatic increase in the number of physicians. The ratio of physicians per 100,000 persons stood at 163 in 1970, compared to 217 in 1982; and the increase continues, with a surplus of physicians in most urban areas. The oversupply of doctors, the high cost of diagnostic and treatment services, and competition for patients has led to the multipractice settings in which physicians share costly equipment and offer diagnostic procedures outside the hospital. Patients are provided with the option of health care delivery in the office, placing the physician in direct competition with the local hospital. Nursing services are returning to their traditional base of home and community, offering a variety of services that until recently were available only in the hospital. These include midwifery, rehabilitation, intravenous therapy, and postsurgical care.

With an understanding of some of the characteristics that influence the cost of health care, examine the displayed material, *Economic Indicators of Health Care Costs.* How do these statements compare to what you have read in recent periodicals and have experienced as a consumer of health care?

Obviously the economics of the health care system have changed, as have the services provided and the consumer's demands for specific services. Before continuing, let's stop and consider a few questions. Based on your knowledge, experiences, and attitudes (all those special features that make you a unique individual), consider the following, then jot down your responses.

- Is health care a right or a function of income?
- Should health care be regulated? If so, by whom? For what purposes?
- How much high technology (*e.g.,* transplant procedures) is needed?
- Who pays for costly health care? Should everyone pay equally? Or only those who use the services?

Reasonable cost, quality, availability, access, and *continuity* are the five most important issues in the delivery of health care services. The goal of the

---

ECONOMIC INDICATORS OF HEALTH CARE COSTS
BETWEEN 1960 AND 1983*

- National health expenditures increased from $27 billion to over $355 billion
- National health expenditures, as a proportion of the gross national product, doubled from 5.3% to 10.8%
- Annual health care expenses per person (paid by individuals or insurance) increased from $146.00 to $1459.00
- Nursing home expenditures increased from 2% to 9%
- Consumer health costs *declined* from 55% to 32%
- Private insurer health costs *increased* from 21% to 26%
- Government health costs *increased* from 9% to 30%

* Data compiled from *Health Care Financing Review* (published by the Health Care Financing Administration, US Government Printing Office). This publication is available in many libraries.

---

health care system is to achieve balance, equity, and efficiency among them. Each issue is influenced by demographic, social, and political forces, including the following factors.

- An aging population with an increased life expectancy (A child born in 1933 had a life expectancy of 49 years; a child born today can expect to live 76 years. Persons over age 65, once 5% of the population, will comprise 20% of the population in the year 2020.)
- A change in the leading causes of death, from infections such as pneumonia and tuberculosis, to chronic conditions, such as heart disease and cancer
- An increasingly specialized health labor force with more than 300 different health provider professions
- Increased regulation and public policy development governing health care delivery
- Increased competition and marketing of health services

Change is constant in the health care system. We've discussed some of these changes. To summarize the overall trend, it can be said that medical care has become increasingly complex. Third-party insurance reimbursement flourished because of the perceived risk of costly hospitalization. People desired more elaborate insurance policies, which, in turn, increased premiums. The government began administering Medicare and Medicaid and became the largest insurer. As a result, consumers paid less of the cost of their health care and insurers paid more; there was little incentive to promote health and to prevent disease. Research investments, with the aid and sanction of government support, generated a steady progression of medical knowledge and advanced technology, most of which remained current for only three or four years. Health care costs skyrocketed. People began to ask how it was to be decided who would receive the expensive high technology, and who would pay the costs. Simultaneously, the rising education level of consumers and their heightened awareness of the association between lifestyle and illnesses (*e.g.,* between smoking and lung cancer, or diet and heart disease) motivated the public to assume a more active role in health maintenance and disease prevention. Health had become a status to be preserved and the public requested health promotion information to use as a guide in making lifestyle decisions.

Concerns that consistent quality of care be provided by professional caregivers and that organizations providing health care have a set of minimum standards for guidance resulted in accreditation and continuing education of caregivers—programs that provided quality, but at increased costs. These programs began to influence health promotion and adaptive lifestyles, representing movement to the goal of prevention of disease and health promotion. The concept of continuity of care suggested that the process of health care should be ongoing, treating the whole person, using something more than a fragmented approach to illness, organs, or body systems. A new era of the ADS had evolved.

ALTERNATIVE DELIVERY SYSTEMS: INNOVATION IN PRACTICE

Alternative delivery systems (ADS) are health care options resulting from public demand, competitive pressures, and escalating health care expenditures. Given the public's demand for options, ADS are replacing the traditional, structured hospital system of health care delivery. Foremost among ADS are the following organizations: preferred provider organizations, health maintenance organizations, emergicenters, surgicenters, wellness programs, home health care, and hospices.

Preferred Provider Organizations

A preferred provider organization (PPO) is a contracted, fixed-fee agreement between an employer and a group of health providers and hospitals for the delivery of health care services to all employees. The PPO offers discounts to employees who use their services. The employer pays for most of the health services provided to the employees through the PPO and pays less for health services provided to employees outside the PPO. Employees pay less if they use the PPO and, because employers have established a fixed fee, their costs do not increase.

Health Maintenance Organizations

First developed in 1930, health maintenance organizations (HMO) have become increasingly popular and, by 1990, an estimated 20% of the United States population will have chosen an HMO for individual or family health care. Many HMOs are corporations of hospital, clinic, and health care providers that offer all health care services for a prepaid, monthly fee. The employer or employee may pay the fee or share the fee payment. Consumers must use the health providers employed by the HMO. Medicare recipients also can choose to enroll in an HMO. Within an HMO, the risk and uncertainty of illness are shared by both health providers and consumers. Illness becomes a "cost" to the HMO rather than the potential income-producing situation under the traditional fee-for-services-when-ill system. Therefore, the focus of HMOs is disease prevention and health promotion with emphasis on primary health care and early screening and detection services. Impressive data exist on the number of hospital days averted and personal productivity increases among consumers who use an HMO.

FREESTANDING EMERGENCY CENTERS

Freestanding emergency centers (sometimes referred to as medical, pediatric, or family-care centers) consist of one or more private physicians practicing independently of hospitals to offer services on a nonappointment basis for episodic illness or injury. The emergency centers are usually located in shopping centers, are open in the evenings and on weekends, and offer accessible care that is affordable. Standard practice is to require immediate payment for services rendered; some emergency centers accept workmen's compensation. Generally, freestanding emergency centers meet the licensing standards required for a doctor's office. The centers use less expensive equipment than would be required by a hospital emergency room and are probably more efficient than traditional hospital emergency rooms, although there is a paucity of research data on this question. The rapid acceptance of emergency centers is explained partially by the high mobility of our society and the fact that many families do not establish a relationship with an individual health provider. Public acceptance and use is seemingly high, based on the continuing growth in numbers of freestanding emergency centers.

AMBULATORY SURGERY CENTERS

Ambulatory surgery centers perform scheduled surgical procedures for patients who do not remain in the center overnight. Such a center can be hospital-based or free-standing, and independently operated or hospital-managed. An estimated 40% of all hospital surgical procedures can be performed on an outpatient basis through day surgery. Insurers are increasingly reluctant to reimburse hospitals for inpatient care associated with surgical procedures that can be performed on an outpatient basis. "Ambulatory surgery center" is a generic term and this type of health service may be termed "day surgery," "outpatient surgery," "in-and-out surgery," or "Surgicenter care."

> NOTE: As with any health-care service, it is the role of the community nurse to determine the scope of services available to community residents, as well as performing general assessment measures of their affordability, acceptability, and accessibility.

As with freestanding emergency centers, there is no single accreditation or licensing body that can collect or provide data on ownership, services offered, usage rates, or growth of ambulatory surgery centers. Factors that may act to inhibit growth of these centers include their slow acceptance by third-party insurers, as well as the sizeable number of physicians who have been reluctant to refer patients. Because of expensive equipment and specialized personnel, ambulatory surgery centers have a high start-up cost. However, supporting factors for continued growth in the number of these centers include increased patient and surgeon convenience; a fixed, predetermined surgical fee schedule; elimination of overnight hospital stays with their associated costs and patient anxiety; and newly modified insurance coverage for outpatient surgery. A limited number of studies related to quality of care indicate that, based on surgical complications, freestanding ambulatory surgery centers provide care that is similar to that received by hospitalized surgical patients.

Wellness Programs

Wellness programs, designed to promote health and prevent disease, gained momentum in the 1970s, initially in response to the business community's recognition of rapidly increasing health costs and rising insurance premiums. Companies must subtract from profits any money paid to workmen's compensation, disability coverage, sick leave, absenteeism, and reduced productivity. Because chronic diseases, such as heart disease, stroke, and cancer, are caused by smoking, poor diet, stress, inactivity, and misuse of alcohol and drugs, it was recognized that changes in lifestyle practices could prevent the occurrence of disease and improve health. To promote health, wellness programs are offered in such areas as stress reduction, smoking cessation, and physical fitness. Special lifestyle modification programs have been devised, implemented, and evaluated by volunteer organizations such as the American Lung Association and the American Cancer Society, as well as private organizations. Public schools, churches, civic associations, and interested citizens have formed self-help and support groups to motivate and encourage individual's decisions to changes lifestyle practices. It has been proven that risk factors and associated chronic diseases can be reduced by changes in lifestyle practices, and that wellness programs can motivate people to change.

Home Health

Home health is the provision of health services to individuals and families in their places of residence for the purpose of promoting, maintaining, or restoring health, or to maximize the level of independence, while minimizing the effects of disability and illness, including terminal illness. Individualized services are planned, coordinated, and made available by providers organized for the delivery of home health care through the use of employed staff, contractual arrangements, or a combination of the two. Nurses perform or supervise most procedures delivered in the home. Home health services can obviate the need for institutional care and can help to contain costs. Home care is for persons of all ages of varying health status; persons who experience chronic developmental and handicapping disabilities that require home-based care; and persons with acute needs such as daily ventilator-assisted care, or involved procedures such as enteral and parenteral feedings, and intravenous medications and monitoring.

In 1980, changes were made in Medicare home-care benefits; these included the elimination of requirements for prior hospitalization, the deductible fees required for home-care services, and the ceiling set on the maximum number of home visits that could be received. In 1982, Congress enacted a hospice option in order to foster community-based care for the terminally ill. Hospice care is a special form of home health care that provides nursing and social services to the terminally ill and their families. It may be delivered in the home or in special care centers that focus on individual care needs. Like home care, hospice care may be organized through employed staff, contractual arrangements, or a combination of both.

THE FUTURE: MORE CHANGE AND MORE CHALLENGES

Each decade has brought a degree of turmoil and uncertainty to health care. The 1950s ushered in the post-war expansion of hospitals and related health facilities that was partially financed through the Hill–Burton Hospital Construction Program. Also contributing to this expansion was the rapid development of third-party health insurance as a reimbursement mechanism. The 1960s saw the introduction of the social and health legislation that resulted in Medicare and Medicaid. It was also during this period that the explosion of research and technology began. The decade of the 1970s saw multiple efforts to contain hospital costs and to regulate the health care system through mandated community involvement in the planning and regulatory process.

The 1980s have witnessed the birth of large for-profit hospital chains, the emphasis on deregulation and competition, and the start of advertising to consumers. Alternative delivery systems proliferated alongside new reimbursement arrangements such as prospective payment systems through DRGs.

Future decades will respond to continuing trends as the "graying of America" gains recognition, requiring special longterm care and less costly care for the 65-and-over age group. Disease prevention through healthy lifestyles and wellness programs will contribute to a healthier population. The consumer will continue to exercise choice in the use of health services and the health providers will shape services accordingly. The public wants convenient and affordable care, and the health care system will respond to this need in new and expanded ways. Community health nursing practice will also change because nursing is part of the health delivery system and must be responsive to community needs. Community nurses can respond optimally to change by understanding the community in which they work—that is, the social, legal, and political forces that shape and affect the health care system, as well as the perceived needs of the health consumers.

BIBLIOGRAPHY

American Medical Association, The American Health Care System 1984. Chicago, American Medical Association, 1984

Barger SG, Hillman DG, Garland HR: The PPO Handbook. Rockville, Maryland, Aspen Systems Corporation, 1985

Hawkins JBW, Higgins LP: Nursing and the American Health Care Delivery System. New York, Tiresias Press, 1982

Health Care Financing Administration: Health Care Financing Review. Washington, DC HCFA Pub. Government Printing Office, 6:2(Winter), 1984

Kress J, Senger J: HMO Handbook. Rockville, Maryland, Aspen Systems Corporation, 1975

National Center for Health Statistics: Health, United States, 1983. DHHS Pub No (PHS) 84-1232, Public Health Service. Washington, US Government Printing Office, 1983

Scientific American Inc: Life and Death and Medicine. San Francisco, Freeman, 1973

Williams SJ, Torrens PR (eds): Introduction to Health Services, 2nd ed. New York, John Wiley & Sons, 1984

Yaggy D, Anlyan W (eds): Financing Health Care: Competition Versus Regulation. Cambridge, Massachusetts, Ballinger Publishing, 1982

2

Epidemiology, Demography, and Research

OBJECTIVES

In order to assess and diagnose community health needs, and to plan, implement, and evaluate programs to meet those needs, the community health nurse requires an understanding of basic concepts in epidemiology, demography, and research. After studying this chapter, you will be able to

- describe the purposes of epidemiology, demography, and research
- interpret and use basic epidemiologic, demographic, and statistical measures of community health
- compare, contrast, and use various epidemiologic approaches to study community health
- apply principles of epidemiology, demography, and research to your practice of community health nursing

The author would like to express her appreciation to the students and faculty at Emory University for their comments and encouragement during the preparation of this chapter. Special thanks also go to Dorothy M. Tuttle, PH.D., the mentor for my community health practice, for her invaluable editorial expertise and guidance.

INTRODUCTION

Epidemiology and *demography* are sciences used to study population health; *research* is a structured process used to acquire new knowledge or verify existing information. To restore, maintain, and promote the health of populations, the community health nurse integrates and applies concepts from these fields at the primary, secondary, and tertiary levels of prevention. The purpose of this chapter is to first explore the meaning and usefulness of these concepts then apply them to an actual community health investigation that was carried out by a community health nurse.

Research

Research is a systematic process for obtaining new knowledge through verifiable examination of data and empirical testing of hypotheses. The term "research" may conjure images of the laboratory scientist applying treatments to material in test tubes, the medical researcher developing new drugs, or the clinical nurse researcher testing innovative methods of nursing care for hospitalized clients. However, the research interests of the community health nurse are likely to be quite different, relating to the health of population groups as they exist in natural settings. Nevertheless, the research *process* is similar regardless of the topic being studied. Critical thinking, the quality of questioning, examining, and verifying statements before accepting them as "true" is a crucial element of research in all fields. This chapter explains why research is essential to community health nursing practice.

Demography

Demography (literally "writing about the people," from the Greek *demos* [people], and *graphos* [writing]) is the science of human populations, and in its strictest sense is concerned with population size, characteristics, and change. Examples of demographic studies—that is, *demographic research*—are enumerations, descriptions, and comparisons of populations according to age, race, sex, socioeconomic status, geographic distribution and migration, and birth, death, marriage, and divorce patterns. Demographic studies often have health implications that may or may not be addressed by the investigators. The census of the United States population is an example of an extremely comprehensive descriptive demographic study that is conducted every ten years.

Epidemiology

Epidemiology ("the study of what is upon the people," from the Greek *logos* [study], *demos* [people], and *epi* [upon]) is the science of population health. Epidemiology incorporates concepts from demography and research as they relate to health and illness, and investigates the characteristics, distribution, and determinants of health conditions in human populations. The student facing the task of learning epidemiologic concepts may be comforted to realize that epidemiology overlaps demography; epidemiologic methods are also research methods, and the critical thinking skills required in epidemiology are the same as those learned in research. The study of epidemiology can be exciting; sometimes it takes on the intrigue of a detective story as the investigator tracks the factors associated with morbidity and mortality (illness and death). In fact, a number of novels describing epidemiologic studies have become quite popular including *The Black Death* by Cravens and Mair (1977), *The Andromeda Strain* by Crichton (1969), and *The Scourge* by Dunne (1978).

Early epidemiologic investigations were concerned chiefly with the control of epidemics of communicable disease. (An *epidemic* is an outbreak of illness beyond the levels usually expected in a population; it need not be a communicable disease.) John Snow's study of a cholera epidemic in London in 1853 is a classic in epidemiologic history. At that time, the mode of transmission of cholera was unknown, but Snow suspected it could be spread by fecal contamination of water. Applying epidemiologic principles, Snow determined that the death rates from cholera were highest in households served by the Southwark and Vauxhall water pumping system, and lowest in households served by other water suppliers. Snow learned that the Southwark and Vauxhall water came from portions of the Thames River in which London sewage had been discharged. Thus, this early epidemiologist was able to identify a water-borne mode of transmission of cholera and determine measures to control its spread.

Contemporary Community Health Research and Practice

Today, advanced and refined epidemiologic and demographic measures and research methods are used not only to study diseases such as the contemporary disorders of toxic shock syndrome (TSS) and acquired immune deficiency syndrome (AIDS), but also to investigate environmental conditions, health services, lifestyles, health-promotion strategies, and other factors that may influence health. This chapter considers aspects of epidemiology, demography, and research that are useful for the practice of community health nursing in this modern, expanded context.

Levels of Prevention in Community Health Practice

Before beginning the discussion of specific measures of community health, consider the concept of *prevention,* an important component of community health nursing practice. In popular terminology, prevention means warding off an event before it occurs. In contemporary community health practice, prevention has a broader scope. Let us examine the *levels of prevention* for community health practice: primary, secondary, and tertiary.

Primary prevention involves true avoidance of the occurrence of an illness or adverse health condition through general health-promotion activities and specific protective actions. Primary prevention encompasses a vast array of areas, including nutrition, hygiene, sanitation, immunization, environmental protection, and general health education, to name but a few; these areas clearly are important components of community health nursing practice. Research into the causes of health problems provides the basis for primary prevention. For example, just as John Snow's 1853 investigation of cholera deaths paved the way for provision of pure water to the residents of London, modern research into motor-vehicle-accident deaths has led to seat belts, air bags, and motorcycle helmets.

Secondary prevention is the early detection and treatment of illnesses or adverse health conditions. Secondary prevention may result in the cure of illnesses that otherwise would become incurable at later stages, the prevention of complications and disability, and the confinement of the spread of communicable diseases. An important aspect of secondary prevention is *screening,* the detection of disease in asymptomatic individuals. For example, the community health nurse may be involved in screening for tuberculosis, diabetes, glaucoma, hypertension, and *in situ* cervical carcinoma. Screening methods, too, are developed through research.

Tertiary prevention is employed after diseases or events have already resulted in damage to individuals. The purpose of tertiary prevention is to limit disability and to rehabilitate or restore the affected individuals to their maximum possible capacities. Examples of tertiary prevention include provision of "meals on wheels" for the homebound, physical therapy services for stroke victims, vocational retraining for handicapped individuals, mental health counseling for rape victims, and peer support groups for persons coping with cancer. The community health nurse may be involved in tertiary prevention in terms of direct care, referral, or planning for community needs.

It is clear that community health nursing interventions may be at primary, secondary, or tertiary levels of prevention. In order to plan appropriate methods of prevention for the community, the nurse must be able to assess the health of the community. The following sections cover some basic epidemiologic, demographic, and research concepts and measures for assessing community health.

DESCRIPTIVE MEASURES OF HEALTH

Demographic Measures

In describing and seeking to explain human health conditions, it is helpful to relate human characteristics or phenomena to patterns of illness and wellness. These human characteristics may be referred to as *demographic descriptors* or *demographics.* Examples of commonly used demographic descriptors are age, race, sex, ethnicity, marital status, income, and educational level.

These and many other demographic characteristics may affect health outcomes directly or indirectly. For example, teenagers are more likely than older persons to have automobile accidents; men are more likely than women to develop heart disease; and blacks are more likely than whites to give birth to low-birth-weight infants. In planning a study of community health, it is important to determine, through a review of related literature, which specific demographic characteristics or factors are likely to influence the health outcome being studied. This enables the community health investigator to formulate a plan of study that ensures collection of data regarding these factors in the particular population of interest.

Incidence and Prevalence

Although modern epidemiology encompasses conditions of wellness as well as illness, wellness is difficult to measure. Therefore, many measures of "health" are expressed in terms of *morbidity,* (illness) and *mortality* (death). Incidence and prevalence, two of these traditional measures, are necessary for appropriate assessment of community health, and can be adapted to health conditions other than illness and death.

Incidence

The *incidence* of a disease or health condition refers to the number of persons in a population who develop the disease or condition during a specified period of time. The calculation of incidence, therefore, generally requires that a population be followed over a period of time, in what is called a *prospective* (forward-looking) study. Prospective studies and measures of incidence are particularly useful in assessing health risks in populations.

Prevalence

The *prevalence* of a disease or condition refers to the total number of persons in the population who have the disease or condition at a particular time. Thus, prevalence may be calculated in a "one-shot" *cross-sectional* ("slice of time") or *retrospective* (backward-looking) study.

Interpretation of incidence and prevalence

Measures of incidence and prevalence provide different information and have different health implications. An increase in the prevalence of cancer may have both positive and negative implications as it simply means that there are more persons with cancer in the population. This might be the result of an increase in the incidence of cancer, that is, an increase in new cases. Or, it might be the result of health improvements that allow persons with cancer to live longer. In either case, the community may need to direct resources toward cancer. However, if knowledge of incidence is lacking, community health professionals will have difficulty determining whether resources should be allocated toward research into the cause of a cancer outbreak, toward cancer prevention programs, or toward cancer treatment services.

Rates

Incidence and prevalence usually are expressed as mathematical measures called *rates*. In order to understand rates, remember that epidemiology is the study of population health, not individual health. Therefore epidemiologic measures must do more than simply count the number of individual occurrences of a particular health condition; they must relate these occurrences to the population base. Rates do exactly this. They express a mathematical relationship in which the *numerator* is the number of persons experiencing an occurrence of the condition, and the *denominator* is the *population at risk,* the total number of persons who have the possibility of experiencing an occurrence of the condition. Rates therefore provide an estimate of the risk of occurrence of the illness or health condition, and are essential for meaningful measurement of population health.

Calculation of rates

Rates are calculated in this general format.

$$\text{rate} = \frac{\text{number of persons experiencing condition}}{\text{population at risk for experiencing condition}} \times K$$

K is a constant (usually 1000 or 100,000) that allows the rate, which may be a very small number, to be expressed in a meaningful way. Let us apply this general formula to the calculation of the infant mortality rate, which estimates an infant's risk of dying during the first year of life.

Example of a rate: The infant mortality rate

The infant mortality rate (IMR) usually is calculated on a calendar-year basis. The number of infant deaths (deaths before the age of one year) during the year is divided by the number of live births (infants born alive) during the year. The numerator represents the number of infants experiencing the "condition" of dying during the first year of life, and the denominator represents the population of infants at risk for dying during the first year of life.

In 1983 the United States reported a total of 3,614,000 live births and 39,400 infant deaths (National Center for Health Statistics, 1984). Applying the formula for a rate, we divide 39,400 by 3,614,000 and find that 0.0109 of the infants died during the first year of life. Because it is difficult to relate to 0.0109 of an infant, we multiply by a constant, in this case 1000, and find that 10.9 infants per 1000 live births died during the first year of life; that is, the infant mortality rate for 1983 was 10.9 infant deaths per 1000 live births.

Use of rates in community health assessment

In preparing an assessment of infant health in a state, county, or smaller area, a similar rate would be calculated for the selected community, and compared with that of the United States as a whole or with that of another community to help us determine whether our rate was high or low. The calculation of rates enables researchers to compare health events and conditions that occur in different populations.

> NOTE: Rates, like most statistical measures, are less reliable when based on small numbers. You will need to bear this in mind when you assess relatively infrequent events or conditions, or communities with small populations.

Rate versus proportion: The importance of the denominator

Another word of caution: a rate should be distinguished from a simple proportion in which the denominator is not the population at risk. For example, the death rate from cancer is not the same as the proportion of deaths caused by cancer. In each, the numerator is the absolute number of deaths caused by cancer. However, the denominators differ. In the death rate (or mortality rate), the denominator is all persons at risk of dying from cancer. Therefore, the cancer death rate is an expression of the risk of dying from cancer. In the proportion of deaths, also called *proportionate mortality,* the denominator is the total number of deaths from all causes; these deaths are not the population at risk of dying of cancer. Therefore, the proportionate cancer mortality simply describes the proportion of deaths attributable to cancer. Lacking an appropriate "population at risk" denominator, the proportionate mortality cannot be used to infer the risk of dying from cancer. In community health, the importance of appropriate denominators cannot be overemphasized.

Commonly used rates

Table 2-1 summarizes a number of rates that should be understood by the community health nurse. Note that the measures of natality and mortality are, in essence, measures of incidence of the conditions of "being born" and "dying." Note also the various ways in which the denominator, or population at risk, is determined in different rates.

Limitations of calendar-year calculations of rates

Be aware of the limitations of assessing risk through calendar year calculations of rates. In the example of the infant mortality rate, you already may have considered that some of the infants who died during the calendar year 1983 actually were born in 1982 and thus were not part of the 1983 population at

---

TABLE 2-1.   COMMONLY USED RATES

Measures of Natality

$$\text{Crude birth rate} = \frac{\text{Number of live births during time interval}}{\text{Estimated mid-interval population}} \times 1000$$

$$\text{Fertility rate} = \frac{\text{Number of live births during time interval}}{\text{Number of women ages 15–44 at mid-interval}} \times 1000$$

Measures of Morbidity and Mortality

$$\text{Incidence rate} = \frac{\text{Number of new cases of specified health condition during time interval}}{\text{Estimated mid-interval population at risk}} \times 1000$$

$$\text{Prevalence rate} = \frac{\text{Number of current cases of specified health condition at a given point in time}}{\text{Estimated population at risk at same point in time}} \times 1000$$

$$\text{Crude death rate} = \frac{\text{Number of deaths during time interval}}{\text{Estimated mid-interval population}} \times 1000$$

$$\text{Specific death rate} = \frac{\text{Number of deaths in subgroup during time interval}}{\text{Estimated mid-interval population of subgroup}} \times 100{,}000$$

$$\text{Cause-specific death rate} = \frac{\text{Number of deaths from specified cause during time interval}}{\text{Estimated mid-interval population}} \times 100{,}000$$

$$\text{Infant mortality rate} = \frac{\text{Number of deaths of infants <1 year during time interval}}{\text{Total live births during time interval}} \times 1000$$

$$\text{Neonatal mortality rate} = \frac{\text{Number of deaths of infants <28 days during time interval}}{\text{Total live births during time interval}} \times 1000$$

$$\text{Postneonatal mortality rate} = \frac{\text{Number of deaths of infants} \geq 28 \text{ days but <1 year during time interval}}{\text{Total live births during time interval}} \times 1000$$

---

risk, and some of the infants who were born in 1983 might yet die in 1984 and not be reflected in the 1983 infant mortality rate. Also, in calculating rates that require population totals for the year, it is obvious that populations may increase or decrease during a calendar year. In such cases, the midyear population estimate generally is used because the population at risk can not be determined exactly. A prospective study that follows a *cohort,* or specified group, forward into time can help overcome some of the limitations of the conventionally calculated calendar-year rate.

Crude and specific rates

Rates that are computed for a population as a whole are called *crude rates.* Subgroups of a population may have differences in health outcome that are not revealed by the crude rates. For example, the 1983 crude mortality rate of 8.6 deaths per 1000 persons for the United States population as a whole completely obscures the much higher rate of 154.2 deaths per 1000 for persons 85 years of age and older (National Center for Health Statistics, 1984). Rates that are calculated for subgroups or specific conditions are referred to as *specific rates,* and can be computed for any specific condition or population subgroup as long as appropriate numerator and denominator data are available. Most frequently, specific rates are computed according to demographic characteristics such as age, race, or sex. If the health outcome being studied is likely to vary according to a particular demographic characteristic or combination of characteristics, it is useful to compute specific rates for the characteristic or characteristics in subgroups of the population. Specific rates help identify groups at increased risk within the population and also facilitate comparisons between populations that have different demographic compositions.

Adjusted rates

In comparing populations with different distributions of a characteristic that is known to affect the particular health condition being studied, the use of *adjusted rates* also may be advisable. An adjusted rate is a summary measure that statistically removes the effect of the difference in the distributions of that characteristic in the populations. A rate can be adjusted for age, race, sex, or any factor or combination of factors known to affect it. In essence, rate adjustment produces an estimate of what the crude rate would be if the different populations were identical in respect to the factor for which adjustment is made.

Interpretation of adjusted rates

Adjusted rates are helpful in making community comparisons, but they are *imaginary rates* and must be interpreted with care, as can be seen in the following illustration. A study of infant mortality in one community showed that the neonatal mortality rate (NMR) for blacks was 14.3 deaths per 1000 live births, compared to 8.2 deaths per 1000 live births for whites (Selby *et al,* 1984). Adjustment for low birth weight, a factor known to adversely affect infant outcome, resulted in a reduction of the black NMR to 6.3 deaths per 1000 live births, while the white NMR remained 8.2 (Selby, 1982). Did this indicate that neonatal mortality was a greater problem for whites than for blacks? Certainly not! The rate of 14.3 was real; the rate of 6.3 was fictitious. However, the adjusted rate provided important information, showing that most of the high neonatal mortality in the black population was accounted for by a high proportion of infants of low birth weight, who as a subgroup had high death rates. If you were in charge of planning health services to reduce infant mortality in this community, to which group would you allocate resources?

ANALYTIC MEASURES OF HEALTH

As you have learned, rates are used to describe and compare the risks of dying, becoming ill, or developing other health conditions. In studying community health, it is also desirable to determine if health conditions or problems are associated with, or related to, other factors in the community. The associated or related factors often point the way to preventive actions, (*e.g.,* the linking of cigarette smoking with lung cancer and other disorders). To investigate potential relationships, analytic measures of community health are required. In this section four analytic measures of health will be discussed: relative risk, odds ratio, attributable risk, and attributable risk percent.

Relative Risk

To determine if a relationship or association exists between a health condition and a suspected factor, it is necessary to compare the risk of developing the health condition in populations *exposed* to the factor with populations *not exposed* to the factor. The *relative risk* does exactly this by expressing the ratio of the incidence rate of those exposed and those not exposed to the suspected factor.

$$RR \text{ (relative risk)} = \frac{\text{incidence rate among those exposed}}{\text{incidence rate among those not exposed}}$$

Interpretation of relative risk

In essence, the relative risk answers two questions

1. Is the rate in the exposed population higher than the rate in the nonexposed population?
2. If so, how many times higher?

A high relative risk in the exposed population suggests that the factor is indeed a *risk factor* in the development of the disease or health condition.

Internal and external risk factors

The concept of relative risk generally is understood readily by students when one group of people clearly is exposed and another is not exposed to an external agent such as cigarette smoke, industrial noise, a chemical pollutant, or a drug. However, students sometimes become confused when seeing relative risks applied to internal, unchangeable factors such as age, race, or sex. Nevertheless, as can be seen in the following example, persons are also "exposed" to intrinsic factors that may carry as much risk as extrinsic ones.

Example of relative risk: Homicide

A study in Atlanta, Georgia, showed that the annual homicide victimization rate (incidence rate) among blacks (those "exposed" to the intrinsic condition of being black) who were age 16 or over was 10.5 per 10,000 persons (Centerwall, 1984). The annual homicide victimization rate among whites (those "not exposed" to the intrinsic condition of being black) was 2.1 per 10,000 persons. Calculating the relative risk from these figures, it can be seen that

$$RR = \frac{10.5 \text{ per } 10,000}{2.1 \text{ per } 10,000} = 4.9$$

In other words, the annual homicide victimization rate for blacks was nearly five times greater than for whites. Clearly, race is a risk factor in homicide, and although the risk factor itself cannot be altered, the information provided by this analysis can be used to direct policies and plan protective services for the population at greatest risk.

Odds Ratio

Calculation of the relative risk is straightforward when incidence rates are available. Unfortunately, not all studies can be carried out prospectively as is required for the computation of incidence rates. However, in a retrospective study the relative risk can be approximated by the *odds ratio,* a simple mathematical ratio of the odds in favor of having the condition when the suspected factor is present and the odds in favor of having the condition when the factor is absent.

Calculation of the odds ratio: Relationship to the relative risk

The calculation of the odds ratio and its relationship to the relative risk is best explained by use of the cross-tabulation in Table 2-2. If this were a prospective study, the relative risk would be calculated as follows

$$RR = \frac{\text{rate in those exposed}}{\text{rate in those not exposed}}$$

$$\text{rate in those exposed} = \frac{a}{a+b}$$

$$\text{rate in those not exposed} = \frac{c}{c+d}$$

$$\text{Therefore, } RR = \frac{a}{a+b} \div \frac{c}{c+d} = \frac{a(c+d)}{c(a+b)}$$

TABLE 2-2. CROSSTABULATION FOR CALCULATION OF ODDS RATIO

	Health Condition		
	Present	*Absent*	*Total*
Exposed to factor	a	b	a + b
Not exposed to factor	c	d	c + d
Total	a + c	b + d	a + b + c + d

Usually the number of persons affected by the condition, $a + c$, is a relatively small portion of the population at risk, $a + b + c + d$. When this is the case, it can be seen from the table that d will approximately equal $c + d$, and b will approximately equal $a + b$. In this case, the odds ratio can be used to approximate the relative risk. Substituting in the relative risk formula above

$$\text{if } d = c + d$$

$$\text{and } b = a + b$$

$$\text{then } \frac{a(c + d)}{c(a + b)} = \frac{ad}{bc} = \text{odds ratio}$$

Example of the odds ratio: Toxic shock syndrome (TSS)

The odds ratio sometimes is referred to as the *risk ratio* and is used when incidence rates, and thus true relative risks, cannot be calculated. In studying TSS, a severe illness involving high fever, vomiting, diarrhea, rash, and hypotension or shock (Centers for Disease Control, 1980a), it was neither practical nor ethical to consider cases only on a prospective basis. Therefore, existing cases were compared retrospectively with non-cases, or *controls*. Early studies noted an association between TSS and menstruation and tampon use, and suggested that users of Rely, a specific brand of super-absorbent tampon, might be at particularly high risk. To clarify the issue, investigators analyzed data from a sample of TSS cases and controls, all of whom used tampons. Let us use the TSS data in Table 2-3 to calculate the odds ratio for users of Rely brand tampon.

$$\text{odds ratio} = \frac{ad}{bc} = \frac{30(84)}{30(12)} = 7$$

In other words, users of the Rely brand were seven times more likely to develop TSS than were users of other brands of tampons. The Rely brand was voluntarily withdrawn from the marketplace by the manufacturer.

Relative Risk and Odds Ratio: Caution in Interpretation

A word of caution: regard a high odds ratio or relative risk with appropriate concern, but do not allow the finding to obscure the potential involvement of

TABLE 2-3.   TOXIC SHOCK SYNDROME CASES AMONG
             146 TAMPON USERS

Tampon Use	Toxic Shock Syndrome		
	Present	*Absent*	*Total*
Rely brand tampon	30	30	60
Other brand of tampon	12	84	96
Total	42	114	146

(Data from: Centers for Disease Control: Follow-up on toxic shock syndrome.
MMWR 29(37):441–444, 1980)

factors other than the one being studied. Beginning researchers sometimes
are overly impressed with their mathematical calculations, they forget to look
at the situation in the context of the real world, and thus neglect to pursue
their research a step further.

For instance, refer again to Table 2-3. Note that 12 persons in the sample
had TSS even though they did not use the Rely brand tampons. In other words,
this product was not the sole cause of TSS. Subsequent research has suggested
that certain super-absorbent materials in Rely brand and other tampons or
certain aspects of tampon use may foster the growth of *staphylococcus aureus,*
the probable ultimate-causal organism in TSS (Centers for Disease Control,
1980a, 1980b, 1981a, 1983; Davis *et al,* 1980).

Attributable Risk

Another analytic measure of risk is the *attributable risk,* or difference between
the incidence rates in those exposed and those not exposed to the risk factor.

$$\text{attributable risk} = \text{incidence rate in exposed group} - (minus)\ \text{incidence rate in nonexposed group}$$

This measure, also called the *risk difference,* estimates the excess risk attributable to the factor being studied, and demonstrates the potential reduction in
the incidence rate if the factor were eliminated.

Example of attributable risk: Coronary heart disease

The U.S. Public Health Service has studied a combination of three potentially
controllable coronary-heart-disease risk factors: cigarette smoking, hypercho-

lesterolemia, and hypertension (Centers for Disease Control, 1984). When all three of these risk factors are present in the population, the incidence rate for myocardial infarction or sudden death from coronary heart disease has been estimated to be 189 cases per 1000 persons; when absent, 23 cases per 1000 persons. Using these rates, the risk attributable to the three risk factors is

$$\text{attributable risk} = 189 - 23 = 166 \text{ cases per 1000 population}$$

That is, 166 cases of myocardial infarction or sudden death from coronary heart disease per 1000 population could be prevented if the three risk factors could be eliminated.

Attributable Risk Percent

The *attributable risk percent* further quantifies attributable risk to estimate the proportion of new cases of the disease or health condition that could be prevented if the risk factor were eliminated.

$$\text{attributable risk percent} = \frac{\text{attributable risk}}{\text{incidence rate in exposed group}} \times 100$$

Example of attributable risk percent: Coronary heart disease

Looking at the triad of coronary-heart-disease risk factors discussed previously, it can be seen that

$$\text{attributable risk percent} = \frac{166}{189} \times 100 = 0.878 \times 100 = 87.8$$

This means that 87.8% of the new cases of myocardial infarction and sudden death from coronary heart disease could be prevented if smoking, hypercholesterolemia, and hypertension were eliminated from the population. Does this information help you determine what our public health priorities should be in relation to coronary heart disease?

CAUSE AND ASSOCIATION

Associations Between Variables

Ultimately, community health professionals hope to determine causes of various health conditions so steps can be taken to improve health. However, in view of the complexity of the human body and human behavior, establishing causality is extremely difficult. Therefore, investigations of population health generally examine relationships or *associations* between variables. The *variables* are the characteristics or phenomena (such as age, occupation, or exposure to chemicals) and the health conditions (for instance, cancer) being studied.

Association is not causation

If an association is found between variables, it means the variables tend to occur or change together, but it does not necessarily indicate that one of the variables causes the other. For example, high cancer mortality has been shown to be associated with old age; that is, as age increases, cancer mortality also increases. This does not mean that old age itself causes cancer deaths. Very strict criteria must be applied before associations can be considered causal. These criteria are discussed in this chapter in the section "Criteria for Determining Causation."

Variables and constants

An important requirement in any study is that the factors studied must have the potential to vary from person to person. If a factor cannot vary, it is not a *variable,* but a *constant.* It is impossible to establish an association between a constant and a variable because the constant, by definition, cannot change when the variable changes.

Example of variables and constants: Sex and Condition X

Let us consider a hypothetical study in which the variables of interest are sex and a particular human condition, which will be called "Condition X." The study must consider both aspects of the variable *sex,* (*i.e.,* men and women) and both aspects of the variable Condition X (*i.e.,* persons with the condition and persons without the condition); otherwise, these factors are constants, not variables. In practice, this is the same as saying that the study must use comparison groups. In epidemiologic studies, comparison groups often are referred to as *control groups* or *controls.* This crucial aspect may be better understood through Tables 2-4 and 2-5.

Table 2-4 shows that 800 men and 200 women have the characteristic or state of Condition X. As can be seen, 80% of the subjects with Condition X are men and 20% are women. It would be tempting to say that Condition X is related to sex, with men having a greater possibility of having the condition.

TABLE 2-4.   SEX OF 1000 PERSONS WITH CONDITION X

	Number of Persons	% of Total
Male	800	80
Female	200	20
Total	1000	100

However, this conclusion is impossible to infer from this study. The investigation was designed without a control group, so 100% of the subjects, both men and women, were required to have Condition X in order to be included in the study. That is, Condition X was not permitted to be a variable, so the possibility of finding a relationship between Condition X and any variable was eliminated.

Likewise, if the study had examined only men or only women with and without Condition X, the possibility of finding an association between sex and anything else would have been eliminated. Without including "the other aspect of the variable," sex would cease to be a variable in this study.

Example of association: Sex and Condition X

The investigation of Condition X begs for crucial information: what proportion of men and what proportion of women did not have the condition? Suppose that the setting for this study was a construction company in which there are 3200 male and 200 female employees. Data from these employees would allow calculation of "the other aspect of the variable" for Condition X (*i.e.,* persons without Condition X).

By including data for the unaffected employees, Table 2-5 now shows that only 25% (800 out of 3200) of the men have Condition X, whereas 100% (200

TABLE 2-5.   RELATIONSHIP BETWEEN SEX
AND CONDITION X

	Male	Female	Total
With Condition X	800	200	1000
Without Condition X	2400	0	2400
Total	3200	200	3400

out of 200) of the women have the condition. In this case, a statistical test could be applied to determine if there is an association between Condition X and sex. It would be discovered that a relationship exists. However, the association is completely opposite from that suggested by the original study.

Lest you be concerned for the women, Condition X was defined in this study as "working primarily indoors." This variable could have been any human condition from cancer to shyness to ingrown toenails, as long as the investigator was able to establish its presence or absence.

Confounding variables

Because an association has been identified between the variables, can it be said that one variable causes the other? In the example of Condition X, an association was found between sex and working indoors, with 100% of the women working indoors, compared to only 25% of the men. Does this mean that one's sex causes one to work indoors? Certainly the fact that some of the men also work indoors creates room to doubt that sex is the sole cause. Also, common sense and knowledge of employment practices would lead to the idea that women might tend to apply for white-collar positions, which happen to be indoors, rather than for blue-collar heavy-construction positions, which happen to be outdoors. In other words, the specific job of the employee may have intervened in our study and *confounded* the results. Any extrinsic factor that may influence a study's results is referred to as an extraneous, intervening, or *confounding variable*.

Criteria for Determining Causation

Because of the possibility of confounded results, very strict criteria for determining causation have been established. If an association is found, it must be evaluated against all of these criteria; the more criteria that are fulfilled, the more likely it is that the association is causal. However, an association may meet all of the criteria for causation and later be shown to be spurious because of other factors that were not considered at the time that the study was done. For this reason, epidemiologists interpret their results with great caution, and rarely consider a cause "proven." The five most widely used criteria for evaluating causation are described below.

The association should be strong

This can be measured statistically by a ratio that compares the morbidity or mortality rate for persons who have the proposed causal factor with the rate for those who do not have the factor. This ratio, discussed earlier, is the relative risk or odds ratio; the higher the relative risk or odds ratio, the stronger the association. As we saw in the investigation of TSS, use of the relative risk and odds ratio led to the identification of tampon users as persons at high risk for the syndrome (Centers for Disease Control, 1980a, 1980b, 1981).

The association should be consistent

The same association must be found repeatedly in other studies, in other settings, and with other methods. Numerous studies, over many years, associated cigarette smoking and certain diseases before the U.S. Surgeon General (1964) could declare with certitude that smoking was a causal factor in cancer or, more recently, cardiovascular disease (Office on Smoking and Health, 1983).

The association should be temporally correct

The hypothesized cause of the health condition must occur prior to the onset of the condition. On the surface this may seem obvious, as in the case of prenatal care, which clearly precedes birth outcome in time. Nevertheless, a "which came first, the chicken or the egg?" debate followed early studies, as researchers considered the question, "Do women have good birth outcomes because they had prenatal care, or do women who are going to have good birth outcomes choose prenatal care?" Careful study design, with adequate controls for other significant variables, has led to general agreement that prenatal care is important. However, the "chicken or the egg" issue must be considered in all studies.

The association should be specific

The hypothesized cause of the health condition should be associated with relatively few health conditions. If the association is with many variables, it is likely to be spurious. For instance, speaking Finnish is likely to be associated with cardiovascular disease; it is also likely to be associated with *any* characteristic of the Finns. The Finns do have a high incidence of cardiovascular disease (McAlister *et al,* 1981; Puska *et al.* 1981), but this, obviously, is not likely to be caused by Finnish speech.

The criterion of specificity must be tempered with the knowledge that certain factors have been shown to have multiple effects. For example, cigarette smoking has been linked to lung cancer, chronic obstructive pulmonary disease, cardiovascular disease, low birth weight, and a number of other conditions (Office of the Assistant Secretary for Health, 1980).

The association should be plausible and consistent with existing knowledge

The association should be logical in respect to what is currently known. The example of the association between cardiovascular disease and the Finnish language clearly is illogical in terms of any plausible physiologic mechanism. However, other associations may not be consistent with existing knowledge simply because "existing knowledge" is not as advanced as the new discovery. Nevertheless, an association that contradicts current scientific views should be evaluated very carefully.

EPIDEMIOLOGIC APPROACHES TO COMMUNITY HEALTH RESEARCH

In studying the determinants of population health, community health investigators may be guided by epidemiologic models. This section describes four epidemiologic models and portrays how four researchers, each guided by a different model, might approach the same problem.

The problem to be considered is an increase in the infant mortality rate in a hypothetical community. The infant mortality rate is a particularly important health index and should be understood even by health professionals whose main concern is not maternal or child health. Because infant mortality is influenced by a variety of biological and environmental factors affecting the infant and mother, the infant mortality rate provides both a direct measure of infant health and an indirect measure of community health as a whole.

Epidemiologic Triangle

The *epidemiologic triangle,* also called the *agent–host–environment model,* is a traditional view of health and disease as a composite of the agent, host, and environment. The *agent,* in the traditional sense, is an organism capable of causing disease in humans. The *host* is the human population at risk of developing the disease. The *environment* is a combination of physical, biological, and social factors that surround and influence both the agent and the host. According to this model, health and illness can be understood by examining characteristics of, changes in, and interactions among the three components.

The epidemiologic triangle, in its normal state of equilibrium, is depicted in Figure 2-1. Equilibrium does not signify optimum health, but simply the usual pattern of illness and health. Any change in characteristics of the agent, host, or environment will result in disequilibrium (*i.e.,* a change in the usual pattern).

The epidemiologic triangle also may be described as a see-saw (Roht *et al,* 1982), as shown in Figure 2-2. The top diagram shows the agent, host, and environment in perfect balance, the community's usual pattern. The middle diagram shows conditions favoring the agent, so that the host experiences increased illness. The bottom diagram shows conditions favoring the host, who now experiences decreased illness.

How would the epidemiologic triangle, or agent–host–environment model guide the investigation of increased infant mortality? To understand this, it is necessary to consider the three facets of the model.

Agent

At first glance, it might be concluded from this portion of the model that the researcher needs to focus on types of infections (agents) that might cause deaths in infants. However, other "agents" also cause infant deaths. The major causes of infant mortality in the United States include prematurity and low birth weight, birth injuries and birth anoxia, congenital malformations, sudden infant death syndrome (SIDS), accidents, and homicides. Therefore, the com-

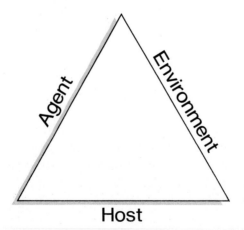

Figure 2-1.   The epidemiologic triangle is the traditional view of health and disease, showing them as a composite state of three variables.

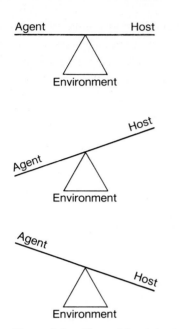

Figure 2-2. The epidemiologic triangle recast as a see-saw image. (Adapted from Roht LH, Selwyn BJ, Holguin AH, Christensen BL: Principles of Epidemiology: A Self Teaching Guide. New York, Academic Press, 1982)

munity health investigator will try to determine whether there has been a change or increase in infant deaths from any of these "agents."

Host

The investigator also will want to know the characteristics of the host, which in this case is the infant population. This involves examination of infant birth characteristics and mortality patterns in terms of race, sex, birth place, birth weight, and age at death. All of these characteristics have been shown to be important risk factors of infant mortality. By investigating these factors in the community, it may be possible to identify groups of infants who are particularly at increased risk of dying.

Environment

Finally, the environment must be assessed. The mother is a significant part of the infant's prenatal and postnatal environment. Therefore, the community health investigator will analyze birth and infant mortality patterns according to factors such as maternal age, marital status, parity (number of previous live births), prenatal care, education or socioeconomic status, race, and ethnicity. Analysis of these factors, which also have been shown to be related to infant survival, will help provide further identification of at-risk groups. Other conditions in the environment also need to be considered. For instance, has migration into the community from other areas increased? Has adult morbidity or mortality, particularly among pregnant women, increased? Have there been changes in health services, policies, personnel, funding, or other factors that could influence infant health?

Practical application

The analysis of these three areas, the agent, host, and environment, should provide information regarding groups at risk for increased infant mortality, and may point the way toward a program aimed at reducing that risk. Thus, the epidemiologic triangle, although it was designed with a communicable disease orientation, can provide a useful guide for study of the multifaceted problem of infant mortality, as well as for other health problems.

The Person–Place–Time Model

Another approach to epidemiologic study is one in which the health condition is described in terms of *person, place, and time* (Roht *et al,* 1982).

Person

Characteristics of persons with the particular condition and those without the condition are compared. In the study of infant mortality, both infant and maternal factors must be considered traits of "person." Thus, the investigator using the person–place–time model will examine infant mortality according to infant race, sex, birth weight, age at death, and cause of death, as well as maternal age, marital status, parity, prenatal care, ethnicity, and socioeconomic status.

Place

The place or location of occurrence is defined and described. The aspects of location to be considered will differ in each study. For example, is it rural or urban, a long-established community or a newly constructed suburb? Is it a manufacturing concern or a university, a low-income housing project or a wealthy neighborhood? These characteristics of location will be compared with characteristics of other locations as they relate to the health condition being studied. In a study of infant mortality, the researcher will be concerned with characteristics of the infant's place of birth and death. Is the increase in mortality among infants born in hospitals or at home? Are specific geographic areas of the community affected? Have there been any changes in the community environment that might influence infant health?

Time

The occurrence of the health condition is described in terms of time (*e.g.,* hours, days, weeks, months, seasons, or years). Patterns or trends may emerge from this description. In infant mortality, the causes of death and methods of prevention of death are quite different for the neonatal and postneonatal time periods, with neonatal deaths tending to have their roots in the prenatal period and postneonatal deaths being related more to immediate environmental conditions. Therefore, the investigator will be particularly interested in analysis of infant deaths according to age at death.

Similarity to epidemiologic triangle

The issues addressed when studying infant mortality according to the person–place–time model are similar to those investigated using the agent–host–environment model; only the approach is different.

The Web Of Causation

Multiple causation

The *web of causation* (MacMahon *et al,* 1970) views a health condition not as the result of individual factors, but of complex interrelations among multiple factors. That is, one factor may lead to others, which in turn lead to others, all of which may interact with one another to produce the health condition.

Synergism

This model also accommodates the concept of *synergism,* wherein the whole is more than the sum of its separate parts. For example, the combined effects of cigarette smoking, hypercholesteremia, and hypertension, discussed earlier in this chapter, are acknowledged to be more deleterious to health than the sum of the individual effects of these three cardiovascular risk factors (Centers for Disease Control, 1984).

Comprehensive scope

In the investigation of infant mortality, use of the web of causation may result in a more expansive study than one guided by either of the models previously discussed. Ideally, the investigator using this model first identifies all factors related to infant mortality; this encompasses all the aspects previously considered under agent, host, and environment, and person, place, and time. Next, the investigator identifies factors that are related to each of these factors. These two very comprehensive steps provide the outline for the web of causation for infant mortality. Finally, the researcher examines the relationships among all the identified components of the web, and attempts to determine the most feasible point of intervention. This analysis may involve sophisticated statistical techniques to help determine which of the factors are related most strongly to infant mortality.

Practical application

This all-encompassing approach clearly addresses the concept of causation in a manner consistent with current knowledge of human health. Nevertheless, it may be overwhelming to carry out in everyday practice. In fact, it is more usual for an investigator to examine only a portion of the web, acknowledging that other relationships exist. Thorough examination of one portion of the web may provide sufficient information for initiation of useful actions. Figure 2-3 depicts a proposed web of causation for infant mortality, based on information readily available from birth and death records.

The Community Syndrome

The *community syndrome model* (Kark, 1981), like the web of causation, acknowledges the multifaceted nature of human health conditions and stresses the interactions and synergism of the factors. The community syndrome model includes specific factors, but also takes into account broader community factors that are often overlooked in studies of health. The business cycle, agricultural conditions, and unemployment levels are but a few of the more global factors that might be included in a study guided by this model.

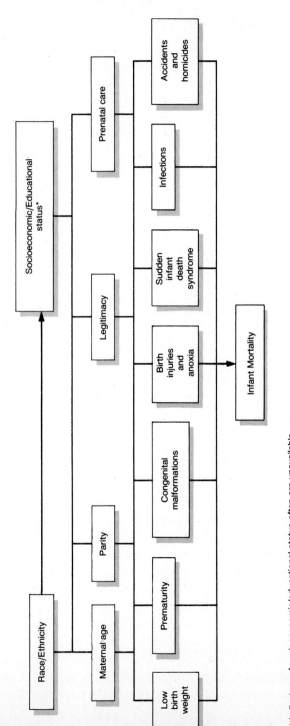

* Indicators of socioeconomic/educational status often are unavailable.

Figure 2-3. A proposed web of causation for infant mortality, based on information available from birth and death certificates.

Practical application

Figure 2-4 illustrates how a community health investigator might view infant mortality as part of a community syndrome of economic recession and unemployment. This particular depiction of the community syndrome model is a combination of specific and global factors related to infant health. The specific factors are similar to those considered in the three models discussed previously; these factors can guide the investigation and subsequent intervention. The global factors are more difficult to measure and act upon, but they place infant mortality in the context of the real world, and provide direction for broader community action.

SCREENING
FOR HEALTH CONDITIONS

Thus far we have focused on methods and approaches for investigating community health problems and assessing risks of morbidity and mortality. It has been shown that such investigation and assessment helps determine causal factors in illness and identifies groups at risk for particular health conditions. The information gained from such studies can be used to plan methods of prevention and intervention. In this section basic principles of *screening* will be discussed; a method of secondary prevention (early intervention), which may be used in population groups that have been identified as being at high risk for a particular health condition. The community health nurse is involved in selecting screening tests and administering screening programs.

Purpose of Screening

Screening is an effort to detect unrecognized or preclinical illness through testing of large groups of asymptomatic individuals. Screening tests are not intended to be diagnostic. Their purpose is to rapidly and economically identify persons who have a high probability of having (or developing) a particular illness so that these persons can be referred for definitive diagnosis and treatment.

Considerations in Deciding to Screen

Screening goes further than identification of groups at risk for illness; it also identifies *individuals* who may actually have the illness. As such, screening

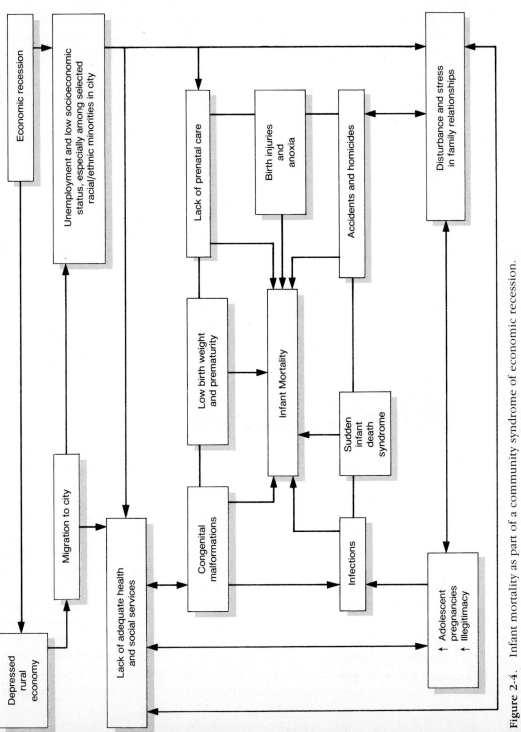

Figure 2-4. Infant mortality as part of a community syndrome of economic recession.

carries an ethical commitment to follow up on these individuals; that is, to provide these individuals with access to diagnostic and treatment services. If screening procedures are incorporated into a research project, arrangements must be made for appropriate referral for such services.

In general, screening should be attempted only if

- Early diagnosis and treatment can favorably alter the course of the illness
- Definitive diagnosis and treatment facilities are available, either through the screening agency or through referral
- The group being screened is at risk for the illness, (*i.e.,* the group is likely to have a high prevalence of the illness)
- The screening procedures are reliable and valid

Screening Test Reliability

Intra-observer and inter-observer reliability

Reliability refers to the consistency or repeatability of the test results. Reliability usually is measured in two ways. In *intra-observer reliability* or *intra-observer agreement,* the screening test must yield the same results when it is repeated on the same individual, under the same conditions, by the *same* investigator or observer. In *inter-observer reliability* or *inter-observer agreement,* the test must yield consistent results when it is repeated on the same individual, under the same conditions, by *separate* investigators or observers.

Ideally, reliability should be 100%. In practice, it may be lower. The community health nurse may be involved in determining the acceptable level of reliability for a particular screening test, and ensuring the highest possible level of reliability in practice.

Possible causes of poor reliability

Lack of reliability may suggest that the screening criteria are inadequately formulated. If so, the screening procedure may require clarification or revision before it is initiated.

Another common cause of poor reliability is the observers' being insufficiently skilled in the use of the test. A good screening program will include a training component. The need for this may seem obvious in community screening programs that use the services of volunteers and nonprofessionals, but even professional health care providers should be required to demonstrate proficiency in screening test procedures, which sometimes differ from the procedures in routine clinical practice. Including required training for all screening personnel may minimize potential personal embarrassment and diplomatic difficulties among the professional staff, while ensuring reliability of the screening program.

Screening Test Validity

Sensitivity and specificity

The *validity* of a screening test refers to its ability to do what it purports to do: distinguish correctly between those individuals who have the illness and those who do not. Validity is measured by the test's sensitivity and specificity, as shown in Table 2-6.

   Sensitivity is the ability to correctly identify individuals who have the disease; that is, to call a *true positive,* "positive." A test with high sensitivity will have few *false negatives.*

TABLE 2-6. SENSITIVITY AND SPECIFICITY OF A SCREENING TEST

Screening Test Results	Reality	
	Diseased	*Not Diseased*
Positive	True positive	False positive
Negative	False negative	True negative
Total	Total diseased	Total not diseased

$$\text{Sensitivity (true positive rate)} = \frac{\text{True positives}}{\text{Total diseased}}$$

$$\text{Specificity (true negative rate)} = \frac{\text{True negatives}}{\text{Total not diseased}}$$

$$\text{False negative rate} = \frac{\text{False negatives}}{\text{Total diseased}} \ or \ 1 - \text{Sensitivity}$$

$$\text{False positive rate} = \frac{\text{False positives}}{\text{Total not diseased}} \ or \ 1 - \text{Specificity}$$

Specificity is the ability to correctly identify individuals who do not have the disease, or to call a *true negative,* "negative." A test with high specificity has few *false positives.*

Screening tests or screening protocols developed by clinical researchers or commercial organizations may vary greatly in sensitivity and specificity. In planning and administering screening programs, the community health nurse must make informed decisions regarding the validity of the screening procedures.

Relationship between sensitivity and specificity

Ideally, for a screening test to be valid, its sensitivity and specificity should be 100%. However, as you can see from Table 2-6, sensitivity, or the *true positive rate,* is the complement of the *false negative rate,* and specificity, or the *true negative rate,* is the complement of the *false positive rate.* Thus, as sensitivity increases, specificity decreases. Therefore, decisions regarding screening test validity may require uncomfortable compromises, as you will see from the following examples.

Sensitivity and specificity: Practical and ethical considerations

Suppose we are screening for a deadly disease curable only if detected early, and have a choice between a test with high sensitivity and low specificity, and one with high specificity and low sensitivity. Which should be chosen? In order to save the most lives, high sensitivity is required; that is, a low rate of false negatives (people who have the disease, but are not detected by the screening test). However, in selecting the test with high sensitivity, its low specificity means a high rate of false positives (people who do not have the disease, but whom the screening test identifies as having the disease). That is, many people will be needlessly alarmed and unnecessary expenses will be incurred in over-referral for nonexistent disease. Which test would you choose?

Now suppose we are screening for the same disease, but the diagnostic and treatment facilities in the community are already overloaded, and further budget cuts are projected. The test with high specificity is desirable in order to minimize the unnecessary referral of false positives. However, because of the low sensitivity of this test, the benefits of a low false positive rate will have to be weighed against the ethics of a high false negative rate. Is it morally justifiable to lull the undetected diseased persons into a false—and potentially fatal—sense of security? Which test would you choose now?

Decisions regarding test validity may be complex, and involve seeking the most favorable balance of sensitivity and specificity. Sometimes sensitivity and specificity can be improved by adjusting the screening process (*e.g.,* adding another test or changing the level at which the test is considered positive). At other times, evaluating sensitivity and specificity may result in abandoning a screening program because the economic costs of over-referral, or the ethical considerations of under-referral, are judged to outweigh the program's usefulness.

An understanding of the principles discussed in this section will enable you to be an informed participant in decisions regarding community screening. You may wish to pursue further reading on this topic; for example, Mausner *et al* (1984) or Roht *et al* (1982).

COMMUNITY HEALTH RESEARCH

In this chapter it has been shown that investigation of community health problems is a vital component of community health nursing. The community health nurse acts as a community health researcher, as well as a health care provider.

Purposes of Community Health Research

Community health (or epidemiologic) research traditionally is considered to have two major purposes: to describe, and explain the health conditions of populations. The author of this chapter believes that the following four categories* more completely describe the purposes and scope of contemporary research in community health.

1. *Description* of the health conditions of aggregates
2. *Identification* of groups at risk for certain health conditions
3. *Explanation* of the health conditions of aggregates, through exploration of association and potential causation
4. *Evaluation* of the usefulness of interventions for improving the health of aggregates

---

*If you previously have learned the two traditional descriptive/explanatory categories, you may find it helpful to think of these four categories as more specific divisions of the traditional ones. That is, the traditional *descriptive* category includes *description* and *identification;* the traditional *explanatory* category includes *explanation* and *evaluation.*

This list of the four major purposes shows how research serves as a guide to the practice of community health nursing. Note from Table 2-7 how the purposes of community health research relate to the nursing process.

Focus of Community Health Research

Clearly, the emphasis in community health research is the health of the aggregate. Community health research is practical; it is used to identify and solve everyday problems in community health practice. Inherent in community health practice is the consideration of "the greatest good for the greatest number." For this reason, community health research usually does not focus on extremely rare health conditions, unless these conditions are expected to affect the health of society as a whole. Thus, for a practicing community health nurse, research priorities are likely to be related to the major causes of morbidity and mortality in a community, rather than to such relatively unknown conditions as myositis ossificans progressiva or relapsing nodular nonsuppurative panniculitis. However, in certain geographic areas, it might be very important to research a relatively uncommon condition such as dengue fever because of its potential for becoming epidemic in a community.

As one would expect, community health research also focuses on the levels of prevention considered in community health practice. That is, the emphasis is on promoting optimum health at primary, secondary, and tertiary levels of prevention, but rarely on high-technology techniques for prolonging life such as organ transplantation. However, community health researchers might examine organ transplantation programs in the context of the overall impact of these programs on the health of the community or nation (*e.g.,* regarding allocation of scarce resources).

TABLE 2-7.   RELATIONSHIP BETWEEN COMMUNITY
             HEALTH RESEARCH PURPOSES AND THE
             COMMUNITY HEALTH NURSING PROCESS

Community Health Research Purposes			Community Health Nursing Process
Description of aggregate	—	is	— Assessment
Identification of at-risk groups	—	aids	— Diagnosis
Explanation of causes	—	guides	— Planning/Implementation
Evaluation of intervention	—	is	— Evaluation

STEPS IN THE RESEARCH PROCESS

1. Identify an area of interest.
2. Review the literature to formulate a problem statement based on theory and research.
3. State the assumptions.
4. Formulate the research questions or hypotheses.
5. Operationalize the variables.
6. Plan the methodology.
   Select the research design.
   Select the sample.
   Select or design the data collection instruments and procedures.
   Plan the data analysis.
7. State the limitations of the study.
8. Ensure protection of human subjects.
9. Perform the pilot study.
10. Implement the methodology.
11. Interpret the results.
12. Communicate the results.

The Research Process

As described earlier, community health research is a process that uses demographic and epidemiologic principles. The research process is the same whether the research is in community health, high-technology medical intervention, or hospital nursing practice. The steps in the research process are outlined in the displayed material. Should you require a more in-depth review of research principles and methods, consult a research textbook, such as Abdellah *et al* (1979), Fox (1982), or Polit and Hungler (1983).

As we discuss the steps in the research process, we will demonstrate their application in a study of infant mortality, a health concern with which you have developed some familiarity. We will trace a particular study by a community health nurse will be traced from its earliest inception through its planning, implementation, and publication (Selby, 1982; Selby *et al,* 1984).

Step 1: Identify an area of interest

In community health nursing practice, you will encounter many unanswered questions and unsolved problems. In the first step of the research process, identify an area about which you would like to learn more. Feeling an interest in the subject is very important because research requires both thoroughness and perseverance. At this stage of the research process, do not be too concerned with the possibility that the chosen area is impossible to effectively research. If you are sincerely interested in finding an answer to a question or a solution to a problem in your practice, you should pursue the topic. Most questions of this nature are resolved in the second step of the research process.

Nevertheless, be aware that research involves empirically demonstrable findings, not value judgments. For example, research cannot determine whether abortion is morally or ethically good or bad. Research can be done on the social, economic, and health effects of abortion, but value judgments about the morality or ethics of abortion must be made outside the realm of research.

Application

How was the area of interest identified in the Selby study of infant mortality? A community health nurse with a pediatric nurse practitioner specialty moved from a midwestern state to Harris County, Texas, which includes and surrounds the city of Houston. Harris County, located approximately 300 miles from the Mexican border, has a large Mexican-American population. From her practice, the community health nurse noted that Mexican-Americans as a group seemed to be of low socioeconomic status, have large families, lack prenatal care, and, generally, have poorer health than persons of other ethnic groups. From her knowledge of infant-mortality risk factors, she thought Mexican-Americans probably also had a high infant-mortality rate. However, she did not know whether her personal impressions were valid. She was *interested* in learning more about Mexican-Americans and infant mortality in her new community.

Step 2: Review the literature and formulate a problem statement based on theory and research

This step is carried out at the library. In many cases, a preliminary *literature review* satisfies the need for knowledge on a topic, and further research is unnecessary. At other times, the literature raises as many questions as it answers, and a more comprehensive search is necessary in order to formulate a specific, researchable, theory-based problem statement.

As you review the literature for *theory* and *research* related to the selected health condition, the *problem statement,* or purpose of the proposed study, may undergo many revisions. It will become clear if the health condition is of sufficient importance to warrant research and if there is a need for such research. While studying theories and critiquing earlier research, a tentative methodology for the needed research will take shape, and it will be possible to evaluate whether or not the proposed research is feasible for you to undertake.

Application

In the infant mortality study, the community health nurse learned (as you have in this chapter) that many factors affect infant mortality. Guided by the theoretical or conceptual base of the *web of causation* model, the nurse noted that a number of infant-mortality risk factors were readily available on birth certificates in Texas: race; birth weight; gestational age; birth order; place of birth; and mother's age, marital status, and prenatal care. The age at death and cause of death also were available on infants' death certificates.

The community health nurse also learned that the poor health status of Mexican-American adults was documented (Lyndon B. Johnson School of Public Affairs, 1979) but the health status of Mexican-American infants was unclear. Mexican-Americans appeared to have a disproportionate share of infant-mortality risk factors: low socioeconomic and educational status, high fertility and large family size, and absent or inadequate prenatal care (Jaffe *et al*, 1980; Lee *et al*, 1981; Teller *et al*, 1974). Within the Mexican-American population, first-generation immigrants seemed to have the most unfavorable distribution of risk factors (Jaffe *et al*, 1980; Lee *et al*, 1981).

Nevertheless, the reported infant-mortality rates for Mexican-Americans in Texas were relatively favorable (Burris, 1974; Gee *et al*, 1976; Lyndon B. Johnson School of Public Affairs, 1979; Powell-Griner *et al*, 1982; Teller *et al*, 1974). The unusually low infant-mortality rates were largely attributed to idiosyncracies in birth and death registration in rural areas along the Texas–Mexico border (Powell-Griner *et al*, 1982; Teller *et al*, 1974).

In all of the studies reviewed, Mexican-Americans were identified by the *Spanish surname* criterion; for example, a Texas resident with a Spanish last name was judged to be of Mexican descent. This was necessary because Mexican-American ethnicity was not documented on birth or death certificates. However, use of the Spanish surname criterion could have resulted in misclassification because not all persons with Spanish last names are Mexican-Americans.

The community health nurse was not able to find out what the infant-mortality rate for Mexican-Americans was in Harris County. She did learn that birth and death certificates were coded by the state health department according to Spanish or non-Spanish surname and, according to the U.S. Bureau of the Census (1973), over 90% of the foreign-born Spanish-surname population of Texas were born in Mexico. Furthermore, birth certificates included information on the mother's and father's place of birth (United States or foreign).

The literature also showed that it was possible to link birth and death certificates on computer tape so that variables from both records could be analyzed. Linked birth and death records also make a prospective or cohort study possible because the births can be followed statistically forward into time. When the infant-mortality rate is calculated by the cohort method, the denominator of the rate is the actual population at risk for death; in the conventional method, the denominator is a calendar-year estimate.

Based on her review of theory and research in the literature, the community health nurse formulated this comprehensive *problem statement:* The purpose of this study is to answer the question: What are the infant, neonatal, and postneonatal mortality rates in relation to birth weight, birth order, maternal age, and prenatal care, for the Mexican-immigrant population of Harris County, Texas, in relation to other ethnic groups?

Step 3: State the assumptions

Assumptions are ideas that are presumed to be true, but for which the researcher has no proof. Assumptions should be derived from theory or research, and they should be stated clearly.

Application

The community health nurse identified two important *assumptions* in the proposed infant-mortality study.

1. The foreign-born Spanish surname population of Harris County is composed mainly of Mexican immigrants.
2. The cohort method of calculating the infant mortality rate is more likely than the conventional method to estimate the risk of infant death.

Review information presented from the literature review. Do you think these assumptions were justified?

Step 4: Formulate the research questions or hypotheses

The *research questions* further delineate the problem statement and specify which questions will need to be answered in order to address the problem statement. If a research question asks about relationships between variables, a *hypothesis,* or projected answer to the research question, may be formulated. A hypothesis is a statement that can be tested statistically. In general, a hypothesis will not be formulated for a study that does not presume to test for the statistical significance of a relationship.

Application

Because of the complexity of infant mortality, the community health nurse's proposed study had many *research questions.* Four are listed below.

1. What are the cohort infant-mortality rates for Spanish-surname white infants of foreign-born parents in relation to time of first prenatal care?
2. What are the cohort infant-mortality rates for Spanish-surname white infants of U.S.-born parents in relation to time of first prenatal care?
3. What are the cohort infant-mortality rates for non-Spanish-surname white infants in relation to time of first prenatal care?
4. What are the cohort infant-mortality rates for black infants in relation to time of first prenatal care?

These four questions called for descriptive answers, rather than testing relationships between variables, so no *hypotheses* were formulated. From your understanding of comparison groups, can you see why the community health nurse included infants of diverse ethnic groups in a study focusing on Mexican-American infant mortality?

Step 5: Operationalize the variables

It is necessary to specify the variables that must be measured to answer the research questions or test the hypotheses. The variables must be *operationalized;* that is, defined explicitly to ensure consistency in data collection and to enable other researchers to replicate a study.

The *operational definitions* must take into account the desired *level of measurement* for each variable. The levels of measurement are reviewed below.

1. *Nominal:* The lowest (weakest) level, in which data are categorized into mutually exclusive groups (*e.g.,* sex or ethnicity).
2. *Ordinal:* A higher level, in which data are categorized into mutually exclusive groups and placed in rank order (*e.g.,* "satisfaction," rated on a scale from very satisfied to very dissatisfied).

3. *Interval* or *ratio:* The highest levels, in which data are categorized into mutually exclusive groups and placed in order on a continuum that includes zero as a possible value (*e.g.,* age in years, diastolic blood pressure in torr).

Application

In her study of infant mortality, the community health nurse *operationalized* the variables for her four research questions as follows

1. *Ethnicity:* A cultural/racial identifier, recorded on the infant's live birth record as "Spanish-surname white," "non-Spanish-surname white," "black," or "other." This is a *nominal* level variable by definition.
2. *Parental nativity:* Place of birth of infant's parents, recorded on the infant's live birth record as "U.S." or "foreign." For this study, parental nativity was categorized as "U.S.-born" (both parents born in the United States) or "foreign-born" (one or both parents foreign-born). This also is a *nominal* level variable.
3. *Time of first prenatal care:* Month of gestation at which first prenatal visit occurred, as recorded on the infant's live birth certificate by month or as "none," and categorized for this study as "first trimester," "second trimester," "third trimester," and "no care." These categories, although they are numerical, are at best ordinal; that is, it is implied that prenatal care that begins in the first trimester is the most preferrable situation (even though this may not be true if prenatal care is not continued after the first visit), and that "no (prenatal) care" is the least desirable situation. Because even the ordinal nature of this variable is questionable, this variable was treated as *nominal* in this study.
4. *Infant mortality:* Death during the first year of life. Infant death will be documented by the presence of a death certificate indicating the live-born infant's age at death to be less than one year. The absence of an infant death certificate indicates survival to one year. Therefore, this is a *nominal* level variable (death versus survival). Risk of infant mortality will be estimated by specific cohort infant-mortality rates (IMRs) to be calculated by the formula

$$IMR = \frac{\text{infant deaths in specific cohort group}}{\text{total live births in specific cohort group}} \times 1000$$

Do you think that these operational definitions ensure that the terms in the research questions were defined consistently from case to case? If not, the eventual study data, based on approximately 70,000 cases, would not be reliable. Can you imagine expending such effort on 70,000 cases, only to produce results that are of questionable value?

Step 6: Plan the methodology

To plan the methodology for your project, select the research design, select the sample, select or design the data collection instruments and procedures, and plan the data analysis. Begin this process by selecting the research design.

Step 6A: Select the research design

In research, the design can be categorized as experimental, quasi-experimental, or nonexperimental. The choice of research design will be determined by the purposes of the research, as well as by real life resources and constraints.

Experimental design

Experimental research requires adherence to all of the following conditions

1. *Manipulation* of the *independent variable* (the presumed causal variable, or the variable that influences the other, *dependent variable*), through intervention or treatment
2. *Control* for confounding variables through use of a comparison or *control group* to which the intervention or treatment is not applied, and through careful monitoring of the study
3. *Randomization,* or *random assignment,* of subjects to the treatment or control groups

The true experiment is the hallmark of excellence in research design. However, in community health, experimental research sometimes is impossible, unethical, infeasible, or simply unnecessary. It is valuable to compare the requirements for experimental research to the four purposes of community health research: description, identification, explanation, and evaluation.

If the purpose of the research is to *describe* a human population or *identify* a population at risk, manipulation of the independent variable usually is impossible and unnecessary. For instance, it is impossible to manipulate a person's heredity or age, race, or sex; and it is unnecessary when the research goal is only to learn what a characteristic's relationship is to a health condition. Therefore, experimental design is inappropriate for such research.

If the research purpose is to *explain* the cause of a human health condition, manipulation of the independent variable often is unethical, even if it is possible; so is random assignment to exposure or nonexposure to the variable. For example, it is impossible to, in good conscience, force a group of persons to consume large doses of saccharin, and forbid consumption to another group, in order to determine the dose at which saccharin is carcinogenic in humans. For such reasons, experimental research rarely is used for determining causal relationships in community health conditions.

However, if the purpose of the research is to *evaluate* an intervention or treatment for a human health condition, experimental research may be highly desirable. The intervention or treatment constitutes the manipulation; its use, of course, must be justified by earlier explanatory research. Adhering to the other requirements for experimental research, namely, randomization and use of a control group, will help ensure that the intervention, rather than a confounding variable, leads to the improvement—or lack of improvement—in health.

As you develop programs to address needs in your community health practice, you must plan how to evaluate their impact. The principles of experimental research are excellent for this purpose. For further review of experimental research, consult the nursing research textbooks cited in the references, including Abdellah, 1979; Cook, 1979; and Fox, 1982.

Quasi-experimental design

Experimental research is not always feasible or practical in program evaluation because of the constraints imposed by real life. In this situation, the best choice may be *quasi-experimental* research. Quasi-experimental design may be employed in any situation in which

1. Experimental research is desirable
2. Manipulation of the independent variable (*i.e.,* the treatment or intervention) is feasible
3. Either randomization or use of a control group, or both, is not feasible

In essence, quasi-experimentation is faulty experimental research and thus is considerably less reliable than a true experiment. However, careful attention to other methodological aspects of the study can make quasi-experimental design a viable option in program evaluation. If you are responsible for health program planning, you may wish to pursue further reading in quasi-experimentation (*e.g.,* Cook *et al,* 1979).

Nonexperimental design

Most community health research is *nonexperimental.* If your practice involves *describing* populations, *identifying* populations at risk, or *explaining* possible causes of health conditions, you will be doing and interpreting nonexperimental research.

Nonexperimental research is used whenever manipulation of variables is impossible, unethical, infeasible, or unnecessary. All of the research studies presented thus far in this chapter are examples of nonexperimental research. As you have seen, nonexperimental research can produce excellent results when sound epidemiologic principles are applied.

Nonexperimental research usually is categorized according to its time perspective: *retrospective,* in which data for a particular health condition are examined in relation to past events, or *prospective,* in which data are collected on an ongoing basis to be examined in relation to a possible future health condition. Sometimes nonexperimental research also is categorized as *cross-sectional,* meaning that data are collected for a "slice of time," which may be in the present or the past. In epidemiologic research, cross-sectional studies usually are included in the retrospective category because, even when they involve surveying a present population, they generally consider past as well as present events.

Prospective research. A well-designed nonexperimental prospective study approximates an experiment as closely as can be done without actual manipulation of variables. A prospective study begins with a group of people, or cohort, exposed to a particular event (the independent variable); the event may be as dramatic as the radiation leak at the Three Mile Island nuclear reactor in the 1970s, or it may be as mundane as being born in a particular year. This event may be seen as a naturally occurring equivalent of manipulation of the independent variable. The study then follows the cohort forward in time to see whether the independent variable results in the health condition under study. Ideally, the study also follows a similar group of people who were not exposed to the event (a type of control group), in order to make comparisons. A nonexperimental prospective study cannot use randomization of subjects to groups, because the change in the independent variable occurs before the groups are identified.

In this chapter, you have learned that prospective designs are advantageous because they allow incidence and relative risk to be calculated. You will find that all of the epidemiologic principles you have studied will help you conduct or interpret prospective research. Of course, you always are encouraged to expand your knowledge through further study of epidemiology texts such as MacMahon *et al* (1970), Mausner *et al* (1984), Roht *et al* (1982), or Slome *et al* (1982).

Despite the many advantages of prospective designs, they also have limitations. They usually are not practical for studying rare health conditions or those with a long latency period. Prospective studies tend to be expensive and time-consuming, and they may suffer from the loss or "drop-out" of subjects over time.

Retrospective research: the case-control study. Because of the difficulties involved in prospective research, retrospective studies are used most in community health. In the earlier example of the study of TSS, you were introduced to the *case-control* study, a special type of retrospective study in which persons with a particular health condition (cases) and persons without the health condition (controls) are compared. An attempt is made to look backward in time to determine risk factors and potential causes of the health condition. As you have seen, the case-control study tries to approximate a prospective study by allowing for estimating relative risk using the odds ratio. At the same time, the case-control study has the advantage of being less costly, in terms of time and money, than a prospective study.

As a community health nurse, you may be involved in planning, implementing, or interpreting case-control studies. You are encouraged to do further reading in one of the suggested texts (*e.g.,* Schlesselman 1982).

Application

Figure 2-5 presents a scheme that may help you determine the study design appropriate for various types of community health research. Refer to this figure as we return to our example of Mexican-American infant mortality and observe how the community health nurse determined the appropriate research design for the proposed study.

First, let us analyze the community health nurse's problem statement to determine whether the study purpose was to *describe, identify, explain,* or *evaluate.* To review, the problem statement was, What are the infant, neonatal, and postneonatal mortality rates in relation to birth weight, birth order, maternal age, and prenatal care, for the Mexican immigrant population of Harris County, Texas, in relation to other ethnic groups?

From the problem statement, it is evident that the community health nurse intended to *describe* the Mexican-immigrant population in terms of infant mortality, *identify* whether they were at risk for infant mortality in comparison to other ethnic groups, and possibly *explain* the relationship of infant mortality to the risk factors of birth weight, birth order, maternal age, and prenatal care. She did not plan to *evaluate* an intervention. Therefore, a *nonexperimental* study design was appropriate.

Now let us determine which type of nonexperimental design, retrospective or prospective, was advisable in this situation. The community health nurse was inter-

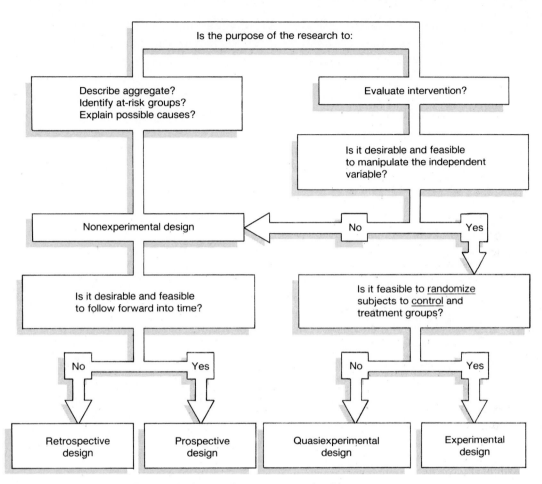

Figure 2-5. Selection of research designs for community health practice.

ested in assessing the infant mortality rates (that is, the *incidence* of infant mortality) among infants of Mexican immigrants. Although prospective designs generally are required for calculating incidence, they are costly in terms of time and money, and rates can be calculated from retrospective calendar year data. However, rates calculated in this manner are not always accurate estimates of incidence because the numerators and denominators may be from different populations. In view of the confusing literature regarding Mexican-American infant mortality, accuracy was considered to be very important in this study. Based on this information, which nonexperimental research design would you choose?

The community health nurse appropriately chose a *prospective* study. Refer again to the information presented from the literature review (Step 2) to see why this was possible and feasible. Birth and infant death records could be matched to create a birth cohort that statistically could be followed forward until the infant reached the age of one year, signified by the absence of an infant death record, or until the infant died during the first year of life, signified by the presence of an infant death record. This special type of prospective study sometimes is called a *prospective study in retrospect* or a *retrospective study, prospectively done.*

Step 6B: Select the sample

Population, sampling frame, sample, subjects, and setting

In selecting the sample, the investigator first must identify the *population* to whom the results are intended to apply. Then the researcher determines the *sampling frame,* which is essentially an operationalized population. That is, the sampling frame is the actual usable data source or listing of the population from which the *sample,* a subset of the population, can be chosen. The *subjects* are the individual members of the sample. The *setting* refers to the geographic or physical location of the sample.

Thus, in a study of sexually active teenage girls, the population might be all adolescent females attending the county teen-family-planning clinics. The sampling frame could be a listing of the names or medical chart numbers of all adolescent females who attended the teen-family-planning clinics in the past year. The sample would be the group of adolescent female subjects (or the medical records of these subjects) actually selected for the study. The setting would be the actual clinic sites attended by the subjects.

Probability sampling

Sampling may be done by a probability or nonprobability method. A *probability sample* is one in which each member of the population has a probability, or chance, of being included in the sample. This is achieved through use of a *table of random numbers* or other probability selection device. Probability sampling helps ensure that the sample is *representative* of the population. Provided the sample size is sufficiently large and the study procedures are valid, this form of sampling allows *generalization* of the results from the sample to the population. Therefore, probability sampling is usually the preferred method.

Nonprobability sampling

A *nonprobability sample* is one in which there is no assurance that each member of the population has a chance of being included in the sample. In nonprobability sampling, the sample is not likely to be representative of the population, and the results cannot be generalized to the population. In community health research, which seeks to make inferences about the health of the community at large, this lack of ability to generalize is an important limitation.

Sampling bias

In research, the possibility of making random and systematic errors that may influence data adversely is a concern. In sampling, the most important error to avoid is systematic error, or *bias. Sampling bias* is the systematic over-representation or under-representation, in the sample, of a specific group from the population. The results from a biased sample are not generalizable to the population. Sampling bias is most likely to occur in nonprobability sampling, but also may occur in probability sampling, either by chance, because of a small sample, or because of inherent biases in the sampling frame or data source.

Data sources

Community health investigation often relies upon existing (*i.e.,* retrospective) data. The source of the existing data can be viewed as the sampling frame. The text below examines several commonly used sources of community health data and considers their quality and completeness.

Census. The decennial census probably is the most comprehensive source of health-related data for the United States. Every ten years, the Bureau of the Census enumerates the United States population and surveys it for basic demographics such as age, race, and sex, and also for numerous other factors, including employment, presence and duration of disability, income, education, family size, type of household, type and age of residence, and presence of indoor plumbing in residence, to name but a few. Because of expense, only a limited number of questions are asked of the entire population; more detailed surveys are taken of selected samples of the population.

Census data are readily available in many public libraries. The *Census of the Population* is published in multivolume sets for the United States as a whole, states, and selected smaller areas. Special *Subject Reports* (*e.g.,* on the Spanish-surname or American-Indian populations) also are published. In noncensus years, segments of the population are surveyed to monitor ongoing demographic trends. These are published as *Current Population Reports.*

In evaluating census data, it is important to note whether the data are from the complete population or from a sample. Generally, total population data are more reliable. However, even these figures are subject to bias. From your own experience in responding to surveys, you probably are aware of one potential source of error: people may answer personal questions dishonestly. Perhaps more significantly, the census is believed to under-represent blacks, Mexican-Americans, low-income inner city residents, and transients. These people are more difficult to locate and enumerate, and tend to be less likely to respond to census surveys.

Vital statistics. Vital statistics are the data on legally registered events (*e.g.,* births, deaths, marriages, divorces) collected on an ongoing basis by government agencies. State health departments usually publish vital statistics annually. The U.S. Public Health Service also gathers data from the states and publishes annual volumes, as well as monthly reports, regarding specific topics.

Beginning researchers tend to consider vital statistics "hallowed," because they are, after all, legal data. However, closer scrutiny reveals that legality does not guarantee validity. Not all births and deaths are registered; those of blacks, Mexican-Americans, and infants who die shortly after birth seem particularly likely to be under-registered (McCarthy *et al,* 1980; Powell-Griner *et al,* 1982; Selby *et al,* 1984; Teller *et al,* 1974). The cause of death recorded on death certificates is noted for inaccuracy (Shryock *et al,* 1980), and discrepancies have been reported in the recording of race on birth and death certificates (Frost *et al,* 1980; Norris *et al,* 1971). In reference to marriages and divorces, the numbers of nonmarried, but cohabiting, couples, and the occasional newspaper reports of newly discovered bigamists, should demonstrate convincingly that these records also are not completely valid measures of reality. At some point in your career, you may wish to explore the voluminous literature regarding bias in vital statistics.

At this point, you may be asking, "Then why use vital statistics at all?" The answer is that, despite their limitations, vital statistics often are the best available data, and much useful information can be gained from them. *All* data sources have potential biases and pitfalls. The investigator must be aware of the limitations that apply to the data being used, interpret the data accordingly, and not ascribe more value to the results than is justified.

Notifiable disease reports. State and local health departments collect morbidity statistics on legally reportable diseases. These statistics are reported to the Centers for Disease Control (CDC) of the U.S. Public Health Service, which analyzes the data. Periodically, the CDC also issues requests for voluntary reporting of nonnotifiable health conditions of special interest; in the early 1980s, water-slide injuries at amusement parks were analyzed. You will find much current information in the excellent CDC publication, the *Morbidity and Mortality Weekly Report* (MMWR).

Nevertheless, be aware that even legally mandated disease reports may not be representative of all cases of the disease; that is, they may not provide valid descriptions of the disease as it exists in the community. In practice, health care providers often fail to report diseases that should be reported, or they do not report them unless they themselves suspect increases in prevalence or incidence.

Medical and hospital records. Medical and hospital records are used extensively in community health research. Unfortunately, these records do not provide a completely valid and representative picture of community health. In the first place, not all clients with health problems present themselves for medical attention, so medical records obviously are biased.

As a nurse, you already have some insights into the quality and completeness—or lack thereof—of medical documentation. A researcher may develop a superbly comprehensive data abstraction form, with clear, explicit operational definitions for each variable; but if each chart says only, "Doing well," the resulting data will be worthless.

The type of population from which the records are taken also will influence the validity of the data for community health. Medical records from a general outpatient practice are more likely to reflect the true state of a disease in the community than are records from a referral or specialist practice; the referred patients usually are sicker. Hospitalized patients, of course, are even more sick.

Hospitalized patients also are more likely to have another illness along with the illness being studied. This phenomenon, called *Berkson's bias,* creates the likelihood of finding a spurious association between the two illnesses. As an example, consider the population of persons with Alzheimer's disease (a neurologically debilitating disorder and major cause of mortality in the elderly) and the population of persons who develop infected leg ulcers. Because of restrictions in their ability to care for themselves, persons with Alzheimer's disease who also develop infected leg ulcers probably are more likely to be hospitalized than persons with either condition alone. Now suppose that the hospital records of Alzheimer's patients are analyzed to try to determine possible causal factors in Alzheimer's. Can you see how this could lead to false associations between Alzheimer's and leg ulcers?

Autopsy records. Autopsy records are not used very often in community health research because of their inherent bias: these patients were so sick that they died. However, this data source is included here because community health professionals must be able to evaluate research that is based on autopsy data.

Autopsies are not performed for all deaths. Therefore, autopsy records include a disproportionate number of persons for whom the cause of death was unknown until after autopsy; that is, these persons had uncommon manifestations of illness. Violent deaths also tend to be over-represented, while deaths of members of religious groups that do not sanction autopsy are under-represented. All of these factors influence the validity and representativeness of the study results.

Protection of human subjects

When selecting the data source and sample, the researcher also must consider measures for protecting the rights of human subjects. To avoid potential violations of human rights, federal guidelines mandate that *informed consent* be obtained from individual subjects involved in research. The components of informed consent are summarized in the displayed material. These components generally are dealt with in a written letter to the potential subjects.

In research not involving direct participation or identification of individuals, the requirements for protection of human subjects may be simplified to include only assurances of *anonymity,* meaning the researcher will not have access to individual identification, or *confidentiality,* meaning the researcher will not disclose individual identification to others not associated with the research project. This frequently is the case in community health research that uses existing data.

Application

In the community health nurse's infant mortality study, the results of her investigation were intended to apply to the *population* of infants born to residents of Harris County, Texas, focusing particularly on Mexican-Americans. Her available *sampling frame,* or source of data, was a computer tape of matched birth and infant death records prepared by the state health department. How did she approach sample selection?

First, she evaluated the data source—the vital statistics computer tape—very carefully. She scrutinized the literature regarding bias in birth and death certificates and made an informed decision to use the data source, despite its limitations, because this source was the best available for the purpose of her study.

Then, she consciously chose a *nonprobability sample* consisting of the computerized records of all (N = 68,584) live-born infants of Spanish-surname white, non-Spanish-surname white, and black ethnicity, born to residents of Harris County,

---

COMPONENTS OF INFORMED CONSENT

---

1. Invitation to participate in study
2. Assurance that subject has right to refuse to participate, and that refusal will not place subject in jeopardy
3. Assurance that subject has the right to withdraw from participation, and that withdrawal will not place subject in jeopardy
4. Explanation of purpose of study
5. Explanation of study procedures (as they relate to subjects)
6. Description of potential risks, discomforts, inconveniences, or threats to dignity involved in study
7. Description of potential benefits of participation in study
8. Description of compensation to be expected, whether monetary or otherwise (if applicable)
9. Disclosure of available alternatives (if applicable)
10. Assurance of confidentiality or anonymity
11. Statement regarding contact person, and an offer to answer questions
12. Language clear, unambiguous, and appropriate for subject's age, educational level, etc.
13. Concluding statement noting that subject indicates by signature (or, in certain studies, return of completed questionnaire) that he/she has read the information and has decided to participate
14. Individual agency may require statement that agency will not provide compensation in case of injury resulting from participation
15. Special restrictions apply to minors or individuals whose ability to give informed consent may be compromised

---

Texas, from January 1, 1974, through December 31, 1975. These were the most recent years for which matched birth and death records were available. Because of changes in the infant mortality rate over time (*i.e.,* the infant mortality rate in the United States tends to improve each year), the nurse judged it to be more important to have current data than to have a probability sample of all infants ever born in the county.

Harris County was chosen as the *setting* mainly because it was the geographic area of interest to the community health nurse. It also had the advantage of being an urban center, with (reportedly) excellent birth and death registration. Additionally, it was considered to be sufficiently far from the Mexican border not to be influenced by the border-related birth and death registration problems cited in the literature.

Protection of human subjects was ensured by the state health department's removal of names and street addresses from the data before making the data tape available to the community health nurse. Data were coded by presence or absence of Spanish surname only.

Step 6C: Select or design the data collection instruments and procedures

Now that the research design and sample have been determined, it is time to plan the methods for obtaining the desired information from the sample. At this point the information desired has already been outlined in the form of operational definitions for the variables of interest. Now, data collection procedures and *instruments,* or devices for gathering data, must be selected or designed to collect data in accordance with the operational definitions.

It has been shown that data sources and sampling methods should be planned to avoid or minimize potential errors in data collection. Obviously, the instruments and procedures also should be designed to avoid errors.

Valid and reliable instruments and procedures help prevent systematic and random error. The concepts of reliability and validity were introduced in the discussion of screening programs. Now, these concepts will be expanded and other aspects of data collection that influence the quality of results will also be considered.

Reliability

As you have learned, *reliability* refers to the consistency of results. Reliability may be expressed as a *correlation coefficient* (r), usually ranging from 0 to 1, or as a *percentage of agreement.* Reliability of 1 or 100% is ideal, but rare; reliability of less than 0.8 or 80% is questionable.

In assessing reliability, you should be aware that the correlation coefficient or percent of reliability is influenced by the sample from which the reliability is calculated (*i.e.,* reliability is *sample specific*). For example, an instrument that has high reliability in a sample of military recruits may be very unreliable in a sample of pregnant teenagers.

In screening tests and procedures, reliability is measured by intra-observer and inter-observer agreement. When using other types of instruments and procedures, reliability usually is measured according to three major aspects: *equivalence, stability,* and *internal consistency.* The aspect of reliability to be addressed will depend upon the type and purpose of the instrument or procedure.

Equivalence. Essentially, this aspect of reliability examines whether different researchers using the same instrument on the same subjects under the same conditions will measure the same characteristic, or if different instruments used on the same subjects under the same conditions will measure the same characteristic.

The first type of equivalence is the same as inter-observer agreement; it also is referred to as *inter-rater reliability.* As you have learned, this type of reliability is expressed as a correlation or percentage of agreement between the observers or raters. Inter-rater reliability is necessary if more than one person will collect data. As you learned in the discussion of screening tests, inter-rater reliability can be enhanced by proper training of the persons who will administer the instruments or procedures.

The second type of equivalence is necessary if two different instruments are to be used for measuring the same characteristic. This sometimes is the case in pretest and posttest studies for program evaluation. Although most often the pretest and posttest are identical, in some cases the researcher may want the tests to be different, but still measure the same concept. In this case, before the study can be conducted, *parallel forms reliability* must be calculated, that is, a correlation or percentage of agreement of responses between the two data collection forms, administered simultaneously to one sample.

Stability. Stability refers to the ability of the instrument or procedure to give the same results on repeated use.

For a data collection form used by the researcher, stability may be measured by *intra-rater reliability,* the equivalent of intra-observer agreement for a screening test. For example, in assessing the stability of a form for abstracting data from medical records, the researcher will use the form on a sample of records; a week to ten days later, the researcher will repeat the process and determine a correlation or percentage of agreement between the two sets of results. This method also will help identify particular items on the form that are unclear. Like inter-rater reliability, this type of reliability can be enhanced by training the rater.

For a data collection form to be used by the subjects, stability may be measured by *test–retest reliability.* The questionnaire or scale is administered to a sample of subjects; a week to ten days later, it is re-administered to the same group, and a correlation or percentage of agreement of responses will be calculated. This method, like the intra-rater method, also helps identify individual items in need of revision.

Stability is not an appropriate aspect of reliability to measure in cases in which the measured characteristic or concept is expected to change over time.

If the trait itself is not stable, the data collection device is not expected to yield stable results on re-administration. An example is the concept of state anxiety, a psychological condition that may vary from moment to moment, depending on the situation (Spielberger, *et al,* 1968).

Internal consistency. Internal consistency refers to the ability of the various subparts of the instrument to measure the same characteristic or concept. This type of reliability is important in attitudinal scales or knowledge tests in which the purpose is to provide an overall estimate of a single characteristic.

If you are involved in developing instruments for evaluation of community health programs intended to change attitudes or increase knowledge, you will need to be familiar with the various techniques for calculating coefficients of reliability for such scales and tests. These include the *coefficient alpha* (Cronbach's alpha), *split-half* or *odd-even* method with correction by the *Spearman–Brown prophecy formula,* and the *Kuder–Richardson 20* (KR-20). In general, the internal consistency of attitudinal scales may be evaluated by the coefficient alpha or split-half/odd-even method; knowledge tests with right or wrong answers may be evaluated by the KR-20 or split-half/odd-even method. Calculation of these coefficients is explained by Polit *et al* (1983).

Measurement of internal consistency generally is not appropriate unless the various items in an instrument are intended to measure the same concept (*i.e.,* to be homogeneous). However, sometimes a researcher will be concerned that a particular variable may not be measured accurately. In this case, a special measure of internal consistency may be added to the instrument. For example, in an attitudinal scale, the same item might appear twice. In a questionnaire asking for the respondent's age, the researcher might have two separate questions

How old are you? ＿＿＿ years
What is your birthdate?

The researcher then determines whether the two responses yield consistent results. If they do not, the reliability of the variable is questionable.

Validity

The discussion of screening tests has shown that *validity* refers to the ability of a test or instrument to measure what it purports to measure. In research, if the instruments consist of screening tests, their validity is assessed through evaluation of sensitivity and specificity. Most often, however, research involves the use of instruments other than screening tests. For these other instruments, validity may be assessed and categorized according to *face, content, criterion-related,* and *construct* validity.

Face validity. Some researchers contend that face validity is a legitimate form of validity. In epidemiologic circles, however, face validity is referred to, "tongue-in-cheek," as "faith validity." Essentially, face validity simply means that the instrument appears valid to the researcher. In your research, you are urged not to consider this a true form of validity. It is presented here so you will evaluate skeptically any study that reports only face validity for its instruments.

Content validity. The presence of content validity in an instrument indicates the individual items in the instrument are representative of the concept(s) to be measured. This type of validity, generally considered the weakest true form of validity, is easily achieved and should be documented for any data abstracting form, questionnaire, attitude scale, or knowledge test. To obtain content validity, the proposed instrument is submitted to a number of experts in the field, referred to as a *panel of experts.* These experts critique the instrument and may suggest revisions before they agree that the items are representative of the concept(s) being measured.

Criterion-related validity. This type of validity is more difficult to achieve. Essentially, criterion-related validity measures the correlation between the proposed instrument and another, supposedly valid, measure of the same concept. The other measure, or *criterion,* may be a more-established instrument or any other valid method of measuring the concept. For example, in designing an instrument to assess the seriousness or "staging" of a particular illness in a patient population, a researcher might correlate the results obtained by the proposed instrument with those obtained when a medical expert does the assessment personally.

   The difficulty with criterion-related validity comes in deciding upon the criterion against which the proposed instrument is to be measured. If the criterion itself is not valid, the validity of the proposed instrument cannot be determined. In the example given above, the medical expert conceivably *could* make mistakes in the assessments.

Construct validity. Construct validity is intended to ensure that the instrument measures the concept it is supposed to measure, and not something else. This is the highest form of validity; essentially, it states that the instrument truly is valid.

Construct validity is difficult to establish; it can rarely be done on the basis of one study. Discussion of the various techniques for determining this type of validity is beyond the scope of this text. These techniques include the *known-groups method,* the *multi-trait multi-method matrix,* and *factor analysis.* As you grow in research experience and expertise, you may wish to consider these methods.

Considerations in choosing a method for determining validity and reliability

The methods for determining validity (Table 2-8) are hierarchical; that is, each succeeding level is a higher form of validity. Therefore, in your research you will want to begin with the easiest method and advance to the highest level possible for your instrument, given your real-life resources and constraints. In no case settle for less than content validity.

On the other hand, the techniques for establishing reliability

TABLE 2-8.   GUIDE TO TECHNIQUES FOR DETERMINING INSTRUMENT VALIDITY

Type	Key Question	Technique	Comments
Face	Does the instrument appear to be logical?	Researcher decision	Alone, this is *not* a legitimate form of validity
Content	Are the individual items representative of the concept?	Panel of experts	Weakest form of true validity Relatively simple to achieve
Criterion-related	Is there a high correlation between this measure and another measure of the same concept?	Correlation coefficient (between the 2 measures)	Difficult to decide on appropriate criterion If another valid measure is already available, is there a legitimate reason for not using the other measure?
Construct*	Does the instrument truly measure the concept and not something else?	Known groups	Assumption is made about characteristics of the known groups Least difficult of 3 construct validity techniques
		Multi-trait multi-method matrix	Requires 2 or more methods and concepts Requires some statistical sophistication
		Factor analysis	Requires some statistical sophistication

* Construct validity is the highest form of validity

(Table 2-9) are not hierarchical; they simply are different. You will need to choose the technique or techniques appropriate for your particular instrument and purpose.

Other considerations: documentation of procedures

A final aspect of quality assurance in data collection is the need for explicit *documentation* of procedures. This was alluded to previously in the discussion of operational definitions. Not only must each variable be defined, each aspect of the study must be described in sufficient detail to permit replication. This allows future researchers to confirm the findings of the study in different populations, locations, or times. In community health practice, appropriate documentation also ensures that even if there are changes in personnel the research can continue without a compromise in reliability or validity.

Application

In the community health nurse's infant-mortality study, the *instruments* and *procedures* she chose required use of a statistical computer program to select and describe the variables of interest. How did the concepts of validity and reliability apply here?

The community health nurse had a working knowledge of the statistical computer language to be used. Nevertheless, she consulted with computer experts as she translated the operational definitions for the variables into computer procedures and prepared a computer program to extract the sample and describe the variables. As the primary investigator for this project, the nurse was responsible for ensuring validity and reliability.

Therefore, she submitted the completed computer program to two public health professionals with computer expertise. This *panel of experts* reviewed the program, suggested revisions, and finally approved it, attesting to its *content validity*.

The community health nurse could not calculate coefficients of reliability using this procedure. However, reliability was addressed by having a trained computer expert test run the program in accordance with established computing procedures, and by examining a sample of ten cases before performing statistical calculations to ensure that the appropriate variables were being selected. To further ensure reliability, the computer program and all study procedures were *documented* in a written research protocol.

Step 6D: Plan the data analysis

The data analysis, and the manner in which the data will be displayed, should be planned before the data are actually collected. In essence, all of the pre-

TABLE 2-9.   GUIDE TO TECHNIQUES FOR
DETERMINING INSTRUMENT RELIABILITY

Type	Key Questions	Technique	Comments
Equivalence	Do different researchers using the same instrument measure the same characteristic?	Inter-rater reliability	Used when more than one researcher using an instrument that requires subjective judgment
	Do different instruments measure the same characteristic?	Parallel forms reliability	Used when it is advisable to have different items for the pretest and posttest
Stability	Will instrument give the same results on repeat administration?		
	Instrument to be completed by researcher	Intra-rater reliability	Not appropriate if data being measured are not stable over time
	Instrument to be completed by subjects	Test–retest reliability	Short period of time between first and second administration may give falsely high reliability because person completing instrument may simply remember earlier responses
Internal consistency	Do the subparts measure the same characteristic?	For Likert-type scale: Coefficient alpha Split-half or odd/even with correction by Spearman–Brown Prophecy For right/wrong questions: Kuder–Richardson 20 (KR20) Split-half or odd/even with correction by Spearman–Brown Prophecy	This type of reliability is not appropriate unless the various items are intended to measure the *same* concept
	Are individuals responding consistently?	Agreement of responses between 2 items that ask for the same information	Used when researcher is concerned about possibility that a particular item will not be measured accurately

vious steps in the research process—the formulation of the research questions and hypotheses, operational definitions, and research design; the selection of the sample; and the design of the instruments and procedures—are directed toward data analysis. If these steps are planned appropriately, data analysis should proceed relatively smoothly. However, many a poorly designed study has "bitten the dust" after months of data collection because it was discovered, too late, that the data collected could not be analyzed to produce valid results.

Basically, data analysis involves the use of two types of statistics: *descriptive statistics,* which describe and summarize data, and *inferential statistics,* which test for the significance of relationships in the data. All studies require the use of descriptive statistics; only those that test hypotheses require inferential statistics.

Descriptive statistics

Description of the sample. The sample should be described in terms of each important variable. The variables can be summarized by *measures of central tendency* such as the mean, median, and mode, and *measures of variability* such as the standard deviation, range, and proportions or percentages. Analyses of the various levels or categories of a variable in terms of numbers and percentages is referred to as describing the *distribution* of the variable. In epidemiologic studies, it also is helpful to calculate rates, which, of course, are a special type of proportion.

Description of relationships between variables. Relationships between the variables can be described by statistical *measures of association,* or correlation coefficients. In epidemiologic studies, *analytic measures* also may be used such as the relative risk, odds ratio, attributable risk, and attributable risk percent.

Considerations in choosing descriptive statistics. You have learned that the selection of epidemiologic measures such as incidence and prevalence rates, relative risks, odds ratios, and so forth, is determined by the study design (*i.e.,* prospective versus retrospective). As you can see from Table 2-10, the selection of appropriate statistical measures of central tendency, variability, and association is dictated by the level of measurement of each variable; the higher the level of measurement, the greater the possibilities for statistical description.

Of course, the level of measurement is determined in turn by the data collection instrument, which is designed to collect data based on the operational definition of each variable. In other words, if a difficulty arises in plan-

TABLE 2-10.   GUIDE TO SELECTED MEASURES OF
              CENTRAL TENDENCY, VARIABILITY,
              AND ASSOCIATION

	Minimum Level of Measurement Required		
	Nominal	*Ordinal*	*Interval/ratio*
Central tendency	Mode	median	mean
Variability	Percent	range	standard deviation
Association (both variables must be at least the level specified)	Contingency coefficient Lambda Phi coefficient	Spearman rho Kendall tau	Pearson product moment

ning the descriptive data analysis, the origin of the difficulty probably can be found at an earlier step in the research process. You can see, therefore, that it is imperative that data analysis be planned before the data are collected, while the opportunity to make revisions still exists.

Application

In her infant mortality study, the community health nurse examined many variables and relationships between variables. The text below covers how she planned to describe the four variables in the selected research questions. These nominal level variables were ethnicity, parental nativity, time of prenatal care, and infant mortality.

The nurse decided to describe the sample of live births according to the *distribution* of ethnic and parental nativity groups, levels of prenatal care, and deaths. She also planned to describe the distribution of births, deaths, and levels of prenatal care for specific ethnic/parental nativity subgroups (*e.g.,* Spanish-surname foreign-born parentage, Spanish-surname U.S.-born parentage).

In this prospective study, the community health nurse was able to describe the *incidence* of infant mortality by calculating infant mortality *rates* for ethnic groups and ethnic/parental nativity subgroups. In order to compare populations with different levels of prenatal care, she planned to calculate *specific infant-mortality rates* for these groups and subgroups according to levels of prenatal care. Because prenatal care was expected to influence infant mortality, she also intended to use *adjusted rates.* To describe relationships between infant mortality and the selected variables, she planned to calculate *relative risks.*

Inferential statistics

Hypothesis testing. Inferential statistics are used in studies in which a hypothesis is to be tested. The hypothesis may be on an *association between variables* such as tampon-brand usage and the presence of TSS or about a *difference between groups* such as the difference in age between persons with a specific disease and without the disease. The inferential statistic tests if the association or difference is *statistically significant,* or divergent from that expected by chance alone.

Considerations in choosing inferential statistics. Essentially, inferential statistics test for the statistical significance of descriptive statistics. In the case of tampon-brand usage and TSS, an inferential statistic was used to test for the significance of the *odds ratio* for use of Rely brand tampons. In the example of the ages of diseased and nondiseased persons, an inferential statistic could be used to test for the differences between the *mean* ages for diseased and nondiseased persons. It should come as no surprise then that appropriate selection of inferential statistics, like descriptive statistics, is based upon the level of measurement of the variables and the design of the study.

The choice of inferential statistics also is influenced by the characteristics of the study sample. Certain statistical tests are appropriate for one-group, two-group, or multigroup samples. Some tests can be used with small samples; others can be used only with large samples. Some are appropriate for groups measured once; others are for repeated measures.

Table 2-11 is intended as a general guide for the selection of inferential statistics in some of the most common community health research situations. This table considers most of the requirements for the level of measurement, study design, and sample. However, each inferential statistic may have its own additional specifications regarding the nature of the data. Therefore, prior to using a statistical test, consult a statistics textbook in respect to the specific statistic, to avoid using it inappropriately. Several well-regarded statistical texts are listed in the references (Daniel, 1978; Fleiss, 1981; Pagano, 1981; Remington *et al,* 1970).

Application

Because the community health nurse did not intend to test a hypothesis in her infant-mortality study, she did not plan to use inferential statistics.

TABLE 2-11. GUIDE TO SELECTED INFERENTIAL STATISTICS FOR TESTING FOR DIFFERENCES BETWEEN GROUPS

Type(s) of Group(s)	Level of Measurement of Dependent Variable		
	Nominal	*Ordinal*	*Interval/ratio*
One sample (comparing distribution of variable to a hypothesized distribution)	Chi Square for goodness of fit	Sign Test Wilcoxon Matched Pairs Signed-Rank Test	*Means:* Unknown population variance: one-sample t-test, df = n − 1 Known population variance: one-sample Z-test *Proportions:* One-sample Z-test for proportions
Two independent groups	Chi Square Tests Fisher Exact Test	Median Test Mann–Whitney U Test	*Means:* Two-sample t-test for independent samples df = $n_1 + n_2 - 2$ *Proportions:* Two-sample Z-test for proportions
Fewer than two independent groups	Chi Square tests	Extension of Median Test Kruskal–Wallis Test	*Means:* One-way analysis of variance (one-way ANOVA) *(continued)*

Displaying statistics: tables

The table as guide. Tables can facilitate communication of statistical data and, if planned appropriately, can actually guide data collection and analysis. Experienced researchers construct *dummy tables,* or outlines of proposed tables, prior to collecting their data. Then they fill in the data as they proceed with data collection, and analyze and write their results from the completed tables. The tables may be modified for final publication, but the basic data will always be readily accessible during the study.

The table as communicator. Tables are helpful in communicating large amounts of data such as sample characteristics in a succinct manner. In order to communicate clearly, a table must have an explicit title that specifies the

TABLE 2-11.   *(Continued)*

Type(s) of Group(s)	Level of Measurement of Dependent Variable		
	Nominal	*Ordinal*	*Interval/ratio*
One group—before/ after, or two related groups (matched pairs)	McNemar Test	Wilcoxon Matched Pairs Signed-Rank Test	*Difference scores:* Paired t-tests for paired data (t-test for related samples) df = n − 1 where n = number of pairs
One group with fewer than two repeated measures. Or fewer than 2 related groups (matched triplets, etc.)	Cochran Q	Friedman Test	Repeated measures analysis
Two groups before/after	Adaptation of data for Chi Square tests Adaptation of data for Fisher Exact Tests	Adaptation of data for Mann–Whitney U (if scores can be subtracted)	*Mean changes:* Two-sample t-test for independent samples, df = $n_1 + n_2 - 2$ One-way analysis of variance *Means:* Analysis of covariance
Fewer than two groups before/after	Adaptation of data for Chi Square tests	Adaptation of data for Kruskal–Wallis test (if scores can be subtracted)	*Mean changes:* One-way analysis of variance *Means:* Analysis of covariance

Note: Lower level tests may be used for higher level data, but some loss of information may result

(This chart was developed with the assistance of Ronald Forthofer, Ph.D., Professor of Biometry, University of Texas School of Public Health.)

contents of the table. The table should be completely understandable without reference to the text. An excellent guide to table construction is available free of charge from the Centers for Disease Control (1981b, May).

Crosstabulation. A *crosstabulation* is a special type of table that allows for the visual inspection of a relationship between variables. We examined crosstabulations when we looked at the relationship between tampon usage and TSS (see Table 2-3 and discussion under Example of the Odds Ratio: Toxic Shock Syndrome) and the hypothetical relationship between sex and Condition X (see Table 2-5 and Example of Association: Sex and Condition X).

Application

In her infant-mortality study, the community health nurse first planned a series of *dummy tables* to include all the variables for which information was required. As data collection proceeded, she filled in the tables. Because your ability to construct useful tables will be determined by your ability to understand and interpret them, let us examine two of her completed tables.

Table 2-12 describes her sample in terms of prenatal care. Note that this particular table also is a *crosstabulation* of the relationship between prenatal care and ethnicity. Do you see that Spanish-surname whites appear more likely to lack prenatal care than either blacks or non-Spanish-surname whites? Eleven percent of Spanish-surname whites lacked prenatal care, compared with 4.8% of blacks and 2.7% of non-Spanish-surname whites. Study the table until you are comfortable with interpreting percentages in a crosstabulation.

Table 2-13 is a more complex crosstabulation of ethnicity, prenatal care, and postneonatal mortality. In your community health practice, you must be able to interpret such tables. Look particularly at postneonatal mortality for those with no prenatal care. Note that the Spanish-surname postneonatal-mortality rate (1.4 deaths per 1000 live births) and relative risk (0.5) surprisingly is *less* than for blacks (rate 15.9 deaths per 1000 live births; relative risk 5.7) or for non-Spanish-surname whites (rate

TABLE 2-12.   DISTRIBUTION OF TIME OF FIRST
PRENATAL CARE BY ETHNICITY:
1974–1975 SINGLE LIVE BIRTH COHORT,
HARRIS COUNTY, TEXAS

Time of First Prenatal Care	Number of Births	Non-Spanish-Surname White		Spanish-Surname White		Black	
		Number	*Percent*	*Number*	*Percent*	*Number*	*Percent*
First trimester	49,025	32,318	84.2	7,425	56.1	9,282	54.7
Second trimester	13,198	4,000	10.4	3,428	25.9	5,770	34
Third trimester	2,950	963	2.5	909	6.9	1,078	6.4
No prenatal care	3,324	1,055	2.7	1,450	11	819	4.8
Unknown	87	53	0.1	26	0.2	8	0
Total*	68,584	38,389	100%	13,238	100%	16,957	100%

* Percentages may not add up to 100% because of rounding

TABLE 2-13.   POSTNEONATAL MORTALITY RATES AND
RELATIVE RISKS BY TIME OF FIRST
PRENATAL CARE AND ETHNICITY:
1974–1975 SINGLE LIVE BIRTH COHORT,
HARRIS COUNTY, TEXAS

Time of First Prenatal Care	Non-Spanish-Surname White		Spanish-Surname White		Black	
	Rate*	RR†	Rate*	RR†	Rate*	RR†
First trimester	2	0.7	2.7	1	4.5	1.6
Second trimester	4	1.4	3.2	1.1	6.6	2.4
Third trimester	11.4	4.1	7.7‡	2.8	12.1	4.3
No prenatal care	12.3	4.4	1.4‡	0.5	15.9	5.7
Total	2.8	1	3	1.1	6.3	2.3

* Rates = Deaths per 1000 live births

† RR = Relative risk, using non-Spanish-surname white total as standard for appropriate mortality period

‡ Rate based on fewer than 10 deaths

12.3 deaths per 1000 live births; relative risk 4.4). Also observe, from the footnote, the small number of deaths in the no-prenatal-care category for the Spanish-surname population. This perplexing finding is examined more closely further on in this chapter.

Displaying statistics: Figures

Figures or pictorial representations also facilitate communication of statistics. Figures generally are reserved for important concepts or findings. Like tables, they should be planned beforehand to ensure that the required data will be available. Their final form, of course, will be dictated by the actual results.

Types of figures. Different types of figures have different uses. The nature of the data and the purpose of the display will guide the selection of figures. For instance, *bar charts* are helpful in displaying discrete categories of data. *Pie charts* and *histograms* can be used to depict the parts of a whole. *Scatterplots* help show relationships between ordinal or interval/ratio level variables. *Line graphs* are useful in emphasizing trends over time, and *flow charts* help explain sequential steps.

It is important to become familiar with the advantages and disadvantages of these various types of charts and graphs. In community health practice, an effective graphic presentation of a community health problem may make the difference between funding or no funding for a program request. The Centers for Disease Control (1981b, May) provides a free guide to the selection and construction of charts and graphs.

Application

The community health nurse planned numerous figures for her study of infant mortality. Figure 2-6, which consists of two *pie charts,* depicts the differences in the U.S.-born and foreign-born Spanish-surname populations of Texas. The nurse used this figure in designing the research project and, without modification, in a final report. Study the figure a moment. Does it show convincingly that the Spanish-surname population is not homogeneous? Does it demonstrate that the foreign-born Spanish-surname group identifies Mexican immigrants, with better than 90% accuracy?

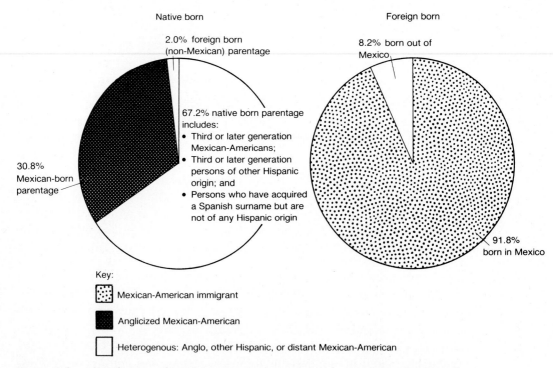

Figure 2-6.   Identification of Mexican-American population by Spanish surname and nativity, Texas 1970. (United States Bureau of the Census: Census of the Population: 1970. Subject Reports. Persons of Spanish Surname, Table 2, p 3. PC(2)1D. Washington DC, United States Government Printing Office, 1973)

The community health nurse planned Figure 2-7, a *bar chart,* prior to the study, but she could not develop its final format until the data was analyzed. Does the chart communicate to you that when the Spanish-surname criterion alone is used to identify Mexican-Americans, as is commonly the case, infant mortality does not appear to be an overwhelming problem in this group? Based on this chart, if you were in charge of health policy, to which group would you direct resources? The community health nurse who conducted this study was quite concerned that resources might not be directed toward the Mexican-American population.

Step 7: State the limitations of the study

By the time the researcher reaches this point, nearly all details of the study have been planned. Given real-life resources and constraints, compromises undoubtedly have been made between what is desired and what is possible; no study design is perfect. The imperfections now must be reviewed as a whole and stated explicitly.

In effect, the statement of limitations serves as a final check on the validity of the study methodology. It provides the researcher with an opportunity to reconsider aspects of the study that should, and still can, be revised; every effort should be made to remedy the limitations before the study is begun. The

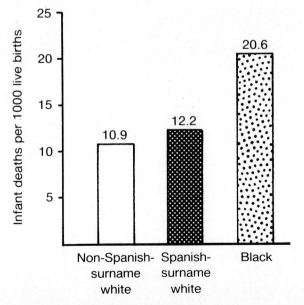

Figure 2-7. Infant mortality rates by ethnicity, 1974–75: single live birth cohort, Harris County, Texas.

statement of limitations also should ensure that the validity of the future results will not be overestimated by the researcher or by others.

Throughout this chapter, limitations have been discussed in terms of individual aspects of study methodology. In identifying the limitations of a study as a whole, it is helpful to consider limitations in terms of threats to the internal and external validity of a study.

Internal validity

Internal validity refers to the validity of the results within the study, or the confidence with which it can be said that the study results can be attributed to the factors considered in the study and not to outside factors that were not considered. In standard research texts, these threats to internal validity usually are categorized as follows

1. *Selection bias*—The study results are attributable to the unusual over-representation or under-representation of certain characteristics in the sample; a specific example is Berkson's bias.
2. *Test effects*—The study results are influenced by the measures used in the study. For example, in a study of blood-pressure medication, improvement in blood pressure may be attributable to changes in health behavior resulting from having the blood pressure measured regularly during the study, rather than to the medication.
3. *History*—The study results are influenced by events that occur outside the realm of the study. For example, in studying Agent Orange and birth defects, research findings are confounded by possible life events and exposures that occurred between the father's exposure to Agent Orange and the subsequent birth of a child with a defect.
4. *Maturation*—The results are influenced by changes that occur owing to time itself. For instance, children normally grow and develop; wounds normally heal; conditions often simply "get better" over time. In a study of a program's impact on infant mortality, the researcher must consider that, without the program, the U.S. infant mortality rate usually improves in each succeeding year.
5. *Mortality*—The results are influenced by the loss of subjects through death, migration, or disinterest. The subjects who remain at the end of the study may be quite different from those who do not.

In stating the limitations of a study in terms of its internal validity, a researcher should describe aspects of research methodology, specific to the proposed study, that fail to control for these threats.

External validity

External validity refers to the validity of the results outside the study; that is, the confidence with which the results from the sample can be generalized to the population. In stating limitations regarding external validity, aspects of the data source and sampling method that limit the generalizability of the findings should be described. If possible, the probable direction of expected bias also should be noted.

Application

The community health nurse's infant-mortality study was a prospective study using a nonprobability sample based on linked live birth and infant death records. The study sought to describe and identify at-risk populations in terms of infant mortality, with a special emphasis on the Mexican-immigrant population. It also was intended to explain possible relationships between infant mortality and a number of variables, including prenatal care.

   The community health nurse listed the limitations specific to her study, as shown below. Study these limitations to see how they relate to the threats to *internal validity* and *external validity*.

1. This study uses linked live birth and infant death certificates to create a prospective data file. Although infant deaths within the United States are required to be reported, this study cannot ascertain infant deaths that occur outside the United States or that occur within the United States but are not reported to the vital registration system. Mexican immigrants probably are more likely to migrate to Mexico and less likely to register infant deaths than other ethnic groups. Therefore, this study is likely to underestimate Mexican-immigrant infant mortality.
2. Identification of infants of the Mexican-immigrant population is determined by foreign-born nativity of Spanish-surname parents. Although census data indicate that over 90% of the Texan-Spanish-surname population were born in Mexico, the group identified in this study as Mexican-immigrant actually may include Spanish-surname immigrants from other countries.
3. The validity of variables recorded on birth and death certificates, particularly the recording of prenatal care by month first begun, may be questionable. Although prenatal care is to be grouped and treated as a nominal level variable to avoid overemphasizing its value, the basic validity of vital statistics is beyond the investigator's control.
4. This study considers only variables available on Texas live birth and infant death records as possible factors in infant mortality. It does not address other factors

known to influence infant mortality, such as socioeconomic and educational status. Therefore, relationships between infant mortality and the selected variables in this study may be confounded by these or other unknown variables.

5. The results from this nonprobability sample cannot be generalized beyond the sample, time period, or geographic location studied.

Step 8: Ensure the protection of human subjects

This step was discussed earlier with sample selection, as it must be addressed when planning the methodology of the study. It is included as a separate step at this point because it usually involves a specific, necessary, but sometimes time-consuming process for which a period of time should be included in the community health nurse researcher's plans.

Generally, assurance of protection of human subjects involves submission of the research proposal and certain required forms to an agency review board. Each agency has its own particular forms and procedures for the review process, and the time required for approval may range from a day or two to a month or more. The review board determines whether the researcher is protecting the safety, confidentiality, and dignity of the subjects in accordance with federally mandated guidelines. The review board is guided in its decision by the requirements for informed consent, which were reviewed in the displayed material on page 65.

Application

How did the community health nurse handle the protection of human subjects in her study of birth and death records? In this case, she did not intend to approach human subjects directly. However, she did plan to examine information about human subjects. Therefore, an assurance of confidentiality or anonymity was necessary. It had been planned to assure subject *anonymity* by the removal of personal identifying data by the state health department before the birth and death records were made available to the research project; the nurse was required to document this in her proposal to the institutional review board of her sponsoring agency. The board reviewed her proposal and approved it.

Step 9: Perform the pilot study

When permission to proceed with the study has been obtained from the designated review board, it may be appropriate to perform a pilot study, particularly if the sample is large. The purpose of a pilot study is to test the research instruments and procedures on a small group before using them on the total sample. The pilot study may reveal unanticipated problems that can be remedied before the instruments and procedures are employed on a large scale. If no problems are identified, the study may proceed as planned.

Application

In the infant mortality study of nearly 70,000 computerized birth records, the community health nurse first tested a sample of ten cases to ensure that the appropriate variables were being selected before statistics were computed.

Step 10: Implement the methodology

By this time, the methodology has been planned and tested. Therefore, this step is straightforward. The researcher uses the appropriate research design, selects the sample, collects data from the sample, and analyzes the data as planned.

Application

The community health nurse implemented the methodology for her infant mortality study as she had planned. She used a computer to select the appropriate sample from the prospective data tape, collect information on appropriate variables, and calculate appropriate descriptive statistics. As the study progressed, she filled in the data in her dummy tables and figures.

Step 11: Interpret the results, and Step 12: Communicate the results

After the data have been collected and analyzed, the results must be interpreted meaningfully and then communicated to the appropriate audiences. Interpretation and communication, of course, are two separate steps in the research process, and they occur at different times (*i.e.,* the results cannot be communicated until they have been interpreted). Nevertheless the steps are intertwined.

When done well, interpretation and communication of community health research findings are a synthesis of the researcher's

1. Comprehension of the basic principles of epidemiology, demography, and research

2. Understanding of the purposes and limitations of the specific statistical measures used in the study
3. Familiarity with all aspects of the data collected for the study
4. Knowledge of theory and past research applicable to the study
5. Awareness of the potential influences of the real world on the study results
6. Awareness of the potential influences of the study results on the real world

It will be shown how the community health nurse researcher attempted to incorporate these aspects into her interpretation and communication of the results from her infant-mortality study. First, however, let us consider each of these six components more closely.

Comprehension of basic principles of epidemiology, demography, and research

The results that come from a study are only as good as the data that go into it. The axiom, "garbage in, garbage out," applies as much to research as to computer operations. Therefore, the results of a study must be interpreted in view of the validity and limitations of the methods used to collect the data, and the findings must be presented to the audience in this light.

In this chapter you have learned some basic principles of epidemiology, demography, and research as they apply to community health research. These principles will help you evaluate and interpret your own community health data and critique the information presented by others. You have had an opportunity to see how these principles were applied to a study of Mexican-American infant mortality; later in the text you will be able to test your ability to evaluate the community health nurse's interpretation of the results of her completed study in view of these principles.

Understanding of the specific statistical measures used

This is part of the researcher's understanding of the basic principles of epidemiology, demography, and research, but it implies more specific knowledge of the statistical measures actually used in the study. This chapter has presented the advantages and disadvantages of some of the most common statistical measures of health; these, and other, measures must be interpreted in respect to their purposes and limitations. Remember, for instance, the example of the high black-infant mortality rate that was adjusted for low birth weight, resulting in a low adjusted rate (see discussion under Interpretation of Adjusted Rates). As you recall, the adjusted rate might have been misinterpreted to suggest that blacks were at *low* risk for infant mortality, when, in fact,

it meant blacks were at *high* risk for infant mortality because of a high proportion of low-birth-weight infants.

In her final report of the Mexican-American infant-mortality study, the
community health nurse could not discuss many of the statistical measures she
used, because of space limitations in the journal in which it was published. As
you read the information presented, consider whether those statistical measures she did include in the report were interpreted correctly.

Familiarity with all aspects of the data

Researchers sometimes make the mistake of focusing on one particularly
interesting finding, to the exclusion of other results. This may lead to misin-
terpretation; the other results may contradict the particular finding or indicate
a trend not apparent from an isolated piece of data. In the community health
nurse's Mexican-American infant-mortality study, you will see that consistent,
unusual trends in rates resulted in an interpretation totally opposite that suggested by individual rates, such as those that were shown in Table 2-13.

Knowledge of theory and past research

You have learned that a research study must be planned in view of existing
theory and research; the results also must be interpreted and explained in this
context. If the findings are not compatible with existing knowledge, the researcher must explore possible reasons for the inconsistencies. The researcher also should address further research needs that have been identified
by the study. As you read the community health nurse's interpretation of the
results of her Mexican-American infant-mortality study, note how her findings
are tied to those of others, and how future research needs are addressed.

Awareness of influences of the real world on the results

It is possible to become so immersed in the results of a study that the context
of the real world is forgotten. The researcher has an obligation to other professionals—and to the community being studied—to be aware of, and report,
real-life influences on the data. For instance, was a particular statistic (*e.g.,*
mean, rate, and so forth) overly influenced by deviant values from one particular segment of the sample? Or, in a multiclinic setting, could the records from
a particular clinic not have been documented as reliably as the rest?

In the community health nurse's infant mortality study, you will see that a
series of paradoxical findings, with a very consistent pattern, suggested to her
that the data were being influenced by something outside the study.

Awareness of influences of the study results on the real world

The researcher also should consider the results in terms of their potential impact on the real world. Sometimes in their preoccupation with statistics, researchers confuse *statistical significance* with real-life or *clinical significance*. With large enough samples, almost any difference may be statistically significant. But, for instance, does it make any real-life difference if one group has a mean diastolic blood pressure of 76 mm. Hg. and another has a mean of 82 mm. Hg., even if the difference is statistically significant? Conversely, a small sample may result in lack of statistical significance, not because there is no true difference, but because the statistics are not sensitive to the difference. For example, in a small study, the difference in diastolic blood pressures between a group with a mean of 84 mm. Hg. and a group with a mean of 98 mm. Hg. might not be statistically significant. The lack of statistical significance should not blind the researcher to the potential need for intervention in the group with the *clinically* higher blood pressure.

The community health nurse did not rely on testing for statistical significance in her infant mortality study. You will see that this in no way undermined the *clinical significance* of her findings.

The researcher's knowledge of the potential influence of the results also will help identify the audience to whom the results should be communicated. The information should be directed toward the groups that can use and apply the results—those who can do something with the new knowledge. In communicating the results, the researcher must consider, and warn against, potential misapplication of the findings by the audience.

The community health nurse presented the findings of her study of infant mortality locally to groups of public health and medical professionals, and nationally to the membership of the American Public Health Association. She formalized the report for publication, emphasizing the most important findings, in the *American Journal of Public Health*. These were audiences whom she believed should hear the message of her data.

Application

Now let us see firsthand how the community health nurse interpreted and communicated the results of her study of Mexican-American infant mortality. Following this chapter, in Appendix A, are excerpts from the *results* and *discussion* sections of the published article, ''Validity of the Spanish surname infant mortality rate as a health status indicator for the Mexican American population'' (Selby *et al*, 1984).

What do you think of the author's interpretations?

SUMMARY

In this chapter you have been introduced to demography, the broad science of populations; epidemiology, the specific science of population health; and research principles applicable to community health. It has been shown that demography, epidemiology, and research principles are interrelated, and are indispensable in community health nursing. In order to advance existing knowledge in the science of demography and epidemiology, upon which community health nursing is based, an understanding of research principles is required; in order to advance nursing knowledge and apply the nursing process in community health, an understanding of demographic and epidemiologic concepts and research principles is necessary.

You have learned that community health research is an integral part of community health nursing practice. Research directs community nursing assessment, diagnosis, planning, implementation, and evaluation. In this chapter, it has been shown how one community health nurse applied the intertwined concepts and principles of demography, epidemiology, and research to investigate a health condition in her community. What began as a clinical concern, an unanswered question about a specific population in the community health nurse's practice, resulted in findings with implications not only for her practice, but potentially for the practice of others as well.

Be assured that you are not yet expected to conduct research with implications for the health of the nation. Nevertheless, after studying this chapter, you should be able to apply epidemiologic, demographic, and research principles to your community health nursing practice. When you are ready to begin a community health research project of your own, the tables and figures in this chapter will help guide you through the research process. For more detailed information on some aspects of epidemiology, demography, or research, you may wish to consult the reference list.

REFERENCES

Abdellah FG, Levine E: *Better Patient Care Through Nursing Research*. New York, Macmillan 1979

Burris JM: (1974). Neonatal and Postneonatal Mortality in a Birth Cohort. Master's thesis, University of Texas School of Public Health, Houston, 1958–1960

Centers for Disease Control: Follow up on toxic shock syndrome. MMWR (September 19):441–445, 1980a

Centers for Disease Control: Toxic shock syndrome—Utah. MMWR: (October 17):495–496, 1980b

Centers for Disease Control: Toxic shock syndrome—United States, 1970—1980. MMWR 30:25–33, 1981a

Centers for Disease Control: Descriptive Statistics: Tables, Graphs, & Charts. Atlanta, Centers for Disease Control, 1981b

Centers for Disease Control: (1983, August 5) Update: Toxic shock syndrome—United States. MMWR 32:398–400, 1983

Centers for Disease Control: Smoking and cardiovascular disease. MMWR 32:677–679, 1984

Centerwall BS: Race, socioeconomic status and domestic homicide, Atlanta, 1971–72. *Amer J Public Health* 74(8):813–815, 1984

Cook TD, Campbell DT: Quasi-experimentation: Design and Analysis Issues for Field Settings. Boston, Houghton Mifflin, 1979

Cravens G, Mair JL: (1977). *The black death.* New York: Dutton

Crichton M: The Andromeda Strain. New York, Alfred A. Knopf, 1969

Daniel WW: Applied Nonparametric Statistics. Boston, Houghton Mifflin, 1978

Davis JP, Chesney PJ, Ward PJ, et al: Toxic shock syndrome: Epidemiologic features, recurrence, risk factors, and prevention. N Engl J Med 303:1429–1435, 1980

Dunne TL: The Scourge. New York, Coward, McCann, & Geohegan, 1978

Fleiss JL: Statistical Methods for Rates and Proportions. New York, John Wiley & Sons, 1981

Fox DJ: Fundamentals of Research in Nursing. Norwalk, Connecticut, Appleton-Century-Crofts, 1982

Frost F, Shy KK: Racial differences between linked birth and infant death records in Washington state. Amer J Public Health 70:974–976, 1980

Gee SC, Lee ES, Forthofer RN: Ethnic differentials in neonatal and postneonatal mortality: A birth cohort analysis by a binary variable multiple regression method. Soc Biol 23:317–325, 1976

Jaffe AJ, Cullen RM, Boswell TD: The Changing Demography of Spanish Americans. New York, Academic Press, 1980

Kark SL: The Practice of Community-oriented Primary Health Care. New York, Appleton-Century-Crofts, 1981

Lee ES, Roberts RE: Ethnic fertility differentials in the southwest. The case of Mexican Americans re-examined. Sociology and Social Research, 65(2):194–210, 1981

Lyndon B. Johnson School of Public Affairs: The Health of Mexican Americans in South Texas. Austin, University of Texas, 1979

MacMahon B, Pugh TF: Epidemiology: Principles and Methods. Boston, Little, Brown & Co, 1970

Mausner JS, Bahn AK: (1984) Epidemiology: An Introductory Text. Philadelphia, WB Saunders, 1974

McAlister A, Puska P, Salonen JT et al: Theory and action for health promotion: Illustrations from the North Karelia Project. Amer J Public Health 72:43–50, 1982

McCarthy BJ, Terry J, Rochat RW et al: The underregistration of neonatal deaths: Georgia 1974–77. Amer J Public Health 70:977–982, 1980

National Center for Health Statistics: Annual summary of births, deaths, marriages, and divorces: United States, 1983. In: *Monthly Vital Statistics Report, 32* (13). DHHS Pub. No. (PHS) 84-1120. Hyattsville, Maryland, Public Health Service, 1984

Norris FD, Shipley PW: A closer look at race differentials in California's infant mortality, 1965–1967. HSMHA Health Reports, 86:810–814, 1971

Office of the Assistant Secretary for Health, U.S. Public Health Service: Promoting Health/Preventing Disease: Objectives for the Nation. Washington DC, U.S. Department of Health and Human Services, Public Health Service, 1980

Office on Smoking and Health: The health consequences of smoking: Cardiovascular disease. A report of the Surgeon General. DHHS Publication No. (PHS) 84-50204. Rockville, Maryland, Public Health Service, 1983

Pagano RR: Understanding Statistics in the Behavioral Sciences. New York, West Publishing, 1981

Polit DF, Hungler BP: Nursing Research: Principles and Methods. Philadelphia, JB Lippincott, 1983

Powell-Griner E, Streck D: A closer examination of neonatal mortality among the Texas Spanish surname population. Amer J Public Health, 72:993–999, 1982

Puska P, Tuomilehto J, Salonen J et al: Community Control of a Cardiovascular Diseases: Evaluation of a Comprehensive Community Programme for Control of Cardiovascular Diseases in North Karelia, Finland, 1972–1977. Copenhagen, Published on behalf of the National Public Health Laboratory of Finland by the World Health Organization, Regional Office for Europe, 1981

Remington RD, Schork MA: Statistics with Application to the Biological and Health Sciences. Englewood Cliffs, New Jersey, Prentice-Hall, 1970

Roht LH, Selwyn BJ, Holguin AH, et al: Principles of Epidemiology: A Self-teaching Guide. New York, Academic Press, 1982

Schlesselman JJ: Case Control Studies: Design, Conduct, Analysis. New York, Oxford University Press, 1982

Selby ML: Infant mortality in the Mexican American community: An analysis of differentials in infant, neonatal, and postneonatal mortality by ethnicity and parental nativity, 1974–75 single live birth cohort, Harris County, Texas. Doctoral dissertation, University of Texas School of Public Health, Houston, 1982

Selby ML, Lee ES, Tuttle DM: Validity of the Spanish surname infant mortality rate as a health status indicator for the Mexican American population. Amer J Public Health 74(9):998–1002, 1984

Shryock HS, Siegel JS, et al: The Methods and Materials of Demography. Washington DC, U.S. Government Printing Office, 1980

Slome C, Brogan DR, Eyres SJ, Lednar W: Basic Epidemiological Methods and Biostatistics: A Workbook. Monterey, California, Wadsworth Health Sciences Div, 1982

Snow J: Snow on Cholera, Being a Reprint of Two Papers by John Snow, M.D., Together with a Biographical Memoir by B. W. Richardson, M.D., and an Introduction by Wade Hampton Frost, M.D., 1936. Reprint. New York, The Commonwealth Fund, 1936

Spielberger C, Gorsuch R, Lushene R: The State-Trait Anxiety Inventory. Palo Alto, California, Consulting Psychologists Press, 1968

Teller C, Clyburn S: Texas population in 1970: Trends in infant mortality. Texas Business Review, 40:240–246, 1974

U.S. Bureau of the Census: Census of the population 1970. Subject reports. Persons of Spanish surname. PC (2)1D. (Table P-7, p 177) Washington DC, U.S. Government Printing Office, 1973

U.S. Surgeon General's Advisory Committee on Smoking and Health: Smoking and health. Report of the Advisory Committee to the Surgeon General of the Public Health Service. Public Health Service Pub. No. 1103. Washington DC, U.S. Government Printing Office, 1964

Appendix A
Validity of the Spanish-Surname Infant Mortality Rate As a Health Status Indicator for the Mexican-American Population

MAIJA L. SELBY,
RN, DR.PH,
EUN SUL LEE, PHD,
DOROTHY M. TUTTLE,
PHD,
HARDY D. LOE, JR.,
MD, MPH

RESULTS

Even though the Spanish-surname population had an excess of births to mothers who were age 35 or older, had three or more previous births, or reported late or no prenatal care (Table 1), Spanish surname neonatal and postneonatal mortality rates were only slightly higher than non-Spanish-surname rates and considerably lower than black rates (Table 2). However, when rates were analyzed by the selected risk factors, several puzzling findings emerged. Among very low birthweight infants, the Spanish-surname group had the highest neonatal mortality rate (NMR) but a postneonatal mortality rate (PNMR) less than that of the non-Spanish-surname group. Spanish-surname infants also had surprisingly low PNMRs for the usually high-risk categories of advanced maternal age, high birth order, and late or absent prenatal

APPENDIX
TABLE 1.   DISTRIBUTION OF SELECTED
RISK FACTORS BY ETHNICITY: 1974–75
SINGLE LIVE BIRTH COHORT, HARRIS
COUNTY, TEXAS

		Ethnicity					
	Total* births	Non-Spanish surname white		Spanish surname white		Black	
Risk Factor	n	n	%	n	%	n	%
Birthweight†							
<3 lb 5 oz	803	290	0.8	119	0.9	394	2.3
3 lb 5 oz–5 lb 8 oz	4,226	1,881	4.9	644	4.9	1,701	10
>5 lb 8 oz	62,879	35,815	93.3	12,342	93.2	14,722	86.8
Unknown	676	403	1.1	133	1	140	0.8
Total‡	68,584	38,389	100%	13,238	100%	16,957	100%
Birth order§							
1st	29,242	17,540	45.7	4,737	35.8	6,965	41.1
2nd or 3rd	31,019	17,855	46.5	5,687	43	7,477	44.1
4th or higher	8,323	2,994	7.8	2,814	21.3	2,515	14.8
Total‡	68,584	38,389	100%	13,238	100%	16,957	100%
Maternal age							
<20 yr	14,418	6,002	15.6	2,888	21.8	5,528	32.6
20–34 yr	51,546	31,105	81	9,629	72.7	10,812	63.8
≥35 yr	2,616	1,279	3.3	721	5.4	616	3.6
Unknown	4	3	0	0	0	1	0
Total‡	68,584	38,389	100%	13,238	100%	16,957	100%
First prenatal care							
1st or 2nd trimester	62,223	36,318	94.6	10,853	82	15,052	88.8
3rd trimester/no care	6,274	2,018	5.3	2,359	17.8	1,897	11.2
Unknown	87	53	0.1	26	0.2	8	0
Total‡	68,584	38,389	100%	13,238	100%	16,957	100%

* 429 births of "other" race/ethnicity excluded

† Birthweights recorded to nearest ounce. Approximate gram equivalents: 3 lb 5 oz = 1500 gm; 5 lb 8 oz = 2500 gm

‡ Percentage totals may not equal 100 due to rounding

§ Birth order = sum of live births, fetal deaths >20 wk gestation, and this birth

APPENDIX

TABLE 2.   NEONATAL AND POSTNEONATAL
MORTALITY RATES BY ETHNICITY
AND SELECTED RISK FACTORS: 1974–75
SINGLE LIVE BIRTH COHORT, HARRIS
COUNTY, TEXAS

Mortality Measures and Risk Factors	Ethnicity		
	Non-Spanish-surname White	*Spanish-surname White*	*Black*
*Neonatal Mortality Rate**	8.2	9.2	14.3
Birthweight†			
<3 lb 5 oz	479.3	613.4	431.5
3 lb 5 oz–5 lb 8 oz	37.2	20.2	17.6
>5 lb 8 oz	2.8	2.8	2.8
Birth order‡			
1st	8.3	9.1	13.3
2nd or 3rd	8	7.6	13.7
4th or higher	8.7	12.8	19.5
Maternal age			
<20 yr	11.0	12.1	15.6
20–34 yr	7.6	8.1	13.8
≥35 yr	8.6	12.5	13
First prenatal care			
1st or 2nd trimester	8	8.8	13.2
3rd trimester/no care	11.4	11.4	23.7

(continued)

care.* The PNMR for Spanish-surname infants whose mothers reported no prenatal care (1.4 deaths/1000 live births) was even lower than for non-Spanish-surname infants of mothers with first trimester care (2 deaths/1000).

Analysis by parental nativity confirmed that the foreign-born Spanish-surname group had the greatest excess of high order births and births to mothers of advanced age or with late or no prenatal care (Table 3). Nevertheless, NMRs for Spanish-surname infants of foreign-born parents were even lower than for non-Spanish-surname infants (Table 4). Closer examination of infants of for-

* These differentials also were true when PNMRs were recomputed by the alternate formula: PNMR = (postneonatal deaths/live births − neonatal deaths) × 1000

APPENDIX
TABLE 2. *(Continued)*

Mortality Measures and Risk Factors	Non-Spanish-surname White	Spanish-surname White	Black
		Ethnicity	
***Postneonatal Mortality Rate*§**	2.8	3	6.3
Birthweight†			
<3 lb 5 oz	37.9	33.6‖	30.5
3 lb 5 oz–5 lb 8 oz	9.6	1.6‖	17
>5 lb 8 oz	2.1	2.8	4.4
Birth order‡			
1st	2.1	3.8	3.5
2nd or 3rd	3.2	2.6	9.1
4th or higher	4	2.5‖	5.6
Maternal age			
<20 yr	5.5	4.8	7.2
20–34 yr	2.1	2.6	5.9
≥35 yr	6.3	1.4‖	3.2‖
First prenatal care			
1st or 2nd trimester	2.3	2.9	5.3
3rd trimester/no care	11.9‖	3.8‖	13.7

* Neonatal mortality rate $= \dfrac{\text{neonatal deaths}}{\text{live births}} \times 1000$

† Birthweights recorded to nearest once. Approximate gram equivalents: 3 lb 5 oz = 1500 gm; 5 lb 8 oz = 2500 gm

‡ Birth order = sum of live births, fetal deaths >20 wk gestation, and this birth

§ Postneonatal mortality rate $= \dfrac{\text{postneonatal deaths}}{\text{live births}} \times 1000$

‖ Rate based on fewer than 10 deaths

eign-born parents showed that very-low-birthweight infants had expectedly high NMRs, but moderately-low-birthweight infants had lower NMRs than other ethnic groups.

The overall PNMR for Spanish-surname infants of foreign-born parents was slightly higher than for infants of US-born parents; this was accounted for by the one-parent foreign-born subgroup, which had a disproportionate number of first births and births to teenage mothers. Infants whose both parents were foreign-born had exceptionally low PNMRs. Over 45% of births in this

APPENDIX

TABLE 3.   DISTRIBUTION OF SELECTED RISK
FACTORS FOR SPANISH-SURNAME
INFANTS BY PARENTAL NATIVITY:
1974–75 SINGLE LIVE BIRTH COHORT,
HARRIS COUNTY, TEXAS

| | | | | Foreign-born Parents | | | |
| | Total Spanish-surname births | Both parents US-born | | One parent foreign-born | | Both parents foreign-born | |
Risk Factor	n	n	%	n	%	n	%
Birthweight*							
<3 lb 5 oz	119	76	1	21	0.7	22	0.8
3 lb 5 oz–5 lb 8 oz	644	393	5.3	143	4.9	108	3.7
>5 lb 8 oz	12,342	6,846	92.4	2,710	93.2	2,786	95.4
Unknown	133	96	1.3	33	1.1	4	0.1
Total†	13,238	7,411	100%	2,907	100%	2,920	100%
Birth order‡							
1st	4,737	2,770	37.4	1,080	37.2	887	30.4
2nd or 3rd	5,687	3,240	43.7	1,256	43.2	1,191	40.8
4th or higher	2,814	1,401	18.9	571	19.6	842	28.8
Total‡	13,238	7,411	100%	2,907	100%	2,920	100%
Maternal age							
<20 yr	2,888	1,948	26.3	562	19.3	378	12.9
20–34 yr	9,629	5,147	69.5	2,171	74.7	2,311	79.1
≥35 yr	721	316	4.3	174	6	231	7.9
Total†	13,238	7,411	100%	2,907	100%	2,920	100%
First prenatal care							
1st or 2nd trimester	10,853	6,266	84.5	2,322	79.9	2,265	77.6
3rd trimester/no care	2,359	1,132	15.3	581	20	646	22.1
Unknown	26	13	0.2	4	0.1	9	0.3
Total†	13,238	7,411	100%	2,907	100%	2,920	100%

* Birthweights recorded to nearest ounce. Approximate gram equivalents: 3 lb 5 oz = 1500 gm; 5 lb 8 oz = 2500 gm

† Percentage total may not equal 100 due to rounding

‡ Birth order = sum of live births, fetal deaths >20 wk gestation, and this birth

immigrant group were of third or higher order; nearly 25% were to mothers 30 years of age or older; and 22% were to mothers who received late or no prenatal care; yet no postneonatal deaths were recorded in these categories.

DISCUSSION

These consistently paradoxical findings lead us to conclude that the Spanish-surname infant-mortality rate is not a valid indicator of health status for the Mexican-American population in Harris County, Texas. It is highly unlikely that the low rates calculated in this study represent a protective factor shared by Mexican Americans, given the IMR of 70 deaths per 1000 live births for the country of Mexico.[1] Rather, our analysis suggests that considerable loss of death data occurs for infants of foreign-born Mexican immigrants even in this urban, nonborder setting. Migration and under-registration of deaths appear to be plausible reasons for the data losses.

The high mobility of the Mexican-American population and the "revolving door" nature of Mexico–United States migration have been documented.[2-4] Therefore, migration to Mexico or to rural areas in the United States where vital registration is less complete could account for the unusual mortality rates. Even where registration is complete, infant deaths are not reported back to the state of birth unless the address given on the death certificate is from the state of birth; time lags and differences in state death certificate reporting may also result in incomplete referral of death records. In this study, indications of data loss were most evident for infants whose parents were both foreign-born. The adverse effects of this ethnic group's low socio-economic status were expected to be most evident in the postneonatal period, yet the PNMRs for this group were exceptionally low, especially for the high-risk categories of high birth order, advanced maternal age, and absent or delayed prenatal care. These high-risk characteristics are not incompatible with those expected in a low socioeconomic status migrant population.

In this study, very-low-birthweight infants of foreign-born Spanish-surname parents had very high neonatal-mortality rates. This 1974–1975 finding in an urban nonborder setting contrasts with that of Powell-Griner and Streck, who found that 1979 NMRs for very-low-birthweight Spanish-surname infants were comparatively low in Texas border counties.[5] Like earlier researchers,[6] they attributed the low rates of underreporting of early infant deaths by undocumented alien parents who fear deportation or by lay midwives who fear prosecution for delivering complicated births. McCarthy *et al* also identified underreporting of very-low-birthweight neonatal deaths as a problem in other

APPENDIX

TABLE 4. NEONATAL AND POSTNEONATAL
MORTALITY RATES FOR SPANISH-
SURNAME INFANTS BY PARENTAL
NATIVITY AND SELECTED RISK FACTORS:
1974–75 SINGLE LIVE BIRTH COHORT,
HARRIS COUNTY, TEXAS

Mortality Measures and Risk Factors	Both parents US-born	Foreign-born Parents		
		Total	One parent foreign-born	Both parents foreign-born
Neonatal Mortality Rate[*]	10.4	7.7	7.6	7.9
Birthweight[†]				
<3 lb 5 oz	605.3	627.9	571.4	681.8
3 lb 5 oz–5 lb 8 oz	25.4	12‖	14.0‖	9.3‖
>5 lb 8 oz	2.9	2.5	3.0‖	2.2‖
Birth order[‡]				
1st	10.8	6.6	5.6‖	7.9‖
2nd or 3rd	8.3	6.5	6.4‖	6.7‖
4th or higher	14.3	11.3	14‖	9.5‖
Maternal age				
<20 yr	14.4	7.4‖	5.3‖	10.6‖
20–34 yr	8.5	7.6	7.8	7.4
≥35 yr	15.8*	9.9‖	11.5‖	8.7‖
First prenatal care				
1st or 2nd trimester	9.1	8.3	7.8	8.8
3rd trimester/no care	17.7	5.7‖	6.9*	4.6‖

(continued)

settings.[7] In our study, moderately low rather than very-low-birthweight infants of foreign-born Spanish-surname parents showed these unusually low NMRs. It is possible that in Harris County, which has a 5000 bed internationally-known medical center, very-low-birthweight infants who are born alive are more likely to be—and thus die—in a hospital, and therefore have death certificates recorded, while moderately low birthweight infants are discharged and/or cared for at home, with their death data being lost through migration or lack of registration. In this case, the singularly high death rate for very-low-birthweight infants may represent the true mortality risk for premature infants of foreign-born Spanish-surname parents. This identifies low birthweight, despite the apparently favorable distribution of birthweights, as a serious health

APPENDIX
TABLE 4. *(Continued)*

Mortality Measures and Risk Factors	Both parents US-born	Foreign-born Parents		
		Total	One parent foreign-born	Both parents foreign-born
Postneonatal Mortality Rate§	2.8	3.3	4.8	1.7‖
Birthweight†				
<3 lb 5 oz	26.3‖	46.5‖	47.6‖	45.5‖
3 lb 5 oz–5 lb 8 oz	2.5‖			
>5 lb 8 oz	2.6	3.1	4.8	1.4‖
Birth order‡				
1st	2.5‖	5.6	6.5‖	4.5‖
2nd or 3rd	2.5‖	2.9‖	4.8‖	0.8‖
4th or higher	4.3‖	0.7‖	1.8‖	
Maternal age				
<20 yr	3.6*	7.4‖	12.4‖	
20–34 yr	2.5	2.7	3.2‖	2.2‖
≥35 yr	3.2‖			
First prenatal care				
1st or 2nd trimester	2.9	2.8	3.4‖	2.2‖
3rd trimester/no care	2.7‖	4.9‖	10.3‖	

* Neonatal mortality rate = $\dfrac{\text{neonatal deaths}}{\text{live births}} \times 1000$

† Birthweights recorded to nearest ounce. Approximate gram equivalents: 3 lb 5 oz = 1500 gm; 5 lb 5 oz = 2500 gm

‡ Birth order = sum of live births, fetal deaths >20 wk gestation, and this birth

§ Postneonatal mortality rate = $\dfrac{\text{postneonatal deaths}}{\text{live births}} \times 1000$

‖ Rate based on fewer than 10 deaths

problem for Mexican Americans; that is, very-low-birthweight Mexican-American infants appear more likely to die than very-low-birthweight infants of other ethnicity. If the very-low-birthweight neonatal mortality rates calculated in this study actually underestimate mortality risk, as data from Powell-Griner and Streck[8] and McCarthy *et al*[7] might indicate, this problem assumes even greater magnitude.

In any case, further research regarding prematurity (as well as other causes of infant death) in the foreign-born Spanish-surname population is required, and examination of fetal deaths, not addressed in this cohort study of live births, is recommended. Spanish-surname parental nativity analysis of births and deaths according to attendant and place of birth* also may provide valuable insights into the possible under-registration of births and deaths in the urban Mexican-American community. Research in other similar geographic areas with larger data sets is recommended to confirm our findings and make meaningful comparisons. Until the issue of Mexican-American infant mortality is resolved, health planners are cautioned not to base policy and programs for the Mexican-American population on the Spanish-surname infant-mortality rate.

REFERENCES

1. US Bureau of the Census: World Population 1979: Recent Demographic Estimates for the Countries and Regions of the World. Washington, DC: Govt Printing Office, 1980, p 334.
2. North DS, Houstoun MF: The characteristics and role of illegal aliens in the US labor market: an exploratory study. Report for US Department of Labor. Washington, DC: Linton and Company, 1976.
3. Roberts K, Conroy ME, King AG, Rizo-Patron J: The Mexican migration numbers game: an analysis of the Lesko estimate of undocumented migration from Mexico to the United States. Bureau of Business Research Report, Austin: University of Texas, April 1978.
4. Weaver T, Downing TE (eds): Mexican Migration. Tucson: University of Arizona, 1976.
5. Powell-Griner E, Streck D: A closer examination of neonatal mortality rates among the Texas Spanish surname population. Am J Public Health 1982;72:993–999.
6. Teller C, Clyburn S: Texas population in 1970: trends in infant mortality. Texas Bus Rev 1974;40:240–246.
7. McCarthy BJ, Terry J, Rochat RW, Quave S, Tyler CW Jr: The underregistration of neonatal deaths: Georgia 1974–77. Am J Public Health 1980;70:977–982.

---

* Due to small subsample size, these variables were not analyzed.

3
The Political Process and Change

OBJECTIVES

Professional community health nurses recognize that many local health issues are directly and profoundly affected by larger policy issues. Consequently, their practice reflects awareness of and responsiveness to legislative action and other means by which health and social policies are set at all levels within the health care system. (American Nursing Association, p. 2, 1986)

This statement from the *Standards of Community Health Nursing Practice* clearly points to the need for community health nurses to be involved in the political process. In this chapter we will discuss the process of change and the use of the political process to effect change in communities. After studying the text, you will be able to

- Describe the political process
- Discuss the community health nurse's role in the political process to effect change
- Explain methods community health nurses can use to become politically active

INTRODUCTION

The community health nurse plays a significant role in determining the success or failure of the initiatives to improve health at the local, state, and national levels. The health care agenda supported by community health nurses will be constantly challenged and altered by the goals, resources, and constraints of the socioeconomic, ideological, and political situations. Nurses' understanding of and involvement in the political situation is essential to effective community health practice.

POLITICS AND PUBLIC POLICY

Politics is an essential part of every organization. Politics plays a part in working for change within our communities in every arena and at all levels of government. To study politics is to study decision making, or, to put it less formally, it is the study of how power, influence, and human behavior affect who gets what, when, and how. A basic definition of politics is "the authoritative allocation of scarce resources" (Kalisch *et al,* 1982, p. 31).

Public policy is a planned course of action taken to address selected issues and concerns. The policy-making process includes four stages: the recognition and definition of a problem, the development of programs and allocation of resources to address the problem, implementation of the programs, and evaluation of the impact of the programs.

Policy decisions regarding health care services and nursing practice are made by elected and appointed officials. Often, these officials are community leaders who do not have any background in health care. They need information from nurses about the ways the health care system really works for clients, providers, and third-party payors. As Diers (1985, p. 433) states,

> *Nurses will have endless opportunities to use our clinical wisdom to influence public policy, especially while policy continues to focus on costs of care. Nurses are the only ones who know what really goes on in hospitals, nursing homes, and other total care institutions. We are also the only ones who know the entire network of services outside of institutions into which people who have needs could be plugged. What we have to learn is how to articulate our clinical knowledge to policymakers.*

CHANGE

Influencing public policy and political outcomes demands an understanding of the change process and the types of change, and requires an appreciation of the different forms of power. Change may be gradual or sudden, but it does not take place unless a crisis occurs, a disequilibrium develops in a system, or there is an expansion of knowledge about a problem. A good example is the recent changes in the Medicare reimbursement system for inpatient hospital care. If the threat of bankruptcy in the Medicare Trust Fund had not existed Congress and the Reagan administration could not have legislated and implemented the prospective payment system for hospital services provided under the Medicare program. Evolutionary change is more easily adapted to, because it is gradual and incremental. Revolutionary change, however, requires more radical alterations in behavior and shifts in values. (See Chapter 8 for further discussion of change theory.)

The first step in the change process is to recognize a problem and define it in terms that can be understood by lay persons. This may mean, for example, that community health nurses concerned for pregnant women who are unable to obtain essential prenatal care because they do not have health insurance will document the problem in their community in order to share the information with policy decision makers and the public. Another example would be school health nurses who document their observation that the immunization levels of children entering school were decreasing because of a lack of access to health care. It is essential that groups and influential persons outside the nursing community recognize and understand the targeted problem. This can be accomplished by developing coalitions of concerned groups and by educating key elected and appointed officials. It should be kept in mind that although anecdotal information is always helpful, quantified analysis is more useful to policymakers.

Every problem has many different solutions that depend on individual and group values and beliefs. Each proposed solution must be analyzed, and positive and negative consequences must be understood and weighed. Past experiences with the same problem or similar problems should be discussed, as well as projections for the future, based on demographics, economics, and current practices. The political feasibility of a solution is also an important consideration. This consists of an understanding of who supports a particular solution, who opposes it, and who is likely to put up active opposition.

In order to develop a consensus on a solution to a given problem, it is first necessary to identify a varied group of citizens who have some interest in the problem. Within the legislative arena a consensus is accomplished by holding public hearings, inviting different organizations to comment on proposed legislative initiatives, and meeting with coalitions of divergent and like-minded interest groups. Changes in public policy can be made through administrative decisions or regulations, which depend on consensus-building among those affected by the proposed change.

Other steps in the change process include developing a plan for the agreed-upon change, implementing the plan, and evaluating its outcome. Each of these steps requires clear objectives regarding what is to be accomplished. When outcome goals can be specified at the beginning of a program, the implementation and evaluation phases of change are more readily accomplished. However, even with a clear set of goals, it is necessary to recognize and deal with the forces both for and against the proposed change.

There are several theories of planned change that are useful in developing strategies for successful change. Lewin (1951) used the force-field analysis to describe driving and restraining forces in studies of how change is accomplished. He used the terms *unfreezing* to describe establishing the need for change and *refreezing* for the process of stabilizing the change after implementation.

In their analysis of change, Chin and Benne (1976) grouped strategies into three categories: *empirical–rational, normative–re-educative,* and *power–coercive.* The empirical–rational approach equates knowledge with power and employs educational efforts to increase individual decision making. Using social beliefs and cultural norms, the normative–re-educative approach persuades people to change behavior based on new norms. An example of changing behavior based on new norms is the changing sexual behavior in response to what is currently known about the epidemiology of AIDS. The third category of change strategies, power–coercive, relies on power, (both legitimate and illegitimate) to force change. Change agents usually rely on a combination of these strategies. Let us look at an example of how the community health nurse can be a change agent through political involvement.

COMMUNITY HEALTH NURSES' INVOLVEMENT IN THE POLITICAL PROCESS

Involvement in the political process by the community health nurse covers several issues related to information and to power. It also involves the nurse in the roles of professional resource, constituent, and support within the community.

Power

Just as community health nurses must understand the distribution of power within a family in order to affect individual and family health behavior, nurses must know the powerbrokers in a community if they are to successfully change public policies for community health. There are many forms of power to be considered such as material wealth, knowledge, and position. Nurses themselves, as the largest group of health care providers, are a powerful group in any community. Another group with power is the growing population of elderly citizens.

By virtue of her expertise in working with families and her understanding of community health problems, the community health nurse is in a pivotal role to effect change and influence decisions regarding health care services. Knowledge of the process of assessing a family or community can be applied to policy development and politics. Just as community health nursing requires familiarity with a community, involvement in the political process requires an understanding of the political system and a familiarity with the elected and appointed officials.

Information

One way to understand political processes is to read newspaper accounts on health issues in order to learn who the key players are in a community. Understanding the issues with which elected officials are concerned is critical. Another approach is to keep in touch with your elected officials and their staff. Community health nurses need to express their concerns early and often— before decisions are made—about the health issues that are important in their districts. The American Nurses' Association (ANA) network of Congressional District Coordinators can be a helpful resource, and a means for making contact with representatives. It can be useful for nurses to make appointments to talk with elected officials and their staffs; meeting with them when they are visiting their home district is most effective. Most politicians want to serve their constituents and value personal contact with the people who keep them in office.

Issues

Many issues that concern officials at the local level have implications for community nursing services. The forum in which these are discussed may be the city council, the county board of health, or the state legislature. Officials must make decisions about resources allocated for childhood immunizations, prenatal care, Medicaid programs, and uncompensated care for the uninsured, as well as nurse practice acts and rules for state insurance. Ambulatory services, home care, and hospice services receive more attention under Medicare and this situation provides opportunities for community health nurses to become involved in decision making at the national level. National policies have direct implications for state block-grant programs such as the preventive health and child health block grants. Community health nurses need to act as advocates for these programs and for other policies, at both the state and federal levels, that are directed toward the prevention of health care problems.

Women's issues are another important area of concern for community health nurses. These include family abusive behavior, child care, and issues of tax reform. The "gender gap" in politics, the observation that women and men have begun to vote differently as groups, is an issue in and of itself. Both political parties now encourage candidates to seek the women's vote and to speak to women's issues. Women's health issues, from prenatal care to retirement and aging, are growing concerns. Women, and among them nurses, are beginning to send a message to policy makers according to Symons (1986, p 77), this message is a directive to "talk to nurses about pay equity, talk to PTAs about student-loan programs, talk to businesswomen about credit barriers, talk to housewives about throw-weights."*

No one person can expect to address all of the issues that have an impact on nursing practice and health care in a community. Based on their experience and areas of interest, community health nurses should select specific areas about which to become knowledgeable. By becoming involved in state nurses' associations, nurses can be kept informed on the current "hot" issues and can ensure that relevant community health issues are an important part of the nursing agenda.

The community health nurse can organize a group of interested people to meet with elected representatives on issues. Before the meeting, she can help the group think through the issues they want to discuss. Each person should be prepared to articulate clearly the arguments that support his or her case. In

---

* *Throw weight:* the weight of nuclear explosive and destructive power that a missile can deliver to its target.

developing these presentations, it is important to remember that knowledge of both sides of an issue is fundamental to the creation of a presentation that is a balanced, rational analysis. The state nurses' associations are a helpful resource on state issues important to nurses and health care, and the associations also can provide current information and background materials on national issues.

Professional Resource

Community health nurses can establish themselves as reliable sources of information for elected officials and the media and popular press. Using the community assessment as a base, health problems can be documented and trend data developed on important issues. Specific examples can be collected and shared with decision makers. This approach was used by community health nurses in a rural area to document how discharge planning under a hospital prospective payment plan resulted in inadequate home care services for the elderly (Kornblatt *et al,* 1984). Community health nurses, working in a local health department, documented the home care requirements of families over a period of time, as well as the situations that resulted from inadequate discharge planning. The problems of providing quality nursing services to Medicare beneficiaries with complex medical care needs were then brought to the attention of public officials through written and oral testimony prior to Congressional public hearings on the impact of hospital prospective payment systems (American Nursing Association, 1985).

Constituent

Elected officials like to hear the opinions of their constituents on current issues. Community health nurses can contact legislators through letters and telephone calls, and can encourage other community members to do the same. Such communication is not only an opportunity to reiterate the merits of the nursing position on an issue, but is important in showing that a number of people are concerned. Passage of legislation at both the state and national levels is a complex process, dependent on the expression of "grass roots" support at every hurdle on a long and difficult road.

Support

Letters and messages to elected officials need to be short and to the point. The rationale for supporting or not supporting proposed legislation or a particular policy should be an expression of the individual writer's conditions and circumstances. For example, this could include the implications of a proposed change, positive or negative, for a given community or age group. Letters should be friendly and should encourage further exchange of information. There is general agreement that threatening messages are not an effective way to communicate rational arguments.

THE LEGISLATIVE PROCESS—
THE FEDERAL PERSPECTIVE

Just as it is important to understand related systems within a community, it is necessary to know the legislative and budgetary systems within the local, state, and national governments. This discussion will focus on the federal system. Although state systems may be similar, they differ slightly in regard to rules and procedures followed and periods of time in session.

> NOTE: The League of Women Voters is an excellent resource for familiarizing yourself with your state and local government.

The United States Congress is divided into two distinct houses with different procedures, rules of conduct, and customs. The Senate consists of 100 Senators, two from each state, who are elected for six-year terms. The House of Representatives has 435 members, who are elected every two years by voters in their geographic districts. The two houses serve different purposes in the representative system. The House of Representative, because of its size, is a more structured body than the Senate. The rules and procedures of the House act to curtail members' actions so that a determined majority is able to work its will. The Senate, on the other hand, is more individualistic, with fewer rules and procedures. A minority group of Senators, or even an individual senator, can defer a legislative action. In the House, members tend to become policy specialists and rely less on staff to advise them. Senators are policy generalists, serving broader constituencies, and relying more on committees and personal staffs to advise them on key issues (Oleszek, 1984).

Any member of the House of Representatives or Senate may introduce legislation. Major legislation is usually introduced in both houses in the form of companion bills. To become law, a bill must be passed in identical form by both the House and the Senate within a two-year congressional session, and be signed by the President. Very few bills introduced ever make it out of the committees they are assigned to; even fewer become public law.

A bill is referred to the appropriate committee, where it is closely studied. The first action taken is usually a request for comments by interested federal agencies. Then, the chairman of the committee will most often refer the bill to a subcommittee for hearings. After considering the bill, the subcommittee reports back to the full committee with its recommendations for action and any proposed amendments. The full committee then votes its recommendation to the House or Senate.

In the House, health legislation is likely to be referred to the Committee on Energy and Commerce and its Subcommittee on Health and the Environment. Issues relating to health insurance such as Medicare and Medicaid are referred to the House Ways and Means Committee, Subcommittee on Health. On the Senate side, the Labor and Human Resources Committee reviews most health care legislation. The Senate Finance Committee's Subcommittee on Health acts on bills dealing with health programs under the Social Security Act.

After a bill is reported back to the house where it originated, it is placed on the calendar. The measure may be debated and acted on quickly or it may never come up for discussion, based on the procedures in the two houses. When a bill has been formally passed by one house, it is sent to the other. The receiving chamber (house) has several options. It can accept the other chamber's language and pass the bill as it is, it can send the bill to committee for further study, or it can reject the bill. If a companion bill is being worked on, the receiving chamber may wait to see its version of the bill in order to compare the contents. It is also possible for one chamber to approve a version of a bill that is vastly different from that passed by the other house, and then substitute its amendments for the language of the other, retaining only the latter's bill designation. If there are only minor differences in the House and Senate versions of the legislation, a set of changes are agreed upon and the bill then is sent to the White House. When there are substantial differences, the bill is usually recommended for review by a committee of Senate and House members to iron out differences. If either house does not agree to a review, the bill dies.

After the bill has been passed by both the House and Senate in identical form, it is sent to the White House for the President's signature. If the President signs it, the bill becomes law. If he does not sign it within ten days and Congress is in session, the bill becomes law without his signature. Should Congress adjourn before the ten days expire, and the President fails to sign the legislation, the result is a *pocket veto*. In the case of a Presidential veto, two-thirds of the members present (who must number a quorum) in both houses must vote to override the veto in order for the legislation to become law.

Application: Center for nursing research

Tracing legislation from the development of the initial idea to enactment of public law is useful for an understanding of the legislative process. In 1983 the Institute of Medicine (IOM) of the National Academy of Science reported that the "federal government's specific nursing research initiative is not at a level of organizational visibility and scientific prestige," and that "the lack of adequate funding for research and the resulting scarcity of talented nurse researchers have inhibited the development of nursing investigations." At the time of this analysis, the House and Senate were considering the authorization of legislation for the National Institutes of Health (NIH).

Rep. Edward Madigan (R-IL), ranking minority leader of the House Committee on Energy and Commerce, Subcommittee on Health and the Environment, introduced an amendment to establish a National Institute of Nursing within the NIH. This legislation was passed on to the full Committee on Energy and Commerce. In the Senate, the Committee on Labor and Human Resources was struggling with companion legislation. Development of consensus was slowed by considerable pressure from groups concerned with animal rights in research and fetal research.

Simultaneously, a number of consumer groups and professional organizations were working to establish an Institute of Arthritis and Musculoskeletal Diseases within the NIH. Sen. Barry Goldwater (R-AZ) introduced separate legislation to establish such an entity. This legislation moved quickly through the Senate and was sent to the House for consideration. Rep. John D. Dingel (D-MI) substituted the House language for the Senate bill, and the measure passed the House. A conference committee was convened and adjusted the differences between the House version and the Senate version (which had proposed only the Arthritis Institute). The reauthorization of NIH. S.540 was passed by both houses and sent to the President for signature just before the end of the 98th Congress. The President vetoed the bill on October 31, 1984.

In the spring of 1985, the House Subcommittee on Health, Energy and Commerce again introduced legislation to reauthorize the NIH with a provision for an Institute of Nursing (HR.2409). This legislation was passed out of committee and was approved by the House. The Senate Committee on Labor and Human Resources introduced companion legislation (S.1309) that did not call for an Institute of Nursing. This legislation was passed unanimously by the Senate on July 19, 1985.

The White House threatened a veto of the legislation because of "micro management" from Congress of issues that should have been left under the authority of the Administration, and stated further that new institutes such as the Institute of Nursing were unnecessary and caused increased administrative expense.

A conference committee again met to iron out differences between the House and Senate versions of the legislation. A major issue was the Institute of Nursing. A compromise was drafted that included a Center for Nursing Research. By the end of

October, both the House and Senate had passed the legislation and the measure was sent once more to the White House.

The President had ten working days in which to sign or veto the legislation. Many groups encouraged their members to write to the President, asking him to sign the legislation. Many members of Congress, both House and Senate, also urged the President to sign the legislation into law.

On November 8, the President vetoed the Health Research Extension Act, the NIH reauthorization that included the Center for Nursing Research. The veto message was sent to the House, which overrode it on November 12, by 380 votes to 32. On the same date, Sen. Orrin Hatch (R-UT) and Sen. Edward Kennedy (D-MA) circulated a letter urging their fellow senators to override the President's veto of the legislation. On November 20, the Senate voted to override the veto, by 84 to 7. The new NIH legislation that included a National Center for Nursing Research was now law.

At every step in the legislative process, state nurses' associations were asked to mobilize their members to write letters to their House and Senate representatives. Nurses who had established communication with their congressmen were asked to make a personal plea. Networks of nurse researchers, educators, and those in specialty practice were also asked to call and write to their elected officials. They did, and their efforts helped to pass the law that established nursing research within the mainstream of biomedical science at NIH.

After authorizing legislation is passed, it must be funded. Efforts had to focus next on the adequate funding of the National Center for Nursing Research and the Administration's plans for implementing the new law. These topics are discussed below.

Budget Process

The congressional budget process is initiated when the President submits his budget to Congress in January. The proposed budget is a major statement of national policy. It expresses the level of financial support that the Administration wishes Congress to approve for federal government activities. In its response to this policy statement, Congress must weigh many competing and conflicting values. These include issues such as increased deficit spending versus a balanced budget, and health and social welfare programs versus national defense spending.

Both the House and the Senate have established budget committees, assisted in their work by the Congressional Budget Office. These committees produce spending resolutions that guide Congress in its efforts to control spending. Spending ceilings are established for broad categories within the budget. The House and Senate Appropriations Committees can shift money among programs within a category, but are expected to keep spending levels within the total designated amount.

The Appropriations Committees determine the actual dollars that will be available in a given fiscal year for each program that Congress has authorized, and refer sections of the budget to the appropriate subcommittees. The Labor, Health and Human Services, and Education Subcommittees are responsible for most of the federal health program budgets. Subcommittee hearings are held each year, allowing government agencies and other concerned parties an opportunity to speak for or against the proposed spending levels.

After the budget discussions are completed, final recommended allowances are made for each program in a "mark-up" session. These recommendations are sent to the House and Senate. Differences between the two houses' recommendations must be negotiated in a conference committee, as is done for authorizing legislation. The Appropriations Bill is then sent to the White House for the President's signature (Santaita, 1985).

The federal budgeting process is lengthy and complex, but it is an important arena for action by community health nurses. This is especially true at the present time because many public health and social welfare programs are currently at risk as the movement to cut deficits while maintaining defense spending gains momentum.

FEDERAL INVOLVEMENT IN HEALTH CARE

The legal basis for federal government involvement in health care is found in the United States Constitution, Article 1, Section 8, which gives the United States Congress the power to promote the "general welfare." The question arises as to how we, as a society, define and determine "general welfare." Both before and since the drafting of the Constitution there have been a variety of views on this question. A better understanding of the tensions experienced by our society today can be gained by examining the differences between Jeffersonian egalitarianism and Hamiltonian libertarianism.

Libertarian philosophers hold individual liberty to be the single, overriding value to which all others are subordinate. Implicit in the libertarian's concept of liberty is the tenet that an individual is entitled to dispose of possessions as he or she sees fit. Thus, to tax one person's wealth in order to finance another person's health care is unjust, as is a policy that compels physicians or privately owned facilities to render health care to certain individuals or groups.

Antithetical to the libertarian credo are the theories of distributive justice espoused by egalitarian philosophers. Equal respect for all individuals and equal opportunity are held as overriding values to which individual liberty is subordinate. Inherent in this philosophy is a requirement that all members of society have equal access to certain basic commodities, namely, education, food, shelter, and health care.

The unique feature of the United States health policy has been the effort to accommodate both philosophies in their purest forms while defining and determining justice and the general welfare. This approach has resulted in an exquisitely expensive medical care system that has certain categorical programs for designated population groups. According to Moccia (1984, p 485), current policies suggest a willingness to sacrifice the nation's health in the cause of individual freedom. Moccia states, "If nursing wishes to sustain a valid social contract, it is clear that we must develop alternatives to the status quo that take into account the interdependent relationship between liberty and equality."

Our legislative bodies, both at the federal and state levels, are complex and multifaceted, as is our society. In a report by the Hastings Center (1985, p. 14) entitled *The Ethics of Legislative Life,* we are reminded of the following

> *Today nearly every facet of social and economic life depends on the effective and judicious functioning of the legislative process. We rely on legislatures to sift and balance conflicting interests, fashioning just and equitable compromises among them for the enhancement of the common good. We rely on legislatures to contain those forces that tend to pull us apart and to nourish those forces that tend to pull us together. In a world of interdependence and technological complexity, we look to legislatures to devise the rules of our collective activity, to guide the allocation of our social and economic resources, and most fundamentally, to help channel the enormous energy and creativity of our people and our civilization toward productive, just, and human ends.*

We live with the consequences of the judgments made by our elected representatives, the budgets they pass, the taxes and laws they adopt, and the regulations they support. Community health nurses, and all nurses, must make their interests known. The current trend is toward more government involvement in health care issues, not less. Political involvement is a means that nurses can use to achieve public policy objectives. And if they wish to have a meaningful role in shaping policy in general—and health care policy in particular—political involvement is an arena more community health nurses will be exploring.

REFERENCES

American Nurses' Association: Standards of Community Health Nursing Practice. Kansas City, Missouri, American Nurses' Association, 1986

American Nurses' Association. (1985). Testimony before the Task Force on Health Committee on the Budget: U.S. House of Representatives on the Impact of the Hospital Prospective Payment System on the Quality of Care Provided to Medicare Beneficiaries.

Chin R, Benne K: General strategies for effecting change in human systems. In Bennis W, Benne K, Chin R (eds): The Planning of Change, 3rd ed, New York, Holt, Rinehart and Winston, 1976

Diers D: Health policy and nursing curricula—a natural fit. Nursing & Health Care 6(8):433, 1985

Hastings Center: The Ethics of Legislative Life. Hastings-on-Hudson, New York, Institute of Society, Ethics and the Life Sciences, 1985

Institute of Medicine: Nursing and Nursing Education: Public Policies and Private Action. Washington DC, National Academy Press, 1983

Kalisch BJ, Kalisch PA: Politics of Nursing. Philadelphia, JB Lippincott, 1982

Kornblatt ES, Fisher ME, MacMillan DJ: Impact of DRGs on home health nursing. Presented at the annual meeting of the American Public Health Association, Washington DC, 1984

Lewin K: Field Theory in Social Science. New York, Harper & Row, 1951

Moccia P: The nurse as policymaker: Toward a free and equal health care system. Nursing & Health Care, 5(9):481, 1984

Oleszek WJ: Congressional Procedures and the Policy Process, 2nd ed. Washington DC, Congressional Quarterly Press, 1984

Santaita BJ: The federal budget process. Nursing Economics, 3 (March–April):103, 1985

Symons J: "Gender gap" widens. U.S. News & World Report, March 12, p 77, 1986

SUGGESTED READINGS

Dodd LC, Oppenheimer BI: Congress Reconsidered, 2nd ed. Washington DC, Congressional Quarterly Press, 1981

Green M: Who Runs Congress? 4th ed. New York, Dell, 1984

Hunter PR, Berger KJ: Nurses and the political arena: Lobbying for professional impact. Nursing Administration Quarterly, 8:66, 1984

Lake RS: Legislators' opinions about nursing: Results of a pilot study. Nursing & Health Care, 5:204, 1984

Mason DJ, Talbott SW: (1985). Political Action Handbook for Nurses. Reading, Massachusetts, Addison-Wesley Publishing Co, 1985

Ornstein NJ, Elder S: Interest Groups, Lobbying and Policymaking. Washington DC, Congressional Quarterly Press, 1978

Remhard S: Financing long-term health care for the elderly: Dismantling the medical model. Public Health Nursing, 3(1):3, 1986

4

Ecological Connections

OBJECTIVES

The community health nurse needs to have an understanding of the principles and applications of human ecology as they affect human health. After studying this chapter you will be able to

- Understand the ecological mechanisms that facilitate the migration of pollutants from their source to human populations
- Apply this ecological knowledge to the promotion of health and the identification of human health problems of environmental origin

INTRODUCTION

No person or community is an independent entity. Each is intimately linked to the environment, frequently in ways we have never imagined. Thus, the environment influences health, directly and through subtle, indirect pathways. Conversely, human activities affect the health of the environmental system. One aspect of *human ecology* is the study of these linkages. This chapter will explore the ways in which interconnections, transport mechanisms, and constant change combine to affect health.

Political action in the United States during the 1970s produced new legislation and strengthened a number of existing laws protecting human populations and the environment. Pollution-control efforts concentrated on reducing the quantities of pollutants emitted by major point sources, such as a smoke-stack or water-discharge pipe. These pollutants affected large numbers of people over broad areas of the nation. The success of these efforts can be gauged by the measurable reduction of the major air and water pollutants that has been achieved in our environment.

The current challenge is to control pollutants from nonpoint sources; pollutants that are released in smaller quantities from innumerable locations. These arise from agricultural activity, urban development, motor vehicle operation, the disposal of solid wastes, among other sources. They are present in our homes and workplaces, as well as at industrial sites. These pollutants may be released in smaller quantities and may affect fewer people than the point-source contaminants, but many are potentially more toxic. Many exhibit carcinogenic, mutagenic, or teratogenic effects.

The carcinogenic potential of hazardous pollutants in air, water, and solid waste is perceived by the public as a major health problem. An effective public policy must be developed to define and reduce any significant risks to public health that may arise from exposure to hazardous substances. Determining *if* and *when* and *how* human exposure to potentially hazardous substances should be regulated will be an essential, yet difficult, governmental task. Risk management decisions are always complex, and almost always involve some degree of uncertainty that cannot be resolved with the available scientific facts.

The difficulties of creating a public policy are further compounded by the observation that everyone does not respond in the *same way* to the *same exposure* to the *same chemical substance*. The effects of a given substance may be magnified in some people by a concurrent exposure to other chemicals, or minimized in other people because of genetic characteristics. The cost of providing complete protection to everyone may not be justified if the benefits accrue to only a small fraction of the exposed population. Further, the existence of health problems unrelated to pollution can complicate evaluation. For instance, in a milieu in which voluntary substance abuse and obesity are major community health problems, it is difficult to determine the limits of regulated exposure to an environmental risk.

In recent history, the interdependency of the human species and the natural world have been too frequently overlooked or ignored. As we seek ways to alleviate problems associated with health, it is imperative to be cognizant of nature's operating principles. The "laws of nature" have not been repealed, and knowledge of these laws is vital to understanding the origin of health problems and in successfully designing strategies to reduce them. The law of gravity is of particular importance to the ecological system. Everything that goes up, including pollutants, must come down, and everything dumped on the surface of the earth must flow downhill. Water and even land masses such as mountains move slowly to the sea. It is imperative that we learn to design with nature, exploiting these principles to advantage, rather than expending resources in a useless struggle, for nature always wins.

It is important to remember three commonsense observations that frequently are overlooked because of their inherent simplicity (Figure 4-1).

Everything is connected to everything else, but some things are connected more tightly than others. This observation is the least obvious and it will be the objective of this chapter to demonstrate its validity. As we go from a climatically controlled workplace to a correspondingly pleasant home, insulated from the vagaries of the weather even while enroute, it is easy to forget that this is a very recent phenomenon, restricted to a minority of the world population. As we select foodstuffs from the bounty of 24-hour supermarkets, we seldom stop to wonder where a particular item came from, what chemical abuses it may have suffered during its growth, harvest or transportation, or what unsuspected surprises may lurk beneath the protective cellophane.

Everything has to go someplace. Although this observation is readily acknowledged, "someplace" is generally considered synonomous with "away" and is not considered to be a problem until the "away" becomes your living space. As human populations and industrial development grow, pollutants are produced in greater quantities and dispersed longer distances. At the same time, unpopulated areas are diminishing. Some pollutants are conspicuous and readily detected. Others, perhaps more insidious, are detected only when sought; the search frequently requiring elaborate instrumentation and methodology.

Everything is constantly changing. While constant change is universally recognized, the nature and rate of change are generally unappreciated. The natural environment undergoes continual change. Some changes seem irreversible, permanent, or barely detectable from our perspective in time (*e.g.,* geologic transformations, and continental drift). Other changes are cyclic (the seasonal climate) or transient (floods or droughts). Changes produced by the actions of human beings have become more prominent. Significant human-induced changes began with the domestication of animals and the development of agriculture. These led to the growth of large human settlements, soon followed by deforestation and the depletion of local resources. The rate of change increased greatly as muscle power was replaced by mechanical power and energy derived from fossil fuels replaced renewable energy resources (wood, wind, and water).

During the last few decades, human impacts have reached an unprecedented intensity and now affect the entire world, owing to a vastly increased population and higher per capita consumption. The nature of change has also

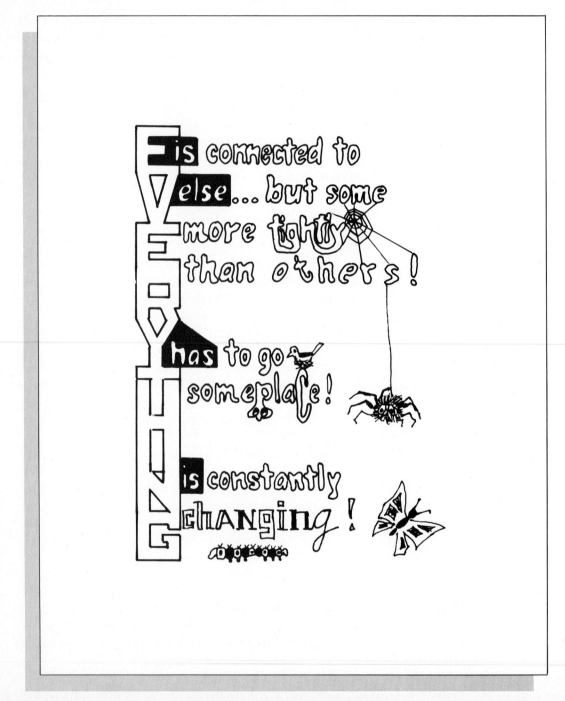

Figure 4-1.   The basic laws of ecology.

been altered as development projects redirect rivers, create lakes, alter sedimentation patterns, introduce new crops, in addition to producing agricultural-industrial air, water, and soil pollution. The desire to control the environment often creates conflicts between our goals and natural environmental patterns. In the quest to increase production people often deflect natural flows of energy, bypass natural processes, sever food chains, simplify natural systems and consume large energy subsidies in order to maintain the equilibria in artificial systems. The pursuit of short-term gains often results in irreversible environmental degradation. Humanity has become a geologic agent and is rapidly altering both the face of the earth and the planet's capacity to support human populations.

When exploring these interconnections it may be useful to remember that only one rule has no exceptions: "There are exceptions to every rule."

ENERGY AND NUTRIENTS

All living organisms require both nutrients with which to build and maintain their bodies and energy to drive the chemical reactions that permit them to function. The nutrients are continuously recycled by way of natural processes and are used over and over again. The energy literally arrives from outer space and cannot be recycled.

The sun is the only significant source of energy in our solar system. A substantial portion of the sunlight that reaches the earth is reflected back into space (the same phenomenon of reflecting light permits viewing of the moon and other planets). The light that is absorbed by the earth is transformed into a lower energy state. Eventually all of this energy will be radiated back into space as heat. Our existence is dependent upon what is done with this energy before it leaves the earth.

This process of absorption is a familiar one because our bodies absorb heat from the sun in the same way. When outdoors in winter we may consciously seek to position ourselves in direct sunlight to warm ourselves by absorbing this free energy, and in summer we seek shade and rapidly overheat when exposed to the sun. Our absorption can be modified through varying the color of our outer garments, using white or light colors to reflect sunlight and black or dark colors to increase absorption.

Consider another example: an automobile parked with all its windows closed. Sunlight passes through the windows and strikes the dashboard, steering wheel, and seat covers. The energy of the sunlight is absorbed and transformed into infrared energy, or heat. This lower form of energy cannot pass through the windows as readily as the visible wavelengths of light. Thus, heat builds up inside the automobile, and those objects that absorbed the most energy have the quickest rise in temperature. The interior of the car will become much warmer than the outside environment and the car will radiate heat long after the source of light is removed at sundown. This is often called the *greenhouse effect.* The earth's unique atmosphere has the same effect. Heat radiating from the surface of the earth is trapped by the atmospheric gases. Uneven heating of the earth's surface (caused by the sun heating (lighting) one side at a time) creates air and water currents. These distribute this heat more evenly, and moderating the extreme temperature fluctuations (that are typical of objects in space that lack an atmosphere such as our moon).

The above examples illustrate two effects of sunlight: a transformation of energy, from visible lightwaves to invisible heat; and a displacement in time and place, with the effects of absorption felt long after the source of illumination is gone, and the heat displaced considerable distances with air and water masses.

Living organisms exist by capturing the physical energy of sunlight and transforming it into the energy of chemical bonds in organic molecules. This process, *photosynthesis,* is unique to green plants. Therefore, humans and all other animals are totally dependent upon the productivity of the plant world for survival. When animals eat green plants they release the energy stored in the chemical bonds and use it to power their own activity. Both plants and animals are capable of respiration, which releases the energy stored in organic molecules.

The laws of thermodynamics apply to these biological energy processes. The first law states that energy may be transformed from one type of energy to another, as from light to chemical bonds to heat, but it is never created or destroyed. The second law specifies that no process involving an energy transformation will occur spontaneously unless there is a degradation from a concentrated form into a dispersed form; that is to say, no energy transformation is 100% efficient (Figure 4-2). Thus, while living organisms are successful in channeling the energy of sunlight into a series of chemical reactions that store and release energy in small, manageable amounts, the end result is always the same—the release of heat to the environment and eventually outer space. We see this process at work constantly, in the metabolic heat of our bodies released in expired air, urine, and feces, or radiated from our body surfaces. The time delay in these biological processes may be considerable, as the amount of energy bound up in organic fuel (such as wood) and fossil fuel (coal, petroleum and natural gas) attest. Primary fuel sources today were produced by biological activity under environmental conditions that no longer exist on earth. It is important to note that biological energy transformation is a flow-through process. Energy enters the earth's environment, is stored and used, and departs in a transformed state. Energy is never cycled.

Nutrients behave in a very different manner. The chemical elements of living organisms circulate from the environment to the organisms and, following death of the organism, back to the environment. These paths, known as biogeochemical cycles, exhibit varying degrees of complexity and time scales. Most elements cycle from a sedimentary reservoir in the earth's crust and a given molecule may have a limited geographic range. A molecule absorbed from the earth may enter plant tissue and persist until the death and decomposition of the plant. If the plant is eaten, the molecule may move a short distance as part of the animal before returning to the earth when the animal decomposes. Other substances cycle as gases from an atmospheric or hydrospheric reservoir and these may be distributed globally, particular examples being nitrogen, oxygen, carbon dioxide, and water.

At this point you may ask what all this has to do with health. The essential point is that human beings have complex and elaborate chemical and homeostatic mechanisms that function to acquire and retain nutrient and energy-containing molecules from the environment. Any toxic or undesirable chemicals that mimic required nutrients or are otherwise incorporated into these natural cycles and pathways will also be transported into our bodies. Frequently it is not a question of whether a given chemical will find its way into our bodies, but rather how long will it take, how much will be acquired, and how long will it persist in both our bodies and the environment. A decade after the pesticide DDT was banned from use in the United States, it is still present in measurable quantities in all people examined.

THE ORGANIZATION OF LIFE

The capture and use of energy by living organisms is accomplished by the high degree of organization characteristic of all levels of the biological world. Subatomic particles combine to form atoms. These atoms link to create molecules. More atoms can be added to produce macromolecules, which are vitally important to organisms. Macromolecules can be assembled into organelles, the essential components of cells. Cells replicate to form a mass of tissue and initiate specialization. Several types of tissue can unite to create an organ. A number of organs can function together as an organ system. The aggregate of the organ systems becomes the free-living organism.

Hierarchal organization continues. A group of individuals of any one kind of organism comprise a population. The composite of all the populations of all the different kinds of organisms occupying a given area comprise a commu-

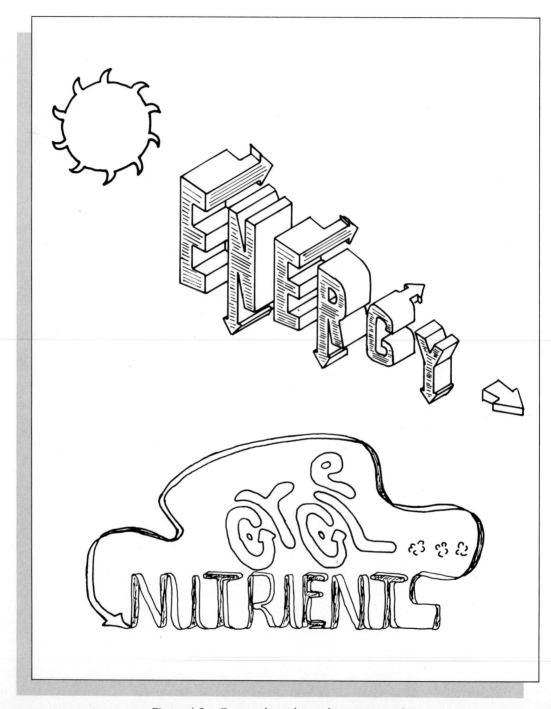

Figure 4-2.   Energy degrades and nutrients cycle.

nity. (Note an essential difference here; health professionals consider only people when describing a community, while ecologists include all organisms.) Since organisms do not live in a vaccuum the physical components of the world must also be considered. The living community functions together with the nonliving (abiotic) environment to form an ecosystem.

The ecosystem is the basic functional unit in ecology. It includes both biotic communities (organisms) and the abiotic environment, each influencing the properties of the other and both necessary for maintenance of life. Within an ecosystem the flow of energy and materials follows distinct pathways. Green plants capture the energy of sunlight and manufacture energy-rich organic compounds. Animals eat the plants or eat other animals that have fed on plants. This transfer of energy from plant to animal to another animal is known as a food chain. At each transfer a large proportion, usually 80% to 90%, of the energy manufactured or eaten by an organism is consumed by that organism in respiration, and is not available for transfer to another animal. Humans and other animals typically consume many different kinds of food. Food chains are rarely simple; they are generally extensively interconnected with one another in a "food web."

The productivity of an ecosystem can be measured by determining the rate at which radiant energy is captured and stored as organic substances that can be used as food materials. High rates of productivity occur when physical factors are favorable and energy subsidies outside the system reduce to cost of maintenance. For example, saltwater marshes have very high productivity because rivers carry nutrients downstream to reach the marsh, and tidal action circulates these materials within the marsh and flushes out the waste products. Thus, water power and tidal energy subsidize productivity of the marsh ecosystem, benefiting marine life from the surrounding area that concentrate their larval and juvenile growth stages in these regions of high productivity. Humans receive direct benefit from this productivity in the form of harvested seafood but frequently view such a marsh as a mosquito-ridden wasteland convenient to the beach, begging to be drained, filled, and covered with condominiums. The subsequent disappearance of the seafood is viewed as another perversity of nature, unconnected to the devastation of the ecosystem.

In complex natural communities organisms whose food is obtained from plants through the same number of steps are considered to belong to the same trophic level. A given species may function at more than one trophic level according to the source of energy actually eaten. For example, humans function at the second level when eating plant material, the third level when consuming beef, and the fifth level when dining on carnivorous fishes such as tuna or salmon. Understanding the trophic concept and energy loss between trophic levels is important when problems of human nutrition are considered.

As food becomes scarce, food chains must be shortened to avoid energy loss. Staple foods are commonly highly productive grasses—cereals, rice, corn, and so forth. It is inefficient to use such plant foods to produce meat for human consumption. Cattle are efficient converters of nonedible grasses (for humans, who lack the necessary digestive enzymes) to meat and have evolved a complex four-chambered stomach (which incorporates decomposing bacteria) for this purpose. Affluent societies circumvent nature's energy-efficient food chains by feeding corn to cattle to increase the fat content of beef intended for human consumption. While more delectable, this marbled beef subsequently creates new health problems.

Food webs and trophic levels are phenomena associated with ecosystems. The physical boundary of a given ecosystem is often indistinct. Even such a discrete habitat as a pond is used by species that alternate between aquatic and terrestrial environments. Minerals can reach the pond from anywhere within its watershed, an area typically much larger than the pond itself. Other chemicals can reach the pond from hundreds of miles away, as the pollutants that create acid rain have taught us. Many food webs overlap several ecosystems. A cursory survey of a pantry shelf or supermarket will easily demonstrate the widespread food-transportation system that has been developed to ship staples, fruits, and delicacies across continents and oceans. Pollutants and toxicants readily accompany these foodstuffs.

Primitive humans were aware of humanity's niche in the biological community and exploited numerous plants and animals in pursuing the hunter–gatherer mode of existence. Agricultural humans focused on a few domesticated species and began to regard other plants and animals as weeds and pests. The increased productivity of cultigens permitted larger human populations but also lead to dependence on a less diverse nutrient base. Technological humans, particularly urbanites, have forgotten their dependence on natural ecosystems and agro-ecosystems. The quest to further increase agricultural production and control pest organisms by chemical means has added new threats to health in the name of feeding human populations.

ECOLOGICAL INTERACTIONS AND HEALTH

Interactions between organisms are particularly important in the cause, transmission, and persistence of disease. Infectious diseases fall into several broad categories, depending upon the number of organisms involved. The simplest consists of only two members, a pathogen and its host. Smallpox is such a system: the pathogen is a virus and a human is the host. Infected individuals that recover are no longer susceptible to reinfection. The immune mecha-nisms can be stimulated with a vaccine and, through this action, the host becomes immune to the pathogen. As the potential host population is reduced (by way of vaccination) the pathogen is unable to persist and eventually will become extinct.

Many diseases include a third party, a vector that transmits the pathogen from host to host without becoming infected itself. The pathogen that causes the bubonic plague is a bacterium that is transmitted to humans, and other animals, through the bite of a flea. The bacterium is maintained in populations of rodents of various kinds. The rodents provide the reservoir wherein the bacillus persists; the fleas are merely vectors of transmission from an infected rodent to an uninfected rodent, or to a human being. Humans are secondary hosts, but when the bacillus is introduced into a crowded human population the results can be devastating, as has been demonstrated by the epidemics that occur every few centuries. These epidemics have disappeared on their own, not as the result of human countermeasures.

POLLUTION

Pollutants are the residues of things humans make, use, and throw away. Nondegradable pollutants either do not degrade or degrade very slowly in the natural environment. Biodegradable pollutants can be rapidly decomposed by natural processes unless input exceeds decomposition or dispersal capacity. Degradable pollutants that provide energy or nutrients may increase the pro-ductivity of an ecosystem by providing a subsidy when the rate of input is moderate. High rates of input can cause productivity to oscillate and additional input may poison the system completely.

When any pollutant is introduced into the environment, we must be concerned about both the *fate* of the pollutant (where it goes and how it gets there) and its *effect* on humans or any of the ecosystems upon which we depend (Figure 4-3). It must always be kept in mind that any effects that pollutants have on other species are early warning symptoms that something is amiss in the ecosystem and that humans may well be the next to be affected. There are five mechanisms of particular concern.

Major Pollutant Mechanisms

Transport

Transport of the pollutant, once introduced into the environment, is generally accomplished by way of wind patterns or through aquatic systems. Pollutants

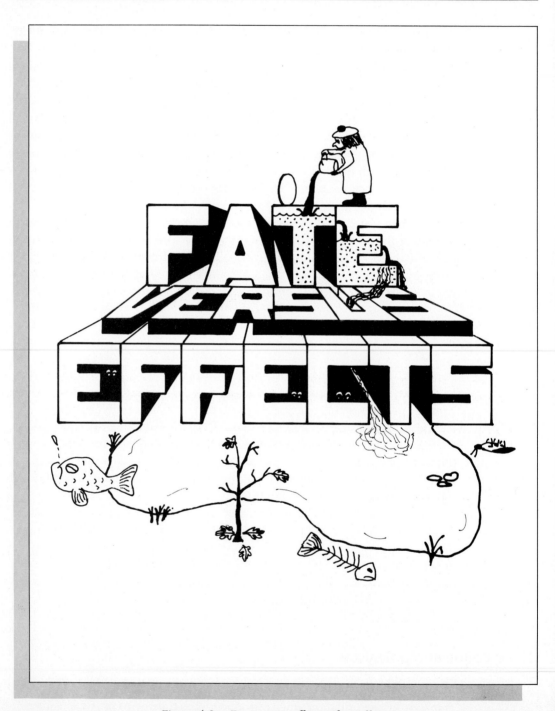

Figure 4-3.   Fate versus effects of a pollutant.

can be dispersed aerially as particulates or in a gaseous state; they can travel long distances before falling to earth as dust, or being carried in rainwater. The construction of taller smokestacks to relieve local pollution generally results in greater dispersal, thus enlarging the area affected without diminishing the amount of pollutant released. Once air pollutants have settled to earth, they frequently continue their movement by moving along waterways. Stormwater runoff can mobilize more suspended particulates following a single heavy rainfall than may be transported during the rest of the year. Dissolved pollutants may be transported long distances before settling onto the bottom sediments through some precipitatory mechanism.

Pollutants generally exert greater influence on aquatic ecosystems than on terrestrial environments. Air pollutants may enter a person's lungs or settle on vegetation and then be eaten with the plants. Water is nature's best solvent and many pollutants go into solution in aquatic ecosystems, so that aquatic animals and plants live in a weakly polluted soup. Many chemicals enter the biota directly through the skin or across gill surfaces, for there is no escape from a dissolved pollutant. The effects of a given one-time polluting event, such as an accidental spill, are also exerted for a longer time in aquatic ecosystems. Not only is a greater portion of the pollution incorporated into and cycled within the biotic nutrient pool, but material that settles into the sediment also can be resuspended and redistributed with every major storm event. The dispersion of pollutants is more restricted in aquatic systems than in terresterial ones because movement is always downstream, until the pollutants reach the ocean. The efficacy of ocean transport has been demonstrated by the ubiquitous spread of several insecticides throughout the world; their area of distribution even includes the Antarctic continent.

Transformation

Transformation of a pollutant within an ecosystem takes place in many ways. Harmful substances can be rendered innocuous or even helpful during the biodegradation process. But occasionally a relatively harmless substance is transformed into a noxious form. A classic example is the transformation of metallic or inorganic mercury, which is relatively immobile, into methylmercury by microorganisms living in aquatic sediments. Methylmercury is readily incorporated into detritous food chains, which may terminate with human consumption of contaminated fish and shellfish, producing the neurological disorder known as the "Minamata disease." Nonbiogenic chemical transformations are more common in the environment; for example, the conversion of sulfur dioxide and nitrous oxides in the atmosphere to form sulfuric and nitric acids and create "acid rain."

Bioaccumulation

Bioaccumulation refers to the introduction of substances into ecological food webs. Chemicals that behave in a manner similar to essential elements are most susceptible to rapid uptake and retention. Chiefly because of the activities of human beings, the ecologist now must be concerned with the cycling of nonessential elements. For example, the radionuclides of strontium and cesium, whose chemical behavior is analogous to calcium and potassium, respectively, are introduced into the environment by nuclear reactors and represent a potential health hazard.

Biomagnification

Biomagnification results when the accumulation of a pollutant greatly exceeds the rate at which it is eliminated from an organism. The pollutant concentrated by organisms at a low trophic level is transmitted to the next level, where it is further concentrated and passed to the third level, and so forth. For example, a pesticide such as DDT is acquired by phytoplankton who may quite innocuously act as tiny scavengers of the pollutant. These are eaten by zooplankton, which in turn are eaten by larger zooplankton, then one or more fishes, and finally consumed by humans or another end chain, end-of-the-line carnivore. At each step the pesticide is sequestered in the fatty tissue of the carrier and stored. The final concentration of pesticide in human beings, osprey, swordfish or whatever may be as much as 30,000 times greater than the original concentration in the water.

Synergism

Synergism is the simultaneous action of separate substances or agencies that together produce a greater total effect than the sum of their individual effects. It is common to discover that a given substance behaves in one fashion in a controlled laboratory environment and quite another when introduced into a natural ecosystem, where it interacts with a number of physical and chemical properties of the environment.

Toxic Substances

In recent years *toxic substances* have received a great deal of attention in governmental regulations and the news media. Any chemical can be toxic, including table salt, sugar, and the chlorine in drinking water. Toxic substances are generally considered to be any chemicals, or mixtures of chemicals, either synthetic or natural, that are poisonous to humans or plants or animals under expected conditions of use and exposure. There are four major categories of toxic substances. *Pesticides* are lethal chemicals specifically designed to kill weeds, fungi, insects, mites, rodents, and other pests. Four pesticides have been banned from further use in the United States: DDT, aldrin, dieldrin, and chlordane. *Industrial chemicals* are particularly numerous and a few have proven especially dangerous (*e.g.,* asbestos, benzene, vinyl chloride, and PCB). A number of *metals* such as arsenic, lead, cadmium, and mercury have proven to be very toxic in the environment. The fourth category includes those substances with isotopes that emit various types of *radiation* such as strontium, cesium, iodine and so forth. There are nearly 60,000 different chemical substances in commercial use in the United States today, manufactured or processed by 12,000 establishments; 98% of these chemicals are safe. Fifty-five thousand firms generated 290 million tons of hazardous waste in 1981. More than 17,000 hazardous waste disposal sites have been identified, and hundreds of these sites represent a substantial threat to human health.

Chemical toxicity occurs when a chemical agent produces detrimental effects in living organisms. The effects of a toxic substance can be immediate or long-term, and can harm selected tissues or the entire organism. Both the toxicity of the substance and the expected exposure to the organism must be considered together to define the risk that can be anticipated.

Pollutants and Human Population Size

All of the environmental processes described above can influence human health. Any pollutant or toxic substance introduced into the environment is subjected to these processes, many of which lead directly to human beings. Pollution of the environment occurs when these pollutants overwhelm the capacity of the environment to assimilate them without being thrown out of balance. Thus, pollution is a rate function involving a quantity of pollutant introduced over a period of time. This is directly correlated to population size.

It can be said that all pollution is the result of population growth. A single family, living on a subsistence level in the wild, burning wood as their fuel and discarding rubbish and human wastes on the landscape, would seldom be a polluting factor in their environment. The population of a small village would denude the landscape of wood fuel, pollute the air with smoke from numerous wood fires, and litter the ground with rubbish and human wastes randomly dispersed. The more numerous inhabitants of cities totally overwhelm the environment with rubbish and human wastes, fostering the development of sewage and garbage disposal systems. Industrial development increases the number of pollutants and environmental insults. Our past practice for handling pollutants has been to just dump them, and take further action only when the natural systems have been overwhelmed. We need to reverse this practice, and remove the bulk of pollutants before inflicting them upon nature. Then the natural ecosystems work for us by removing the final bit of pollution that always proves so difficult and expensive to neutralize.

Demographic changes can rapidly alter the stress inflicted upon the environment. As population grows, the stress increases. If the population moves, both the nature and the intensity of an environmental problem can shift. For example, the recent decline of industrial productivity in the northeastern United States has resulted in a shift in the population caused by the exodus of workers (particularly younger families) and an improvement in the surface water quality. The growth of population in the south, especially the arid southwest, is both increasing water pollution and straining overall water supply.

The solution to one environmental problem may be the creation of another. Pollutants do not disappear. Sulfur that is scrubbed out of powerplant smokestack gases ends up as a sludge stored on the ground, where it may threaten water quality. Pollutants removed from wastewaters by precipitation end up in the bottom sludge, which also requires disposal. If the sludge is burned, the pollutants may be released into the air, to settle and become incorporated into the water or land once again. If the sludge is buried in a landfill, it may threaten surface water or groundwater supplies. Sewage treatment plants that aerate water as part of the process may discharge substantial amounts of volatile toxic substances to the air. *Everything has to go someplace.*

In summary, virtually any pollutant that is introduced into the environment will subsequently be transported away from its point of entry. It may be transformed into another chemical form, either less or more hazardous. It will probably be accumulated by biological organisms and possibly magnified in concentration. It is likely to react with other chemicals or physical processes and produce unanticipated effects. Distinct and efficient chemical cycles and pathways that have evolved over millions of years ensure that toxicants will enter biological systems and eventually reach humans, or other organisms upon which they depend. *Everything is connected to everything else* and *everything has to go someplace.* There is nowhere to hide. The only solution is to stop the pollution.

INTERCONNECTIONS

Humanity's attempts to intervene in natural processes seldom go smoothly, and frequently produce effects far removed from the immediate intervention site. Some of the most profound effects have been experienced in attempts to control or eradicate diseases. The following example reveals some unexpected connections.

Malaria is caused by four species of *Plasmodium,* a single-celled sporozoan parasite. During the first stage of the disease, elongate sporozoites in the blood penetrate cells within the liver. The sporozoites multiply asexually to produce numerous merozoites. During the second stage of the disease the merozoites leave the liver and enter red blood cells. The merozoites reproduce, again asexually, within the red blood cells and erupt, with the progeny invading new red blood cells and continuing the cycle. These eruptions eventually synchronize to 48-hour or 72-hour cycles, depending on the *Plasmodium* species involved. The shock of the simultaneous release of the merozoites can produce chills in the victim, followed by a high fever caused by toxins released with the merozoites. Some merozoites become gametocytes, capable of sexual reproduction.

The human immune system functions by being able to recognize the chemical antigens of an infectious agent and produce specific antibodies to combat it. The malarial pathogen presents three different stages (sporozoite, merozoite, gametocyte) with three different antigens. Antibodies that counter one antigen are not effective against the other two stages. Also, the antibodies will be effective only when the various parasite cells are free in the bloodstream. Once they have entered either liver cells or red blood cells they cannot be attacked by the antibodies. Thus, an effective vaccine would have to work against all three stages.

Mosquitoes are insects found in abundance virtually everywhere in the world. More than 1500 species are known; and a few tropical and subtropical species are involved in the transmission of human diseases. Larval mosquitoes develop in water and many species are quite adaptable in their choice of breeding sites, using water that collects in abandoned tin cans, rubber tires, and so forth. Adult male mosquitoes suck plant juices for their nourishment and do not bite animals. Adult females require a blood meal to provide nutrients for their eggs. Various species bite reptiles, birds, and mammals (including humans) to obtain the blood. When a female *Anopheles* mosquito bites a human who is infected with malaria, the malarial gametocytes may be drawn up into the digestive system of the insect. The gametocytes are transformed into gametes within the stomach of the mosquito, unite to form a zygote, and burrow into the cells in the wall of the stomach. The resulting oocyte produces numerous new sporozoites, which migrate to the salivary glands of the mosquito. When the female mosquito next bites a human, some sporozoites may be injected into the wound by way of saliva. Mosquito saliva contains an anticoagulant to keep the blood flowing until the mosquito has drunk her fill.

This complicated procedure is the only mechanism by which the malaria parasite is transmitted from one human host to another. It cannot be transmitted by direct human contact (although it has been transmitted by means of blood transfusion and intravenous drug abuse), nor is it passed from one mosquito to another. It persists only by using the mosquito vector to complete its complex lifecycle. Malaria is a widespread and debilitating disease. It has been estimated that each year, worldwide, 250 million people fall ill with this disease, and more than one million die. It causes anemia, fever, spleen enlargement, miscarriage, contributes to a high infant mortality, and causes in its victims a greater susceptibility to many kinds of infection. The eradication of malaria has been a top priority goal of the World Health Organization (WHO) for many years.

As the primary host of the malarial parasite, humans represent three distinct populations in the transmission of this disease. There are people who are susceptible to being infected with the disease, those who are already infected, and those who are immune to infection. Newborn infants may acquire some antibodies from their mothers, but these do not persist. Children from one year to four years old are highly susceptible to malaria and constitute most of the deaths from the disease. Older children and adults can develop partial immunity to small numbers of the malarial parasites but when large numbers are present they tend to overrun this limited immunity.

Temporary artificial immunity to malaria can be created with the continuous intake of drugs. The South-American Indians discovered that the bark of the cinchona tree yielded quinine, which was effective in preventing and treating malaria. The famous gin and tonic, made with quinine water, is reputed to have been developed by the British to ameliorate their daily intake of quinine in malarial regions. Quinine was replaced by quinacrine hydrochloride (Atabrine), which had the side effect of coloring the eyes yellow. The drug in present use is chloroquine, which prevents DNA replication and RNA synthesis in the parasitized red blood cells. For prevention and suppression of malaria, chloroquine must be taken on a weekly basis.

Mosquitoes have no immune system to counteract invasion by malaria parasites. Mosquitoes do have high rates of reproduction; uninfected females become infected by biting an infected human. Infected mosquitoes never recover from the infection and continue to transmit the parasite to subsequent victims. Malaria can be maintained in areas of low human population density if the mosquito population density is high. Efforts to eradicate malaria have focused on eradicating the mosquito, or at least lowering mosquito populations to the point where they were no longer effective vectors of the disease.

The weapons of choice for this worldwide campaign were insecticides. A favorite was DDT, a chlorinated hydrocarbon that attacks the central nervous system. Although synthesized in 1874, it was not used as an insecticide until 1939. It is a broad-spectrum pesticide, affecting many organisms in addition to the target species. DDT was used widely during World War II to protect United States troops from malaria, typhus, and other insect-borne diseases. DDT was inexpensive to manufacture and easy to handle. Its long-lasting residual effect was hailed as one of its chief advantages.

Within a dozen years unwelcome side effects began to appear. Eggshell thinning in birds began as early as 1947. Fishes, crabs, shrimps, and oysters accumulated lethal concentrations of DDT even at very low levels of exposure. Citizen opposition to widespread use, particularly aerial spraying, began in 1957. Domestic production of DDT peaked at 188 million pounds annually in 1963, but declined to 60 million pounds in the 1970s. Domestic consumption peaked at 79 million pounds in 1959 and declined to 20 million pounds by 1971. In 1972 the Environmental Protection Agency suspended virtually all uses of DDT in the United States on the grounds that continual use would pose an unacceptable risk to humans and the environment.

DDT was more persistent in some environmental systems than others. Residues in soil degrade slowly. In arid areas, the time required for one half of the DDT to wash out or break down exceeds 20 years. DDT applied to soils can evaporate into the air and move long distances (it has been recorded in Antarctic snow). Rainfall and surface runoff transport DDT to streams, rivers, estuaries, and oceans. DDT breaks down in the environment to DDD or DDE, which are even more potent.

The Food and Drug Administration established a maximum allowable concentration of DDT in foodstuffs at 5 parts per million (ppm). By the 1960s several species of fishes from the Great Lakes and the Atlantic and Pacific Oceans exceeded this level. The National Human Monitoring System was initiated in 1967 and DDT has been found in more than 99% of all human tissues sampled. Total DDT (including DDD and DDE) in human fatty tissues peaked at nearly 9 ppm in 1971. DDT is concentrated in fatty tissues of the body and frequently contaminates milk and dairy products. At one point the DDT content of human milk exceeded the 5 ppm level, rendering breast milk unfit for human consumption. Since DDT was banned in the United States, the level of DDT in food organisms and wildlife has slowly, but steadily, declined. More than a decade later, DDT is detectable in 100% of human adipose tissues analyzed, with a median concentration of 2.5 ppm.

DDT has spread throughout the world and has been found in both arctic fishes and antarctic penguins, far from any site of direct DDT aplication. This is vivid evidence of worldwide environmental transport mechanisms. DDT has been directly implicated in the precipitous decline of brown pelican and peregine falcon populations. Both species occupy positions at the end of long food chains that concentrate DDT at each transfer level. DDT interferes with calcium metabolism, causing the birds to produce eggs with abnormally thin shells that frequently crack during incubation, thus failing to hatch. Both bird species are classified now as endangered. Both reveal only the tip of the iceberg, for the DDT contamination is widespread throughout their food web.

The war against malaria appeared to be succeeding for a number of years, with spectacular reductions being made in the prevalence of the disease. Many agencies and governments felt that the benefits gained far outweighed the environmental costs. However, in recent years the prevalence of malaria has soared to precontrol levels in the very areas that enjoyed the greatest success. The mosquitoes are no longer affected by the insecticides and, in some regions, the malarial organisms no longer respond to chemotherapy. Human endeavors have encountered the reality of biological adaptation.

All organisms exhibit variability. This is recognized readily in humans, for we not only look different as individuals, but our chemical makeup, reaction to drugs, and even taste sensors respond differently to a given stimulus. In a parallel fashion, not all targeted organisms will succumb to a given pesticide. In any large population there always seem to be a few that survive various stressors. Thus, when an area is treated with an insecticide, the majority of the mosquito population, perhaps more than 99%, will die. But the resources that supported that mosquito population may be unaffected, and some of the natural enemies and predators of mosquitoes may also have been killed by a broad-spectrum pesticide. So the few mosquitoes that survive find themselves in an advantageous situation. Their resources are intact, their enemies are gone, and they can reproduce and grow in number as they please. But one significant change has occurred. Assuming that the characteristic that permitted them to survive the pesticide is inheritable, all of their progeny will also possess this characteristic. This means that the new generation will not be susceptible to that pesticide.

This description of adaptation is an oversimplification, but the principal is valid. It is applicable equally to the development of drug or antibiotic resistant strains of micro-organisms. In fact, this has occurred with malaria organisms in some parts of the world, where chloroquine-resistant strains have arisen. Just as the overuse of antibiotics leads to antibiotic-resistant pathogens, the overuse of insecticides leads to insecticide-resistant insects. When the strength and frequency of insecticide applications are increased, insecticide-resistant insects develop all the faster.

Widespread insecticide application can have even broader effects. Malaria was a serious, prevalent disease in Borneo (in some areas over 90% of the population suffered from enlarged spleens). In 1955, WHO began a successful program of malaria control. Two insecticides, DDT and dieldrin, were sprayed inside the thatched-roof houses to eradicate two species of mosquitos that were transmitting the malaria. The insecticides also reduced the populations of small parasites of a moth species. The parasites were killed outright by dieldrin and they avoided thatch that had been sprayed with DDT. Freed from their parasites, the population of moth larvae expanded rapidly and consumed large quantities of thatch in the housetops. The insecticides were also picked up by cockroaches and geckos (small lizards that lived in the houses and fed upon insects). Both cockroaches and geckos were captured and eaten by the domestic cats kept by the villagers. The cats proved to be particularly susceptible to the insecticides and many died.

With the cat population drastically reduced, two species of rats, native to the forests and plantations, then invaded the villages. These rats were potential carriers of plague, typhus, and leptospirosis. Thus, while the villagers had gained protection from malaria, they were subsequently exposed to much more virulent pathogens. To redress this imbalance, surplus cats were transported from urban areas to the villages, some even being packed into special containers and parachuted into remote villages.

These examples demonstrate the reality of extensive ecological interconnections. Environmental transport mechanisms have distributed DDT all over the globe. DDT has been transformed into its breakdown products, DDD and DDE, which are even more dangerous than their precursor. All three forms are accumulated by biological organisms and concentrated as they progress upward in ecological food webs. The concentration of DDT in higher food organisms is commonly 30,000 times greater than the concentration dissolved in water at a given site. Biological populations are both variable in their response to given toxicants and quick to produce toxicant-resistant populations that negate the temporary inroads gained by human actions. Once introduced into the environment, DDT and other pesticides may persist for decades, contaminating and killing numerous nontarget organisms. Humans are not exempt from these processes and toxic chemicals that are released for very commendable reasons may return to haunt us for years to come. The pathways and interconnections are frequently unpredictable, even when the road is paved with good intentions.

Application: A Case Study

Now that we understand what pollutants are and how they reach humans, how can this information be used to solve community health problems? The following scenario is offered as an example of such problem solving. The pollution episode was real; the embellishments and details are fictitious.

The Problem

A graduate nurse has accepted a job with the Department of Public Health in Leadville. The town's primary industry and economic base is a small lead mine and smelter. During her first week on the job, the Director of Public Health informs our nurse that a local group of environmental activists has complained about the insidious, but undefined, health effects of the smelter operation and have demanded that it be closed. The devastating economic impact that such an action would precipitate has prompted the mayor and city council to exert pressure on the health department director. As the latest immigrant from academia, our community health nurse has been selected to design and implement an investigation of the health effects of the smelter. The director's final words to her are, "Do something, even if it is wrong!" Naturally, because this is not a budgeted item, the financial and staff support available to her are limited.

The First Goal

Our nurse decides that her first goal should be to determine if the lead smelter is affecting the health of the local residents. She knows nothing about lead as an environmental toxicant, but she has been trained well in problem solving so she forges ahead with confidence.

Available Information

Our nurse begins by researching the health effects of lead in the environment and the environmental impacts of lead smelter operations. She learns that lead is ubiquitous in nature, being a natural constituent of the earth's crust. Since lead is an element, it cannot be destroyed and may be expected to persist indefinitely in the environment in some form. Current production of lead in the United States is 1.3 million tons per year, of which 50% is used in batteries, 20% in antiknock compounds for gasoline, and 6% in pigments and ceramics.

Lead's primary routes into the human body are ingestion of food and water, and inhalation of atmospheric particles. Rocks and soils usually contain 10 μg to 30 μg of lead per gram of material. Natural groundwaters have 1 μg to 10 μg of lead per liter of water, considerably below the safe drinking water standard of 50 μg per liter. There does not appear to be any biomagnification of lead during the movement of nutrients from soil to groundwater to organic matter in plants. There exists a definite, positive correlation between the concentration of lead in drinking water and the concentration of lead in the blood of humans drinking the water. The amount of lead that will dissolve in water is dependent upon both hardness and *p*H. More lead will dissolve in soft water than in hard water, which contains more dissolved mineral salts. Only 1 μg of lead will dissolve in a liter of moderately alkaline water at *p*H 9, but 10,000 μg of lead will dissolve in a liter of moderately acid water at *p*H 5.5. Seawater contains only 0.03 μg of lead per liter of water, but freshwater ecosystems average 23 μg per liter (ranging from 2 μg to 140 μg).

The toxicity of lead to aquatic animals is affected by the season of the year, water temperature and chemistry, animal size, and length of exposure. Chronic effects can be detected at 7.6 μg per liter, and acute effects at 450 μg per liter. While algae may concentrate lead as much as 31,000 times above ambient water concentrations, there is no evidence of biomagnification in the food chain from aquatic vegetation to fish and shellfish. Fish do not constitute an unusually significant source of lead in the human diet. Bacteria have been reported to convert inorganic lead to organic forms.

Armed with this basic information, our community health nurse can identify and evaluate the ecological mechanisms that may affect lead accumulation by humans. She understands that lead is an ubiquitous but minor component in *biogeochemical cycles,* but these appear to exert only a slight influence upon human lead accumulation. Its ubiquity does create problems in designing epidemiological studies and interpretation of data. In regard to *food chains,* lead adhering to the exterior surfaces of food items is perhaps of more significance than lead contained within the food. Leafy vegetables with extensive surface area would be particularly important in this respect. The transfer of lead between trophic levels does not appear to be significant. Lead is not *biodegradable.*

In regard to environmental *transport,* lead is extremely mobile along both atmospheric and hydrologic pathways and virtually all human lead consumption is the direct result of such movement. Certain bacteria are able to *transform* inorganic lead to organic forms. Lead is also altered photochemically. Neither action is likely to contribute significantly to human accumulation or toxicity. Lead is readily *accumulated* into virtually all living organisms. There is little evidence of increasing *biomagnification* at higher trophic levels. The solubility of lead in water is significantly affected by the *p*H and hardness of the water, so *synergistic* effects are important. The status of essential nutrients such as calcium, iron, phosphorus, fat, and protein affects the extent of gastrointestinal absorption of ingested lead. Pregnant women have increased risk of iron and calcium deficiency and physiological stress, which may lead to a higher risk at a given lead exposure. There is no available information on the *assimilative capacity* of natural ecosystems for lead.

Having now learned more than she ever wanted to know about lead in the environment, our community health nurse queries the appropriate offices of the Environmental Protection Agency (EPA) and the state health department. She learns that air emissions and water effluent from the smelter and mine are continuously monitored and that the lead concentrations of each are below the prescribed federal and state guidelines. The community drinking water is also sampled regularly and always found to contain less than the 50 μg of lead per liter of water permitted. Both agencies report that the smelter has recently upgraded its pollution control devices and that company officials are conscientious in their control efforts. The local health office has received no reports of lead intoxication from the local hospital or private physicians. Thus, on the basis of existing information, there is no indication of a community health problem.

> DECISION POINT: Our health professional realizes that her efforts thus far have only addressed the possibility of *acute* lead *toxicity* in her community. She determines that her next step should be to search for *chronic effects* by means of a limited screening program. This creates several questions. How can she select a target population? How can she reach them? Can she use any existing programs as an avenue of contact?

A *special risk* population is one exhibiting characteristics associated with significantly higher probability of developing a condition, illness, or other abnormal status due to exposure to a given toxic agent. Two such populations are definable for lead; pre-school children and pregnant women. Our nurse's health department already has two programs that can provide ready access to these populations; a Well-Child Clinic and Maternal–Infant Care. Thus, she has two alternatives at this point, but is also operating under certain constraints. The primary goal is still to determine if a health problem exists, so she would not want to begin to use her meager resources until the problem under study is more clearly defined.

Her literature survey identified the highest risk group to be children, age 1 to 6 years. These clients will be the most likely to exhibit the effects of lead toxicity. Pregnant women would require higher levels of lead before exhibiting toxic symptoms. The unborn fetus is perhaps the most susceptible to lead toxicity but also is the most difficult to assess. Infants show less effect than toddlers or preschoolers, perhaps due to their limited mobility and different diet. Thus, the preschool children participating in the Well-Child Care Program at the clinic should be the most rewarding group to investigate.

Survey Data

Our health worker learned from her literature survey that the amount of lead present in a blood sample is a good indication of body lead levels. She accepts 30 μg of lead per 100 ml of blood as her action level, in accordance with the U.S. Surgeon General's recommendation. This is the level at which a child is considered to be in potential danger of developing clinical lead poisoning. She arranges for the analysis of the blood samples and the cooperation of the clinic personnel who run the Well-Child Care Program in obtaining a capillary tube sample of blood from 100 children in their program.

Remembering that each datum of information collected costs additional money to process and analyze, what other information can our nurse justifiably collect with each blood sample? She limits her choices to just six pieces of information. The child's *name* to identify each sample. The child's *address* to determine the relationship of the residence to the smelter location and to aid in relocation of the client. The child's *age* because age is known to correlate to lead uptake and toxicity and it will be a general indicator of the child's activity pattern. The child's *sex* because the sex role of the child may influence lead uptake. The *pica history* of the child; pica is the mouthing of unusual items such as dirt and paint chips, both of which are potential routes of lead ingestion. The *occupation and worksite* of adult members of the household, in order to identify families associated with the smelter.

Survey Results

The collection and analysis of the 100 blood samples produced the following results. All 100 children had detectable levels of lead in their blood; 24 had more than 30 μg of lead per 100 ml of blood, and 10 had more than 80 μg of lead. All children with blood lead at a level greater than 30 μg had one or more household adults employed at the smelter, but not all children with household adults employed at the smelter had blood lead greater than 30 μg.

Action Taken

Having demonstrated that a *chronic* lead toxicity problem existed, the community health nurse notified the health director of the results. She also noted that blood lead levels of 60 μg or more dictated immediate chelating treatment and that levels of 80 μg or more should be accompanied by demonstrable metabolic toxicity. The health director mobilized an immediate treatment program for all children with blood lead levels greater than 60 μg and ordered continuation of the screening program and investigation of the route of lead uptake by the children.

The Second Goal

Our health professional now shifted her focus to determining the route of lead uptake by the affected children. She decided that a matched sample investigation would be most appropriate. She proceeded to match each family of an above-threshold (30 μg) child to a family with a below-threshold child of similar sex and age. She was able to obtain 20 matched pairs in this manner. Having selected the families for further investigation, she had to determine what samples and information to collect.

Second Survey Data

The nurse decided to obtain blood samples from: all of the children in the matched sample, to verify the original blood lead data; all of the involved siblings, to determine if other children in the families had elevated levels; and all household adults, for comparative purposes. Also collected were samples of tap water, house paint, yard soil, and house dust to assist in identifying the source of the lead uptake.

Second Survey Results

The blood levels of the children previously sampled were nearly identical to the original data, verifying the original analyses. The blood levels of siblings were strongly correlated with those of the children originally sampled. The fathers of all children with blood lead levels greater than 80 μg per 100 ml of blood also had blood levels above 80 μg and required chelation treatment. The mothers of all families had blood lead levels below 40 μg. No families inhabited houses with leaded paint. There was no difference in the lead content of yard soil between above-threshold and below-threshold families. Similarly, there was no difference in the lead content of the tap water. All families were serviced from the city water supply and all samples were below the 50 μg per liter limit.

Household dust lead concentrations from above-threshold families averaged 2600 μg of lead per gram of dust; from below-threshold families, 400 μg per gram, with less than a 2% probability that this significant difference was attributable to chance alone. The blood lead level of the children was strongly correlated with the level of lead in household dust. Geographic analysis revealed that all families resided nearly equidistant from the smelter, which was located eight miles from the town. Prevailing winds would transport emissions away from, rather than toward, residential areas. Smelter employees who were members of below-threshold families held administrative or clerical positions and were not directly involved with the smelting process. Smelter employees who were members of the above-threshold families were workmen directly involved with the smelting process.

Interpretation, Verification, and Remedy

Our community health nurse deduced from the second survey results that the origin of the lead affecting the children might be their fathers' workclothes. Subsequent investigation proved this to be the case. The workclothes were worn home and cleansed by the family. The solution to this problem was to provide showers and clothes lockers for the workmen at the plantsite. Workclothes were provided by the company and laundered in a special facility at the site. The homes were thoroughly cleansed and blood lead levels eventually were lowered to and maintained at normal values for that geographic locality. An unidentified health problem was discovered and corrected, without closing down the plant or causing severe economic disruption.

REFLECTIONS

Where does this knowledge of ecological processes leave us? As practitioners of community health, how does this information aid us?

First, be aware that the health of any population can be affected by its surrounding environment. Remember that pollutants can travel long distances undetected. Next, be skeptical of any claims of perfect disposal schemes for pollutants; they do not exist, for when pollutants are removed they must go some place. Water treatment systems usually precipitate pollutants to a bottom sludge. Eventually the sludge must be cleaned out. If it is burned, will the pollutants go back up the smokestack, only to settle into another watershed? If buried in a landfill, will they remain in place or seep into a groundwater reservoir, only to surface at your kitchen faucet? Everything has to go someplace, and it may be difficult to keep it there.

Finally, as a consumer or a public advocate, do not demand perfect disposal schemes. Demand honest and realistic estimates of the risk that invariably accompanies any plan, no matter how appealing. Beware of flowcharts that indicate perfect control of pollutants at all stages of the cycle. Remember that it is people who handle pollutants, and the *people factor* can overwhelm every other part of any plan. It is people who load, transport, and dispose of pollutants. It is people who operate and maintain pollution control systems. It is people who give illegal orders for "midnight dumping and roadside disposal." In some instances, particularly involving the ultimate disposal of nuclear wastes, we may be planning caretaking operations that exceed the realm of past human experience. Our oldest civilizations generally have not persisted for more than 5000 years, and individual nations typically survive for far shorter periods. Can we honestly listen to glib talk of storing radioactive materials that will require maintenance for 10,000 years or longer—and take such plans seriously?

SUGGESTED READINGS

Commoner B: The Closing Circle—Nature, Man and Technology. New York, Bantam
    Books, 1971
Council on Environmental Quality. Environmental Quality. The Annual Report of the
    Council on Environmental Quality, Executive Office of the President (issued an-
    nually since 1970). U.S. Government Printing Office, Washington, DC
Council on Environmental Quality: Environmental Trends. Washington DC, U.S. Gov-
    ernment Printing Office, 1981
Storer JH: The Web of Life. New York, The New American Library, 1953
U.S. Environmental Protection Agency: Quality Criteria for Water. Washington DC, U.S.
    Government Printing Office, 1976
U.S. General Services Administration: Code of Federal Regulations. Title 40—Protec-
    tion of the Environment; Part 50. National Primary and Secondary Ambient Air
    Quality Standards; Part 129. Toxic Pollutant Effluent Standards; Part 141. National
    Interim Primary Drinking Water Regulations; Part 143. National Secondary Drink-
    ing Water Regulations. 1983

5

The Use of Models
in Community
Health Nursing

OBJECTIVES

The use of models to guide nursing practice, education, and research has become an important tool for community health nurses. This chapter focuses on the use of a nursing model to guide practice. At the completion of this chapter you should be able to

- Define "model" and "nursing model"
- Describe the purposes of a nursing model
- Identify nursing models for community health
- Begin to use a nursing model in practice

INTRODUCTION

Although nursing models have been in existence since the beginnings of the nursing profession, it has been only quite recently that they have been explicitly applied to practice. Professional nursing practice is based on scientific knowledge. But boundaries are needed to define areas of concern, and a conceptual map of the nursing process is a necessary guide for action. A *model* provides us with both the map and the boundaries.

MODELS

A conceptual model is the synthesis of a set of concepts and the statements that integrate these concepts into a whole. A *nursing model* can be defined as a frame of reference, a way of looking at nursing, or an image of what nursing encompasses. A nursing model is a representation of nursing, not a reality. Other types of models that are used to represent realities are model airplanes, blueprints, chemical equations, and anatomic models.

A model with which nurses identified for many years was the medical model, that is, a disease-oriented, illness-focused approach to patients, with an emphasis on pathology. However, reliance on the medical model excludes health promotion and the holistic focus that is central to nursing. Additionally, important aspects of care, such as psychological, sociocultural, and spiritual areas, are not included in the medical model. Thus, to effectively administer health care to the whole person, a nursing model should encompass all aspects of health care needs and incorporate long-range goals and planning.

As a representation of reality, a model can take numerous forms. Because they *describe* nursing, all nursing models are narrative; that is, words are the symbols that are used by nurses to define how they view their practice. Two examples of nursing models in community health are the definitions created by the American Nurses' Association (ANA) (1980) and the American Public Health Association (APHA; 1980). A comparison of these models is included in Table 5-1.

Although all nursing models are described in words, many are clarified further through the use of diagrams or illustrations. The use of such images allows the model-builder to show relationships and linkages among the concepts in the model. Diagrams are an efficient and effective way of depicting nursing models. The diagram is often thought of as the model itself with accompanying text then seen as the elaboration or explanation of the model.

The method chosen to depict a nursing model reflects the model-builder's own philosophy and preference. No one method is accepted as the best way to present a model. There are, however, certain components that must be included in any model of nursing. Table 5-2 presents these essential elements.

There is general agreement that four *concepts* are central to the discipline of nursing: *person, environment, health,* and *nursing.* (Concepts are defined as general notions or ideas and are considered to be the building blocks of models.) How each of the four concepts is defined will both dictate the organization of the model and be illustrated in that model. For example, health may be defined on a continuum with wellness at one end and death at the other, as a dichotomy wherein one is seen as well or ill, as the outcome of numerous biopsychosocial and spiritual forces, or as the interaction of these biopsychosocial and spiritual forces. In the medical model health has been defined traditionally as the absence of disease. Figure 5-1 depicts four ways to view health and illustrates these definitions. Notice that the diagrams vary widely, reflecting the fundamental differences among these views of health.

What then are the uses of a model of nursing? Think for a moment of what a nursing model is to you—and how a model might be useful in your practice. Although you may not have formulated your own model of nursing, you have been greatly influenced in your education by the model or models upon which your nursing curriculum is based. Does your faculty subscribe to one particular nursing model? Perhaps you are already familiar with names such as Callista Roy, Dorothea Orem, and Imogene King. Each is considered a nursing theorist and each has developed a nursing model that has been used as a curriculum framework. Just as the choice of a model creates a basis for curriculum planning and decisions, a model can also provide a basis for practice.

What is nursing to you? If you can formulate an answer to that question, you have begun to describe your model of nursing. A nursing model serves the following purposes

- A "map" for the nursing process
  Gives direction for assessment (What do you assess?)
  Guides analysis
  Dictates nursing diagnoses
  Assists in planning
  Facilitates evaluation
- Provides a curriculum outline for education
- Represents a framework for research
- Provides a basis for development of theory

A model is nothing more—or less—than an articulation of nursing. A model not only describes what *is*, but also provides a framework for making decisions about what *could be*.

MODEL EXAMPLES

Two models of community health nursing, the ANA and the APHA models, were introduced earlier in this chapter. All models in existence, (there are hundreds, perhaps thousands) cannot be described in this chapter, but several

(*Text continues on page 148*)

TABLE 5-1.   TWO NARRATIVE MODELS OF COMMUNITY
             HEALTH/PUBLIC HEALTH NURSING

Dimension/Component Name	ANA, DCHN Conceptual Model: Community Health Nursing*	APHA, PHN Section Position Paper: Public Health Nursing†
Definition	Synthesis of nursing practice and public health practice	Synthesis of body of knowledge from the public health sciences and professional nursing theories
Focal system/client	Individuals, families, and groups as they contribute to the health of the population as a whole	A total community or population group: ■ Subgroups in the community that are at high risk of illness, disability, or death ■ Groups, families, individuals
Goal/Purpose	Promoting and preserving the health of populations Prevention of illness, promotion of health for those that are more well than unwell (emphasis on primary care) Holistic approach to care of individuals, families, groups	Improving the health of the community through primary prevention, health promotion; this is the foundation of PHN practice ■ By identifying groups at high risk of illness or disability and directing resources towards these groups ■ Through nursing intervention, working with others, and social action
Scope of practice/role in health care delivery	Distinguishing characteristic is primary care, with emphasis on prevention of illness, and health maintenance and promotion Two major modes of practice have evolved ■ Direct care of individuals, families, and groups ■ Care of the community population as client with consideration of problems as they affect the group, family, or individual	Strong PHN services congruent with the characteristics described is essential ■ Tax-supported agencies with legal mandate to protect health, including unmet population health care needs ■ Programs that serve only specific segments of the population Realistic adaptations are made in accordance with type of community health service provided

(*continued*)

TABLE 5-1. (*Continued*)

Dimension/Component Name	ANA, DCHN Conceptual Model: Community Health Nursing*	APHA, PHN Section Position Paper: Public Health Nursing†
Methods/process	Maximize strength of the individual Standards of community health nursing practice Direct care of individuals, families, and communities Collaboration with individual, family, and community during wellness and illness Consumer viewed as central to influences that facilitate high-level wellness	Identify high-risk groups and work with resources to help them Systematic process ■ Assessment ■ Planning ■ Implementation ■ Evaluation Consumer involvement essential Work with groups, families, and individuals yet function in multidisciplinary teams and programs Coordinate planning and programs Participation of public is basic to success
Settings	Principally primary care settings where clients live, work, play, and attend school	All community-based health programs (*e.g.,* those defined by setting, age groups, and health problems)
Educational preparation	Entry: Baccalaureate in nursing Specialist: Master's in CHN; functional component encompasses further specialization	Entry: Baccalaureate in nursing Specialist: Master's or doctoral preparation with advanced content in nursing theory and practice, and in public health sciences and practice

* American Nurses' Association, Division of Community Health Nursing

† American Public Health Association, Public Health Nursing Section

(Henry OM: Comparison of ANA conceptual model of community health nursing and APHA, PHN Section, position paper on public health nursing. Unpublished materials. Rockville, Maryland, Nursing Practice Branch, Division of Nursing, Bureau of Health Professions, Health Resources and Services Administration, 1981)

TABLE 5-2.   ESSENTIAL UNITS OF A NURSING MODEL

Essential Unit	Description of Unit
A goal of action	The mission or ideal goal of the profession expressed as the end product desired (a state, condition, or situation)
A descriptive term for the patient population	That concept that best isolates who or what is acted upon to achieve a goal, that is, those aspects of the person (as patient) or the organization or those aspects of their functioning towards which attention is to be directed; the target of action
The actor's role	A descriptive label that indicates the nature of the nurse's (the actor's) actions on patients
Source of difficulty	The origin of deviations from the desired state or condition
Intervention focus	The kind of problems found when deviations from the desired state occur; the kinds of disturbances in patients that are to be prevented or treated. Mode is the major means of preventing or treating such problems (the kinds of levers that can be used to change the course of events toward the desired end).
Consequences intended	Outcomes of action that are desired, stated in more abstract or broader terms than the mission or including significant corollaries of the intended outcomes. Unintended outcomes may follow and may or may not be desirable.

(Data from: Riehl JP, Roy C: Conceptual Models for Nursing Practice, 2nd ed, p 2. New York, Appleton-Century-Crofts, 1980) (from unpublished lecture notes of D. Johnson, UCLA, Fall, 1975)

key models will be discussed to provide an overview of the types currently in use. The last to be discussed, the Community-as-Client Model, was developed by the authors and provides the framework for the nursing process chapters that follow. The Bibliography List at the end of the chapter includes readings about each model.

Nightingale Model

Although Florence Nightingale did not show her model in a graphic image (as in Figure 5-2), presenting it in schematic form provides a fine example of the four central concepts and their relationship to each other. In this simple drawing health is seen as a function of the interaction between nursing, person, and the environment. Nursing contributes, directly or indirectly, to the person's ability to regain or maintain health through management of the person's environment. It is likely that this model is the first conceptual model of community health nursing. Nightingale described the focus of nursing activity

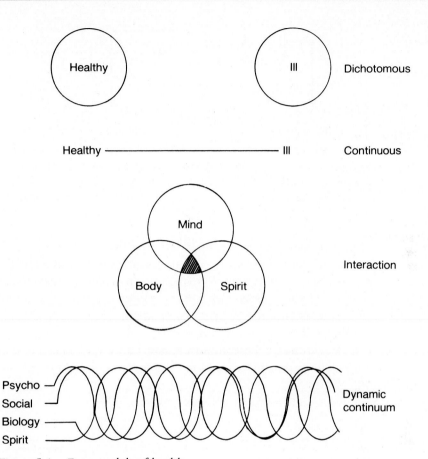

Figure 5-1. Four models of health.

as the proper use of fresh air, light, warmth, cleanliness, and the proper selection of and administration of diet. Consider for a moment how this translates to the community health nurse's concerns, for example, the problems of air pollution, crowding, housing, noise pollution, and nutritional adequacy.

Clark Model

The model developed by Clark (1982) permits the four key concepts of nursing to be viewed from several different levels (Fig. 5-3). At its core, as in Nightingale's model, is the nurse–patient interaction. It is important to understand that the four diagrams are different views of the same model. Note that the arrows illustrate that the relationship between nurse and patient is not

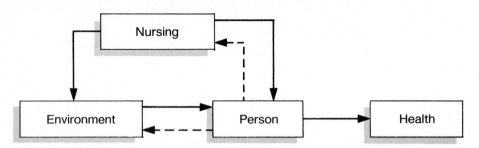

Figure 5-2. Nightingale's model of nursing. (Reed PG, Zurakowski T: Nightingale: A visionary model for nursing. In Fitzpatrick JJ, Whall AL (eds): Conceptual Models of Nursing: Analysis and Application, p 17. Bowie, Maryland, Robert J. Brady, 1983)

unidirectional; feedback is included. Clark's model stresses the reciprocity of the nurse–patient (or nurse–community) relationship as well as the significance of the environment. Note that the environment is shown as surrounding both nurse and patient and that arrows indicate that both are affected by and affect the environment. The stress on the importance of the environment highlights the need for the patient to be an informed and active participant in care. By extension, a community must be informed on health issues in order to participate in health promotion. The interaction also points to the need for

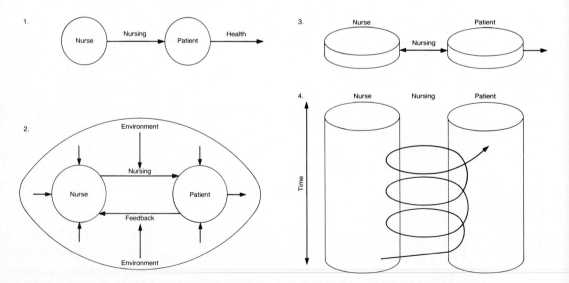

Figure 5-3. A simple model of nursing. (Clark, J: Development of models and theories of the concept of nursing. J Adv Nurs 7(2):129–134, 1982)

political activity by nurses to ensure that social and economic conditions are conducive to health.

Freeman Model

Ruth B. Freeman developed one of the earliest models of community health nursing (Figure 5-4). This model was used in early textbooks to depict areas of responsibility, process, and interaction in community health nursing. Note that although the major concepts are included in the diagram, today it seems incomplete as a model because the relationships among the elements are not

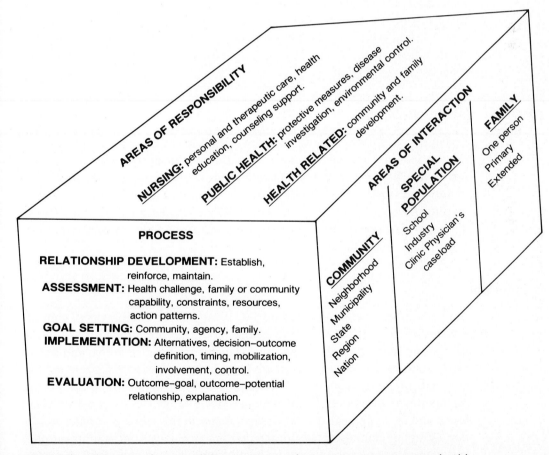

Figure 5-4. The areas of responsibility, process, and interaction in community health nursing. (Freeman RB: Community Health Nursing Practice, p 32. Philadelphia, WB Saunders, 1970)

explicated. However, many community health nursing models are derived from Freeman's work.

White Model

The PHN Conceptual Model, created by White, is based on the premise that community (public) health nursing is necessarily political in nature and that in order to be effective, public health nurses must be politically active (Fig. 5-5). The influence of Freeman can be seen in the use of a cube to depict the scope and priorities of practice.

The scope of practice in this model extends from the individual through aggregates, the community, and beyond. Note that the model is dynamic in that two *processes* can be viewed—the nursing process and the valuing process. Valuing is included in this model to recognize that people are guided by value judgments in all that they do. Think for a moment how your values are reflected in your actions.

Chavigny and Kroske Model

Chavigny and Kroske's model was developed in response to the question of how to measure the effectiveness of public health nursing. Its creators believed that before research on effectiveness could be done, they needed to define the practice. Their model (Figure 5-6) uses a familiar symbol of overlapping rings, a Venn diagram. The seven enclosed areas of the diagram correspond to seven basic concepts that were identified from analysis of several models and definitions.

Braden Model

Braden's conceptual model (Figure 5-7) illustrates the complexity of community health nursing. The outline of the model is formed from three major factors and their interrelationships: social system, practice arena, and behavioral repertory. Within each area are included process factors, structural factors, and interrelationships. For example, in the *practice* arena the *process factors* are organizational (management style), personal (style of performing a role), and interpersonal. The *structural factor* in this arena is conflict resolution (keeping community health nursing practice consistent with its purpose and with roles prescribed for it by health organizations, the ethics of professional discipline, and consumers).

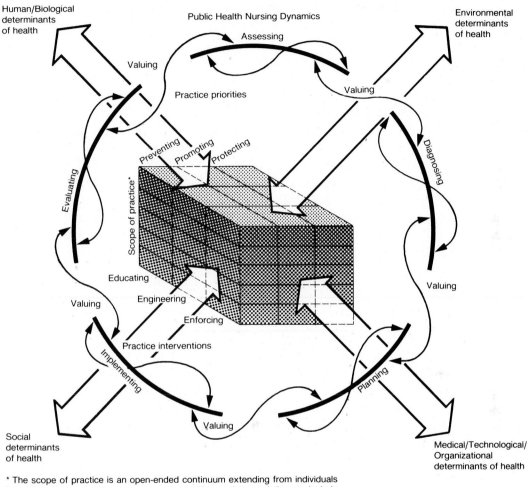

Human/Biological determinants of health

Public Health Nursing Dynamics

Assessing

Valuing

Practice priorities

Valuing

Environmental determinants of health

Preventing Promoting Protecting

Evaluating

Scope of practice*

Diagnosing

Valuing

Educating

Engineering

Enforcing

Valuing

Practice interventions

Implementing

Valuing

Planning

Social determinants of health

Medical/Technological/ Organizational determinants of health

* The scope of practice is an open-ended continuum extending from individuals through such aggregates as groups, communities, entire populations to include the entire globe.

Figure 5-5. A public health nursing conceptual model. (White MS: Construct for public health nursing. Nurs Outlook 30(9):527–530)

NOTE: The preceding models have been presented as illustrations and as the state-of-the-art information available in community health nursing. The descriptions are, of necessity, brief. It is hoped that you will go to the source (listed in the Suggested Readings) for a complete description of each.

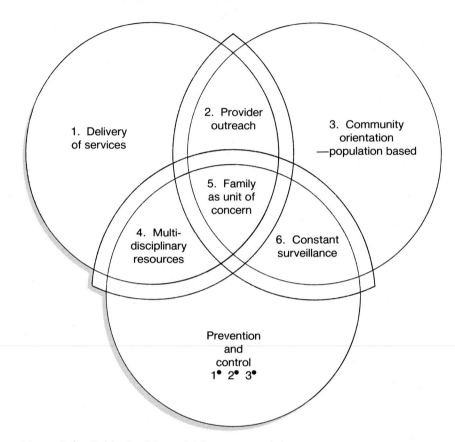

Figure 5-6.   Public health model for practice. (Chavigny KH, Kroske M: Public health nursing in crisis. Nursing Outlook 31(6):312–316)

Community-as-Client Model

Based on Betty Neuman's model (Figure 5-8), the Community-as-Client Model was developed to illustrate the definition of public health nursing that states it to be a synthesis of public health and nursing.

Recall the four central concepts for any nursing model: person, health, environment, and nursing. Each is defined in Table 5-3 to provide a foundation for the more specific description of the Community-as-Client Model.

Now consider the Community-as-Client Model (Figure 5-9). There are two central factors in this model: a focus on the *community* as client (represented by the Community Assessment Wheel at the top of the model) and the use of the *nursing process*. The model is described in some detail to assist you

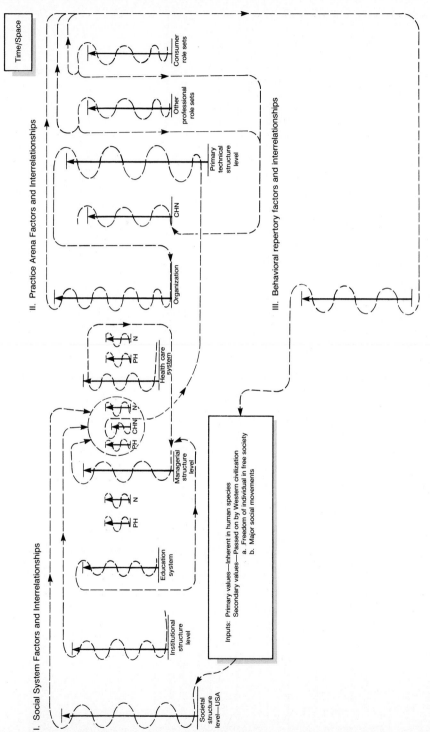

Figure 5-7. A conceptual model for community health nursing. (Braden CJ: The Focus and Limits of Community Health Nursing, p 398. Norwalk, Connecticut, Appleton–Century–Crofts)

155

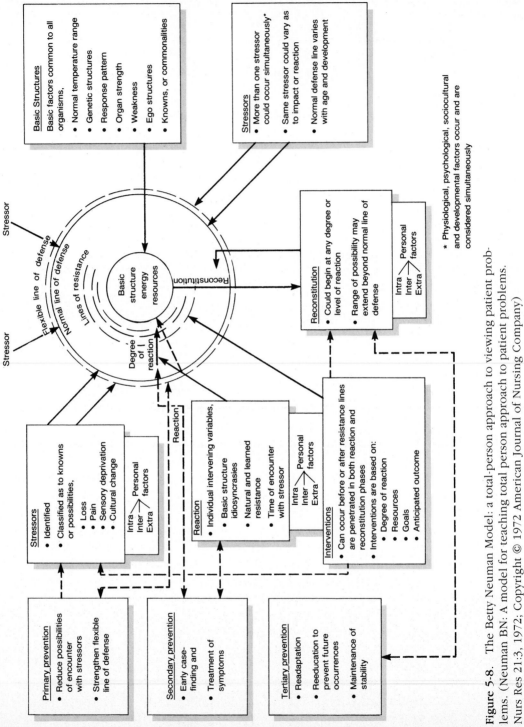

Figure 5-8. The Betty Neuman Model: a total-person approach to viewing patient problems. (Neuman BN: A model for teaching total person approach to patient problems. Nurs Res 21:3, 1972; Copyright © 1972 American Journal of Nursing Company)

TABLE 5-3. DEFINITIONS OF CONCEPTS CENTRAL
TO THE COMMUNITY-AS-CLIENT MODEL

Concepts	Definitions
Person	The community; all persons residing within a defined geopolitical boundary or sharing a common characteristic
Environment	All the conditions, circumstances, and influences surrounding and affecting the development of the community, which is, in and of itself, also a part of the environment
Health	Competence to function; a definable state of equilibrium in which subsystems are in harmony so that the whole can perform at its maximum potential
Nursing	A profession that brings a unique, holistic view to the community and contributes to the health of the community by participating in the community assessment; identifying and diagnosing problems amenable to nursing intervention; planning for the alleviation of community health problems; carrying out nursing interventions in conjunction with others; and evaluating the effect of those interventions on the health of the community

in understanding its parts. In subsequent chapters, the Community-as-Client Model will be applied to a real community.

The focus of the Community-as-Client Model is the community (presented in Figure 5-10 with assessment components highlighted). The *core* represents the *people* that make up the community. Included in the core are the *demographics* of the population as well as the *values, beliefs,* and *history* of the people. As residents of the community, these people are affected by and, in turn, influence the eight subsystems of the community. These subsystems are housing, education, fire and safety, politics and government, health, communication, economics, and recreation.

The solid line surrounding the community represents its *normal line of defense* or the level of health the community has reached over time. The normal line of defense may include characteristics such as a high rate of immunity, low infant mortality, or middle class income level. The normal line of defense includes the usual patterns of coping, along with the problem-solving capabilities: it represents the *health* of the community.

The *flexible line of defense,* depicted as a broken line around the community and its normal line of defense, is a "buffer zone" representing a dynamic level of health resulting from a temporary response to stressors. This temporary response may be a neighborhood mobilization against an environmental

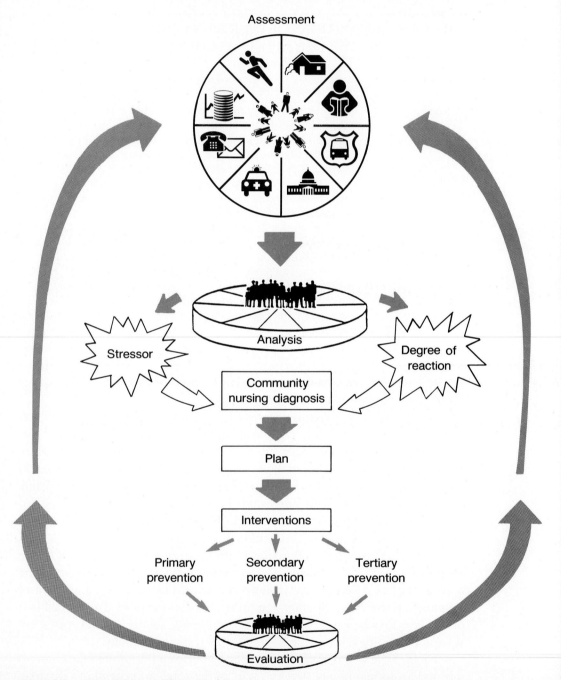

Figure 5-9.   Community-as-Client Model.

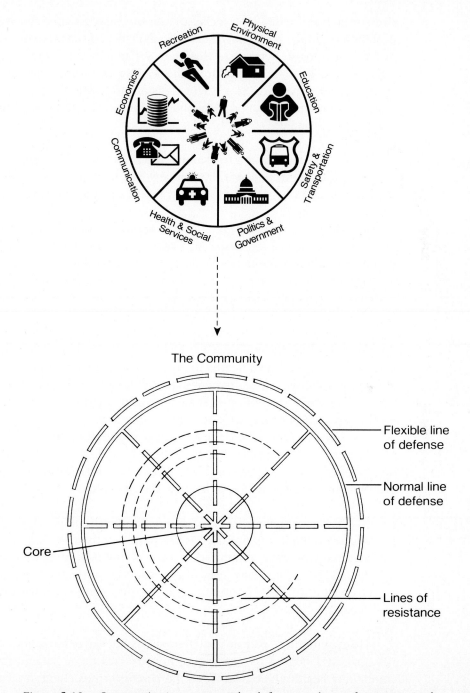

Figure 5-10. Community Assessment Wheel, featuring lines of resistance and defence within the community structure.

stressor such as flooding or a social stressor such as legislative activity aimed at prohibiting "adult" bookstores near schools. The eight subsystems are divided by broken lines to symbolize that they are not discrete and separate, but influence one another. (Recall from the reading on ecology that everything is connected to everything else.) This division both defines the major subsystems of a community and provides the community health nurse with a framework for assessment.

> NOTE: Take a moment to examine the selection of subsystems that have been identified. Can you think of any that have been omitted? Think of your community—what examples of each subsystem can you identify?

Within the community are *lines of resistance,* internal mechanisms that act to defend against stressors. An evening recreational program for youth implemented to decrease vandalism and a free-standing, no-fee health clinic to diagnose and treat sexually transmitted diseases are examples of lines of resistance. Lines of resistance exist throughout each of the subsystems and represent the community's *strengths.*

Stressors are tension-producing stimuli that have the potential of causing disequilibrium in the system. They may originate outside of the community (e.g., air pollution from a nearby industry) or inside the community (*e.g.,* the closing of a clinic). Stressors penetrate the flexible and normal lines of defense, resulting in disruption of the community. Inadequate, inaccessible, or unaffordable services are stressors for a community.

The *degree of reaction* is the amount of disequilibrium or disruption that results from stressors impinging upon the community's lines of defense. The degree of reaction may be reflected in mortality and morbidity rates, unemployment, or crime statistics, to name a few examples.

> NOTE: The outcome of a stressor impinging on a community is not always negative. Often it is positive. For example, in the face of a crisis people may band together, and may develop a community group to deal with the crisis. This group may continue to function after the crisis is over—strengthening the community and continuing to contribute to its "health."

The community's core and subsystems, its lines of defense and resistance, stressors, and degree of reaction comprise assessment parameters for the community health nurse who views the *community* as client. Analyzing data on these parameters leads to the *community nursing diagnosis*. Note the similarities and differences in a nursing diagnosis of an individual and a community nursing diagnosis in Table 5-4.

The community nursing diagnosis gives *direction* to both nursing's goals and interventions. The goal is derived from the stressors and may include the elimination or alleviation of the stressor or strengthening of the community's resistance through strengthening the lines of defense. By stating the degree of reaction, the nurse can plan interventions to strengthen the lines of resistance through one of the prevention modes.

Primary prevention is the nursing implementation that aims at strengthening the lines of defense so that stressors cannot penetrate to cause a reaction, or at interfering with a stressor by taking action against it. An example of primary prevention is the immunization of preschoolers to increase the per-

TABLE 5-4. NURSING DIAGNOSIS: COMPARISON OF INDIVIDUAL AND COMMUNITY FOCUS

Response	System/ Function	Source of Situation	Manifestation of Problem
Individual			
Patient behavior	Biopsychosocial–spiritual	Etiology	Symptoms from head-to-toe assessment
Example: Alteration in status	Oral integrity	Loose-fitting dentures	Oral pain; redness in mucosa; 10-cm open sore, etc.
Community			
Degree of reaction	Community subsystem	Stressor	Systems assessment (*e.g.,* rates)
Example: Increased	Respiratory disease	Air pollution	Increased hospital admissions for respiratory problems; higher rate of chronic obstructive pulmonary disease readmissions

centage of immunized youngsters in the community. *Secondary prevention* is applied after a stressor has penetrated the community. Nursing interventions support the lines of defense and resistance to minimize the degree of reaction to the stressor. Conducting a blood-pressure screening and referral program in an identified high-risk community is an example of secondary prevention. Such a program is aimed at early case finding to reduce the degree of reaction (*e.g.,* the incidence of strokes). *Tertiary prevention* is applied after the stressor penetration and a degree of reaction have occurred. There has been system disequilibrium, and tertiary prevention is aimed at preventing additional disequilibrium and at promoting equilibrium. For example, a school fire has occurred and a large number of children are suffering from shock (physical and psychological). Teams of specialists (including community health nurses) are brought in to provide appropriate therapies and long-term follow-up as needed to reestablish equilibrium in the community.

Feedback from the community provides the basis for evaluation of the community health nurse's interventions. Often the parameters that were used for assessment also are used for evaluation. For example, after the immunization program did the percentage of immunized preschoolers increase? How many persons with hypertension were identified and referred for medical care? What was the long-term effect of the school fire? Were the children re-assimilated into their classes? Were fire codes investigated? Were additional precautions (increased fire drills, replacement of flammable materials) instituted in the schools? Such is the process of working with the community as client. Interconnections, overlap, and interdisciplinary considerations must be the rule rather than the exception.

Consider the Community-as-Client Model (Figure 5-9) once more. The *goal* represented by the model is system equilibrium, a healthy community, and includes the preservation and promotion of community health. The model *target* or "patient" is the total community system, the aggregate, and as such includes individuals and families. The *actor's role* (*i.e.,* the nurse's role) is to help the community to attain, regain, maintain, and promote health. The nurse contributes to the regulation and control of system responses to stressors that are the source of difficulty. The *intervention focus* is the actual or potential disequilibrium or an inability of the community to function. The *intervention mode* is comprised of the three levels of prevention: primary, secondary, and tertiary. The *consequences intended* in this model include a strengthened normal line of defense, an increased resistance to stressors, and a diminished degree of reaction to stressors in the community. A summary of this analysis is provided in Table 5-5.

TABLE 5-5.   COMMUNITY-AS-CLIENT MODEL:
APPLICATION OF ESSENTIAL UNITS
OF A NURSING MODEL

Essential Unit	Community-as-Client Model
Goal	System equilibrium
Target	Total community system
Actor's role	Assist to attain, regain, maintain, and promote health
Source of difficulty	Stressors
Intervention focus	Inability of community to function
Intervention mode	Prevention (primary, secondary, and tertiary levels)
Consequences intended	Strengthen normal line of defense: increase resistance to stressors, decrease degree of reaction

RELATIONSHIP OF MODEL TO THEORY

The primary emphasis in this chapter has been placed on the use of a conceptual model in community health nursing practice. Model development comprises the identification of key concepts, and their placement in a logical order with clear definitions and defined relationships.

Besides meeting criteria of clarity and logic, a model must possess social congruence, social significance, and social utility. That is, the following questions must each receive a positive response in order for the model to be considered successful: Is this what society expects of nursing (congruent with society's expectations)? Does nursing action based on the model make a difference to society? And is this model of value to the profession?

The creation of models is just one step in the process of developing theories for nursing. Until relationships and assumptions of the model are tested through research, there will be no theories to explain or predict nursing practice. Models describe what *is,* while theories may explain why it exists. Models cannot be tested through research—they are too broad and all-encompassing; but theories, which are much more specific, can be tested through research.

NOTE: Think of theories with which you are already familiar, for instance, theories of human behavior from psychology. An example is the stimulus–response theory of the behaviorists. One theory says that if a stimulus is followed by a certain response and the person is rewarded for that response, the behavior will tend to occur again given the same stimulus. Note that with this theory, it is possible to predict and explain behavior.

As you read the next chapters, which illustrate the community-as-client model, and as you practice in community health nursing, consider how a conceptual model guides you in applying the nursing process. When using a defined model for practice you have direction for assessment, guidance in analysis, and assistance in planning and evaluation.

BIBLIOGRAPHY

Adam E: Frontiers of nursing in the 21st Century: Development of models and theories on the concept of nursing. J Adv Nurs 8(1):41–45, 1983

American Nurses' Association: A Conceptual Model of Community Health Nursing. Kansas City, American Nurses Association, 1980

American Public Health Association: The Definition and Role of Public Health Nursing in the Delivery of Health Care (A statement of the Public Health Nursing Section). Washington DC, American Public Health Association, 1980

Braden CJ: The Focus and Limits of Community Health Nursing. East Norwalk, Connecticut, Appleton-Century-Crofts, 1984

Chavigny KH, Kroske M: (1983). Public health nursing in crisis. Nurs Outlook 31(6):312–316, 1983

Clark J: Development of models and theories on the concept of nursing. J Adv Nurs 7(2):129–134, 1982

Clemen SA, Eigsti DG, McGuire SL: Comprehensive Family and Community Health Nursing. New York, McGraw-Hill, 1981

Freeman RB: Community Health Nursing Practice. WB Saunders, Philadelphia, 1970

Henry OM: Comparison of ANA conceptual model of community health nursing and APHA, PHN Section, position paper on public health nursing. Unpublished materials. Rockville, Maryland, Nursing Practice Branch, Division of Nursing, Bureau of Health Professions, Health Resources and Services Administration, 1981

Neuman B: The Neuman Systems Model: Application to nursing education and practice. East Norwalk, Connecticut, Appleton-Century-Crofts, 1982

Pesznecker B, Draye MA, McNeil J: Collaborative practice models in community health nursing. Nurs Outlook 30(5):298–302, 1982

Reed PG, Zurakowski TL: (1983). Nightingale: A visionary model for nursing. In Fitzpatrick JJ, Whall AL (eds): Conceptual Models of Nursing: Analysis and Application. Bowie, Maryland, Robert J. Brady, 1983

Reilly DE: Why a conceptual framework? Nurs Outlook 23(8):566–569, 1975

Riehl JP, Roy C: Conceptual Models for Nursing Practice, 2nd ed. New York, Appleton-Century-Crofts, 1980

Torres G: Florence Nightingale. In Nursing Theories Conference Group: Nursing Theories: The Base for Professional Nursing Practice. Englewood Cliffs, New Jersey, Prentice-Hall, 1980

White MS: Construct for public health nursing. Nurs Outlook 30(9):527–530, 1982

PART II

Application of Concepts
and Theory
to Community Health Nursing

6
Assessment

OBJECTIVES

Preceding chapters have focused on concepts such as health, epidemiology, and ecology; therefore, objectives for those chapters dealt with evaluating your understanding of the concepts. This chapter and the following four chapters focus on the application of the nursing process, and specifically on how the process relates to community health nursing. Consequently, the objectives are practice oriented. The objective for this chapter is

- After studying the text, you will be able to complete a community health assessment

INTRODUCTION

Assessment is the act of becoming acquainted with a community. To direct the assessment process the systems model developed in Chapter Five is used (see Figure 5-9). Recall that a system is a whole that functions because of the interdependence of its parts. A community, too, is a whole entity that functions because of the interdependence of its parts, or *subsystems*. The Community Assessment Wheel (Figure 6-1) identifies eight community subsystems and a community core. To illustrate the process of assessment, a community, Rosemont, was chosen at random and then the systems model has been used to

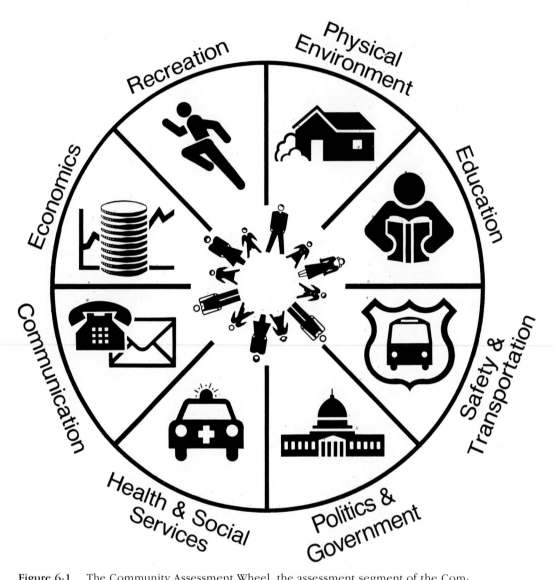

Figure 6-1. The Community Assessment Wheel, the assessment segment of the Community-as-Client Model.

direct and guide an assessment of it. Although we have chosen an urban community defined by census tracts (CT), the assessment wheel can be used to assess any community regardless of size, location, resources, or population characteristics, and can also be used to assess a "community within a community" (for example, a specific school, industry, or business). The process of assessment always remains the same.

COMMUNITY ASSESSMENT

Looking to our Community Assessment Wheel for guidance, eight subsystems surround the community core; therefore we will first assess the community core, then proceed to assess each subsystem. To facilitate the work of data collection, a "guide table" has been presented with each subsystem. Some information on these tables may not be available in your community, may not apply, or may be redundant; Other information, omitted from the areas suggested in the tables, you may decide to include for your community. This is to be expected, for every community is a unique and special entity. It is this uniqueness that we seek to record.

> NOTE: It may be that in your community health nursing course, time limitations will not permit each student to complete an entire community assessment. Therefore, teams of students may be assigned to assess one or two community subsystems. At the end of the course each team will present its assessment and the total community assessment is complete. A similar situation frequently arises in agencies when health providers, who are frequently from a variety of disciplines, are assigned one aspect (one subsystem) of a community to assess; later all the subsystems are assembled and the assessment is complete.

Assessment is a skill that is refined through practice. Everyone feels awkward and unsure as they begin—this is normal. The first step is always the most difficult. It is time to take the first step.

COMMUNITY CORE

The definition of *core* is "that which is essential, basic, and enduring." The core of a community is its people—their history, characteristics, values, and beliefs. The first stage of community assessment is to learn about its people. Table 6-1 is a guide that lists the major components of the community core

TABLE 6-1.   COMMUNITY CORE DATA

Components	Sources of Information
History	Library, Historical Society
Demographics	Census of Population and Housing
Age and sex	Planning Board (local, city, county, state)
characteristics	Chamber of Commerce
Racial distribution	City Hall, City Secretary Archives
Ethnic distribution	
Household types by:	
Family	
Nonfamily	
Group	
Marital status by:	
Single	
Separated	
Widowed	
Divorces	
Vital statistics	State Department of Health (Information
Births	distributed through city and county
Deaths by:	health department)
Age	
Leading causes	
Values/beliefs/religion	Personal Contact
	Windshield Survey (To protect against
	stereotyping, avoid the library for this
	portion of the assessment)

along with locations and sources of information about each component. Because every community is different, information sources available to one community may not be available to another. The text that follows presents core information about Rosemont.

The History of Rosemont

Rosemont includes CT 402 and CT 403. The Rosemont property was originally deeded to a Miss Ima Smith, who received a land grant of 3370 acres in 1827. For almost 100 years the area remained as prairie, dotted with cattle ranches and small farms. In 1920 John Walker and William Bell formed a land corporation and began developing the Smith property. The first area that was improved and deed restricted was named Rosemont after a legendary town in

Scotland. Following development, Rosemont prospered and attracted new-comers to the area. Numerous prominent families made their homes in Rosemont, including a state governor, a Nobel Laureate, and a soon-to-be president of the United States. However, during the economic depression of the 1930s, and the years before and during World War II, a drastic decrease in building activities occurred. Many stately homes deteriorated and either became multi-family dwellings or were left to decay. Eventually economic forces succeeded in breaking deed restrictions and residential areas were forced to accept the introduction of industry and small businesses. As a result, property values plummeted, leaving quaint boutiques and antique shops to exist alongside an increasing number of night clubs and nude-modeling studios.

From 1950 to 1970 Rosemont witnessed the influx of a large population of young adults, commonly referred to as "hippies," who used the large spacious homes for group living. This practice was also taken up by drug addicts and runaways. Rosemont gradually assumed the reputation of tolerating nontraditional lifestyles—a factor that precipitated the more recent influx of a large population of male homosexuals.

Because of lower property values and affordable rent during the mid to late 1970s, large groups of Vietnamese and Mexicans settled in Rosemont. Simultaneously, a trend began that still continues today of established families and single professionals, weary of the lengthy commute from suburbia to the inner city, returning to Rosemont. Today, older homes are being refurbished, businesses revitalized and pride, once lost, is being reclaimed.

Demographics— The People of Rosemont

Tables 6-2 and 6-3 set forth age, sex, race, and ethnicity data for CT 402 and CT 403, as well as for the nearest city and county. (The census lists only numbers of persons; you must calculate percentages.) Tables 6-4 and 6-5 list data on family types and marital status.

NOTE: During the next step of the nursing process (*i.e.*, analysis) you will need city and county population data; therefore, collect all needed data now.

Vital Statistics

Table 6-6 lists birth and death vital statistics for CT 402 and CT 403, as well as the city and county. Using a similar format, Table 6-7 lists the leading causes of death.

TABLE 6-2.   POPULATION AGE AND SEX
             CHARACTERISTICS FOR CT 402, CT 403,
             HAMPTON, AND JEFFERSON COUNTY

Age (Years)	CT 402			CT 403			Hampton		Jefferson County	
	Males	Females	Total %	Males	Females	Total %	Number	Total %	Number	Total %
Under 5 yr	370	362	10.6	29	11	0.6	123,150	7.8	189,246	8.4
5–19	1200	991	31.9	241	195	6.5	377,345	23.9	569,991	25.3
30–34	395	437	12.2	1965	911	42.6	514,705	32.6	716,431	31.8
35–54	837	970	26.2	1758	721	36.7	339,453	21.5	484,380	21.5
55–64	222	370	8.6	221	181	5.9	116,835	7.4	157,705	7
65 and over	270	450	10.5	175	349	7.7	107,361	6.8	135,176	6
Total	3294	3580	100	4389	2368	100	1,578,849	100	2,252,929	100

(Data from 1980 Census of Population and Housing, Selected Characteristics.)

TABLE 6-3.   POPULATION RACE AND ETHNIC
             DISTRIBUTION FOR CT 402,
             CT 403, CITY OF HAMPTON,
             AND JEFFERSON COUNTY*

	CT 402		CT 403		Hampton		Jefferson County	
	Number	Total %	Number	Total %	Number	Total %	Number	Total %
White	852	12.4	5871	88.5	970,489	61.5	1,562,091	69.4
Black	3732	54.3	305	4.6	434,014	27.5	467,177	20.7
Asian/Pacific Islander	1312	19.1	54	0.7	32,335	2.1	45,432	2
Hispanic	625	9.1	321	4.7	131,763	8.3	163,774	7.3
American Indian	242	3.5	38	0.6	3203	0.2	4923	0.2
Other	111	1.6	58	0.9	7045	0.4	9532	0.4
Total	6874	100	6757	100	1,578,849	100	2,252,929	100

* Refer to Chapter Two for explanation of racial classification and changes with 1980 Census.
(Data from 1980 Census of Population and Housing, Selected Characteristics.)

TABLE 6-4.   POPULATION BY FAMILY TYPES, CT 402 and CT 403

	CT 402		CT 403	
	Number	Total %	Number	Total %
Family	5706	83	2443	36.2
Nonfamily	1168	17	4103	60.7
Female-headed household	721		994	
Male-headed household	447		2189	
Group quarters			211	3.1
Total	6874	100	6757	100

(Data from 1980 Census of Population and Housing, Selected Characteristics.)

Values, Beliefs, and Religion

Part of the community core is the values, beliefs, and religious practices of the people. All ethnic and racial groups have values and beliefs that interact with each community system to influence the people's health.

To validate the demographic data, a windshield survey (Table 6-8) is

TABLE 6-5.   PERSONS 15 AND OVER BY SEX AND MARITAL STATUS, CT 402 AND CT 403

Marital Status	CT 402			CT 403		
	Male	Female	Total %	Male	Female	Total %
Single	348	408	15.2	2418	1016	53.5
Married	1510	1498	60.1	796	768	24.4
Separated	120	245	7.2	113	72	2.8
Widowed	52	119	3.4	68	198	4.3
Divorced	294	407	14.1	572	397	15
Total	2324	2677	100	3967	2451	100

(Data from 1980 Census of Population and Housing, Selected Characteristics.)

TABLE 6-6. SELECTED BIRTH AND DEATH VITAL
STATISTICS FOR CT 402, CT 403,
HAMPTON, AND JEFFERSON COUNTY

	CT 402	CT 403	Hampton	Jefferson County
Births	210	117	30,726	56,865
Deaths				
Infant Deaths	7	2	372	698
Neonatal Deaths	5	2	245	471
Fetal Deaths	16	1	387	870
Total Deaths	72	42	9,533	16,440

(Data from State Vital Statistics, 1984. Department of Health.)

needed to establish the presence and geographic location of different racial and ethnic groups. It is during this phase—assessment of the physical system —that we step into the community to learn and experience the values, beliefs, and religious practices of the community.

Notice that Table 6-1 cautions against the use of the library for information about values, beliefs, and religious practices—the reason is that books and articles frequently offer broad generalizations to describe the practices of ethnic and racial groups (*e.g.,* the lifestyles of urban blacks) or discuss one practice of one ethnic group (*e.g.,* breast-feeding practices of Mexican-born hispanics). Each community is unique with values, beliefs, and religious practices that are rooted in tradition and continue to evolve and exist because they meet the community's needs.

PHYSICAL ENVIRONMENT

Just as the physical examination is a critical component of assessing an individual patient, so it is in the assessment of a community. And just as the five senses of the clinician are called into play in the physical exam of a patient, so, too, in the community. Table 6-9 provides the components of the physical

TABLE 6-7. DEATHS BY SELECTED CAUSES
FOR CT 402, CT 403, HAMPTON,
AND JEFFERSON COUNTY

Cause of Death	CT 402		CT 403		Hampton		Jefferson County	
	Number	*Total %*	*Number*	*Total %*	*Number*	*Total %*	*Number*	*Total %*
Heart disease	16	22.2	10	23.8	3186	33.4	5932	36
Malignant neoplasms	17	23.6	11	26.1	2078	21.8	3972	24.2
Cerebrovascular	6	8.3	2	4.7	690	7.3	1213	7.4
Accidents	4	5.6	4	9.5	585	6.2	932	5.7
Emphysema, asthma, bronchitis	0	0	0	0	79	0.8	115	0.7
Diseases of early infancy	7	9.7	1	2.4	248	2.6	501	3
Homicides	6	8.3	1	2.4	592	6.2	831	5.1
Cirrhosis of liver	0	0	1	2.4	163	1.7	253	1.5
Pneumonia	2	2.8	1	2.4	210	2.2	365	2.2
Suicides	3	4.2	1	2.4	195	2	234	1.4
Diabetes mellitus	0	0	2	4.8	139	1.4	305	1.8
Congenital anomalies	0	0	2	4.8	99	1	245	1.5
Nephritis and nephrosis	0	0	0	0	13	0.1	26	0.2
Tuberculosis	1	1.4	0	0	17	0.2	28	0.2
All other causes	10	13.9	6	14.3	1239	13	1488	9.1
Total deaths, all causes	72	100	42	100	9533	100	16,440	100

(Data from Hampton Vital Statistics, City of Hampton Health Department.)

examination, both of an individual and a community, and compares tools and sources of data for each.

Our client, the Rosemont community, is located within the city of Hampton and is in Hampton's central business district. It is bounded by Way Drive on the west, Buff's Bayou on the north, Live Oak Boulevard on the south, and

(*Text continues on page 180*)

TABLE 6-8. WINDSHIELD SURVEY COMPONENTS

Element	Description
Housing and zoning	What is the age of the houses, their architecture, of what materials are they constructed? Are all the neighborhood houses similar in age, architecture? How would you characterize the differences? Are they detached from or connected to others? Do they have space in front and behind? What is their general condition? Are there signs of disrepair—broken doors, windows, leaks, locks missing? Is there central heating, modern plumbing, air conditioning?
Open space	How much open space is there? What is the quality of the space—green parks or rubble-filled lots? What is the lot size of the houses? Lawns? Flower boxes? Do you see trees on the pavements, a green island in the center of the street? Is the open space public or private? Used by whom?
Boundaries	What signs are there of where this neighborhood begins and ends? Are the boundaries natural—a river, a different terrain? physical—a highway, railroad? economic—difference, in real estate, or presence of industrial, commercial units along with residential? The neighborhood has an identity, a name? Do you see it displayed? Are there unofficial names?
"Commons"	What are the neighborhood hangouts? For what groups, at what hours? (*e.g.,* schoolyard, candy store, bar, restaurant, park, 24-hour drugstore?) Does the "commons" have a sense of "territoriality" or is it open to the stranger?
Transportation	How do people get in and out of the neighborhood? Car, bus, bike, walk, etc.? Are the streets and roads conducive to good transportation and also to community life? Is there a major highway near the neighborhood? Whom does it serve? How frequent is public transportation available?
Service centers	Do you see social agencies, clinics, recreation centers, signs of activity at the schools? Are there offices of doctors, dentists? Palmists, spiritualists, etc? Parks? Are they in use?
Stores	Where do residents shop? Shopping centers, neighborhood stores? How do they travel to shop?
Street people	If you are traveling during the day, who do you see on the street? An occasional housewife, a mother with a baby? Do you see anyone you would not expect? Teenagers, unemployed males? Can you spot a welfare worker, an insurance collector, a door-to-door salesman? Is the dress of those you see representative or unexpected? Along with people, what animals do you see? Stray cats, dogs, pedigreed pets, "watchdogs?"
Signs of decay	Is this neighborhood on the way up or down? Is it "alive?" How would you decide? Trash, abandoned cars, political posters, neighborhood meeting posters, real estate signs, abandoned houses, mixed zoning usage?
Race	Are the residents white, black, or is the area integrated?
Ethnicity	Are there indices of ethnicity—food stores, churches, private schools, information in a language other than English?

(*continued*)

TABLE 6-8.   (*Continued*)

Element	Description
Religion	Of what religion are the residents? Do you see evidence of heterogeneity or homogeneity? What denomination are the churches? Do you see evidence of their use other than on Sunday mornings?
Health and morbidity	Do you see evidence of acute or of chronic diseases or conditions? Of accidents, communicable diseases, alcoholism, drug addiction, mental illness, etc.? How far is it to the nearest hospital? Clinic?
Politics	Do you see any political campaign posters? Is there a present headquarters? Do you see any evidence of a predominant party affiliation?
Media	Do you see outdoor TV antennas? What magazines, newspapers do residents read? Do you see *Forward Times, Hampton Post, Enquirer, Readers' Digest* in the stores? What media seem most important to the residents? Radio, TV?

(Adapted from Terry Mizrahi Madison: School of Social Work, Virginia Commonwealth University.)

TABLE 6-9.   **PHYSICAL EXAMINATION COMPONENTS AND SOURCES OF DATA**

Components	Sources of Data	
	Individual	*Community*
Inspection	All senses	All senses
	Otoscope	"Windshield survey"
	Ophthalmoscope	Walk through community
Auscultation	Stethoscope	Listen to Community sounds/residents
Vital signs	Thermometer	Observe climate, terrain, natural boundaries
	Sphygmomanometer	and resources
		"Life" signs such as notices of community meetings; density
Systems review	Head-to-toe	Observe social systems, including housing, businesses, churches, hangouts
Laboratory studies	Blood tests	Almanac; census data
	Xrays	Chamber of Commerce planning studies,
	Scans, other tests	surveys

Hampton Street on the east. Figure 6-2 is a map of the Rosemont community. Using the "windshield survey," (see Table 6-8) as a guide, we step into the community.

Inspection

Rosemont Boulevard bisects the community and serves as a major north–south thoroughfare for residents traveling to or through the community. It is tree-lined and divided by a grassy median in sections. Many businesses, especially restaurants, are located along Rosemont Boulevard. Many of the restaurants

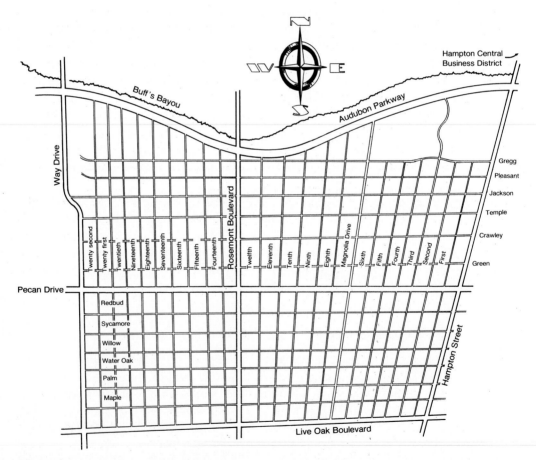

Figure 6-2. Rosemont Community.

are of the "specialty" type that serve quiche, sprout sandwiches, and herbal teas. Other businesses situated along the boulevard are gas stations, office buildings, art-supply stores, a veterinarian, small art galleries, a nursery, one Mexican *barbacoa* stand in a grocery store, florists, a bank, a pharmacy, and various shops specializing in leather goods, books, and handcrafted items. (See the Economics section of this chapter for a summary of business units.)

The major east–west thoroughfare through Rosemont, Pecan Drive, is also lined with businesses and, with fewer trees, presents a more urban face. At the east end can be seen nude modeling studios, small restaurants specializing in various ethnic foods (Greek, Pakistani, Mexican, Vietnamese, Indian, to name a few) and numerous small art shops. The Rosemont Health Center, which is discussed later in this chapter, is located in this area. Further west on this street is a large theater that attracts many "first run" productions. There are a couple of "adult" movie houses and the ubiquitous specialty restaurants (in this section they are of the type that caters to the business or professional crowds—quiet tea rooms that play classical music). Along this street, too, are many large old houses, homes that have been converted into antique shops, flower shops and other small stores. There is no large industry in Rosemont.

Behind the two-business-filled thoroughfares that divide the community, Rosemont can give one the feeling of having entered a different world. The streets are narrower, some are cobbled; old oaks and pecan trees are abundant and, in many areas, the branches of the trees meet over the streets to form protective canopies of green.

The streets (except the thoroughfares) are narrow and most have sidewalks, as is typical of older neighborhoods in Hampton. In general, the streets and sidewalks are in good repair and free from debris; however, because there is little off-street parking, many residents park on the streets, so there is traffic congestion at the times when most residents are home (primarily nights and weekends).

Vital Signs

The climate of Rosemont (and the Hampton Standard Metropolitan Statistical Area [SMSA]) is mild and, according to the Chamber of Commerce (1983), is "moderated by winds from the sea." Summers are hot (the temperature is 90°F or higher, approximately 87 days a year) and humid (averaging 62%), but evenings are cool and there is rarely a hard freeze in the winter. Flora that seem both temperate and tropical abound—live oaks, hibiscus, and pines may grow in one block, for example.

The terrain is generally flat with little variation in grade. It is 20 feet above sea level. The only naturally occurring water in the area is Buff's Bayou, a concrete-lined "river" that serves to carry off excess rain and drainage to reduce chances of flooding in Hampton. The bayou ends in the Hampton Channel that leads to the sea.

Rosemont is the third most densely populated area in Hampton with 14.4 persons per acre. An area in CT 402 that contains the subsidized housing complex is the most densely populated in all of Hampton with 221 persons per acre (1980 Census).

The variety of local stores reflect the diversity of interests in Rosemont. Posters advertising a meeting of the "Gay Political Caucus" share bulletin-board space with senior citizen's meetings, church announcements, educational programs at the community college's "Sunday School," Vietnamese relocation services, the community's "STD Clinic" (specializing in sexually transmitted diseases [STD]) and a musical show by "El Barrio" from the Mexican-American area. Rosemont is a community of rich diversity, a microcosm of Hampton.

The churches of Rosemont also reflect its diversity—virtually all denominations are represented. From the large Methodist and Presbyterian churches on its borders, to the small "storefront" churches for refugees, Rosemont contains resources for all major religious groups.

Systems

Most of Rosemont is developed; there is little space not in use. Four small neighborhood parks, a narrow strip along the bayou, and the land around the Community College are the "greens" available to the community (see map, Figure 6-3), although most houses have well-kept lawns with trees and shrubs. See Table 6-10, which presents land use data on Rosemont.

The majority of houses in Rosemont are old, reflecting the early development of the area. Within certain sections, the houses resemble each other (*e.g.,* all one-story, wood frame with porches); however, there also may be great heterogeneity from one block to the next. In the northeast quadrant is a large subsidized housing area comprised of run-down apartments with broken windows and poorly kept streets, while in the southwest quadrant are houses that have been well-kept and remodeled. Also in the northeast there is a several-block area of what are called "shot-gun" houses (the story is told that one can shoot a shotgun from the front door and the shot will go out the back

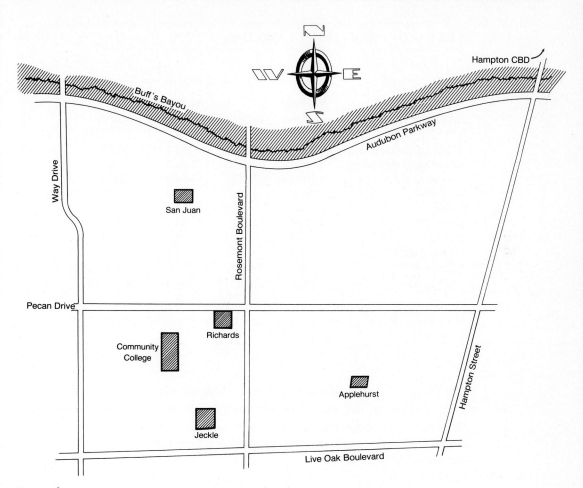

Figure 6-3. Rosemont Community Greens and Parks.

door); placed side-by-side, they are tiny and poorly maintained. See Table 6-11 for housing information.

During the day most of the people seen on the streets move quickly as though on business or an errand and as though they will be "on their way" as soon as their business or errand is complete. Those who could be described as

TABLE 6-10.   ROSEMONT LAND USE

Land Use	CT 402		CT 403	
	Number of Acres	*Total %*	*Number of Acres*	*Total %*
Single family dwellings	161.2	28.03	95.4	31.78
Multi-family dwellings	46.4	8.06	46.5	15.49
Commercial	210.2	36.55	61.2	20.39
Industrial	44.9	7.8	0.2	0.06
Public	6.8	1.18	11.1	3.69
Open	52.9	9.2	53.2	17.72
Water	6.3	1.09	4.7	1.56
Undeveloped	46.3	8.05	14.6	4.86
Right-of-Way	0	0	13.2	4.39
Total Acres	575	100	300.1	100

(Data Book, Rosemont Community Development, City of Hampton. Planning Department, 1980)

'strolling' are elderly persons or young men, usually alone. Few children are seen during the day except in the schoolyards, which are not on the main thoroughfares. Dogs are heard to bark as one walks through the neighborhoods and cats sun themselves in windows; however, few pets run loose in the area.

TABLE 6-11.   AVERAGE VALUE OF HOUSING AND RENT
FOR YEARS 1970 AND 1980

	CT 403		CT 402		Hampton	
	1970	*1980*	*1970*	*1980*	*1970*	*1980*
Average value of housing	$16,900	$58,432	$17,800	$25,777	$18,300	$49,630
Average rent	$48 mo	$259 mo	$95 mo	$243 mo	$109 mo	$244 mo

(Data from 1980 Census of Population and Housing, Bureau of Census)

At night Rosemont assumes a different flavor along Pecan Drive: all the restaurants are open and many have outdoor patios for serving. Smells of fajitas, curry, exotic spices and charbroiling fill the air. "The Strip," as Pecan Drive is called, comes alive with sounds of disco, punk and rock'n roll, along with the stroking of a sitar or quiet strumming of a guitar.

Most of the clients in these restaurants and nude modeling "studios," according to residents, come from outside of Rosemont. Many are attracted by the food, and some by the free-wheeling sex that is reputed to be available in the area.

Many of the residents express disdain for the Strip, calling it a "tourist attraction," and they feel that it is contributing to the deterioration of Rosemont. They state that "outsiders" and "cowboys" exploit and prey on unsuspecting tourists and that the unsavory reputation of the area is not the fault of the people who live there. An absence of zoning laws has facilitated the establishment of some of the less-than-desirable businesses in the area.

The physical examination of Rosemont reveals it to be a community of contrasts: churches and nude modeling studios, subsidized city housing units and restored homes from a more affluent time, old people and young, white and black (and all shades between), quiet tree-lined streets and busy thoroughfares, sedate tea rooms and garish adult movie theaters, families and singles, and the rich and poor.

HEALTH AND SOCIAL SERVICES

One method of classifying health and social services is to differentiate between facilities located outside community (*extra-community*) versus those within the community (*intra-community*). Once the health and social service facilities are identified, group them into categories, perhaps by type of service offered (*e.g.,* hospitals, clinics, extended care), by size, or by public versus private usage. Table 6-12 suggests a classification system, as well as possible major components of each facility requiring assessment.

Extra-community Health Facilities

Hospitals

Jefferson County has 50 hospitals with 12,321 beds of which 4321 are in the Hampton Medical Center—a complex that includes all medical subspecialties,

TABLE 6-12. HEALTH AND SOCIAL SERVICES

Component	Sources of Information
Health Services	
Extra-community *or* Intra-community facilities. Once identified, group into categories (*e.g.,* hospitals and clinics, home health care, extended care facilities, public health services, emergency care)	Chamber of Commerce
	Planning Board (county, city)
	Phone directory
	Talk to residents
For each facility, collect data on	Interview administrator or
1. Services (fees, hours, new services planned and those discontinued)	someone on the staff
	Facility annual report
2. Resources (personnel, space, budget, record system)	
3. Characteristics of users (geographic distribution, demographic profile, transportation source)	
4. Statistics (number of persons served daily, weekly, monthly)	
5. Adequacy, accessibility, and acceptability of facility according to users and providers	
Social Services	
Extra-community *or* intra-community facilities. Once identified, group into categories (*e.g.,* counseling and support, clothing, food, shelter, and special needs)	Chamber of Commerce
	United Way Directory
	Phone directory
For each facility collect data on the areas 1–5 listed above	

as well as sophisticated diagnostic and treatment services. The Medical Center is located seven miles from Rosemont. All patients admitted to the Medical Center must be referred by a physician; self-referral is not permitted. (Self-referral allows the individual independently to choose and acquire medical care.) Although existence of the Medical Center is common knowledge among Rosemont residents, few persons know anyone that has sought or received care. Numerous private hospitals are located in Jefferson County, most being in Hampton. All private hospitals require payment for services rendered to third-party reimbursements. (Third-party reimbursement means payment for services by an entity other than the patient. For example, Medicare, Medicaid, insurance, and workman's compensation are third-party reimbursers.) In addition to private hospitals, most communities use tax revenues to support at least one hospital for the general public—in Jefferson County, the public hospital is Jefferson Memorial.

Jefferson Memorial is a full-service facility located five miles south of Rosemont. Care units and clinics at Memorial include: medical, surgical, pediatrics, maternity, gynecology, trauma and burns, psychiatry, and emergency rooms. Persons can self-refer to Jefferson Memorial. According to the director of the emergency room (ER), 290 persons are seen daily in the ER (approximately 100,000 persons annually). Of these, some 40% are admitted. Follow-up care is provided by Memorial's outpatient clinics. Memorial is supported by city and county taxes, as well as by fees collected for services. The base charge for an ER visit classified as minor is $42.60, a visit deemed major costs $87.20. Health provider fees, as well as treatments and diagnostic services are in addition to the base fee. All fees are on a sliding scale according to income and family size. Rosemont residents use Memorial, but complain of lengthy waits of up to eight hours and of having to undergo repeated assessments as they are moved from one health provider to another. Hospital personnel recognize the lengthy waiting period and fragmentation of care, but cite budget constraints and high staff turnover as major obstacles to improving care. No services have been discontinued at Memorial, and no new services or staff positions are budgeted for the next two years.

Private care providers, group practices, and specialty clinics

A full selection of general medical and specialty care is available in Jefferson County through private practitioners, group practices, and specialty clinics. Payment is usually third-party reimbursement. Two health maintenance organizations (HMOs) are located in Jefferson County. Rosemont residents with adequate finances use a variety of private practitioners and specialty clinics. The residents usually self-refer themselves following a favorable recommendation from a neighbor, friend, or work colleague.

Public health services: The health department

To monitor, maintain, and promote the public's health, each state has a state health department and accompanying regional, county, and sometimes city health departments. National, state, and local tax revenues are used to support public health services. There exists a Hampton Health Department, as well as a Jefferson County Health Department. Because Rosemont is within the city limits of Hampton, the services of the Hampton Health Department are assessed.

The Hampton Health Department offers all medical outpatient services through its seven satellite clinics. The Sunvalley Clinic, located six miles from Rosemont, provides the following services

- Immunizations
- Well and ill infant, child, adolescent, and adult care

- Antepartal/postpartal care
- Family planning
- Nutrition counseling
- Screening and testing for genetic and acquired conditions, such as sickle cell anemia, diabetes, phenylketonuria (PKU)
- Dental assessment, cleaning, and restoration
- Mental health counseling and referral
- Health education
- Maternal and infant home visitation following early hospital discharge (defined as earlier than 48 hours)
- Child abuse, battered spouse, and abandoned person
- Counseling and referral

Additional services include a pharmacy, laboratory, and radiation department. Payment for most services is on a sliding scale; remaining services are free to all city residents. Free services include immunizations, as well as screening and treatment for STDs. The majority of Rosemont residents who use the health department attend antepartal or postpartum clinics. The staff nurse in the maternity clinic estimates that of the 75 women seen in the prenatal clinic each week, 20 to 25 are Rosemont residents.

The major service-delivery problem cited by nurses in the maternity clinics is the long waiting period (frequently 8 to 10 weeks) between a woman's initial request for an appointment and the scheduled appointment date. Because many women wait until they are six or seven months pregnant to request antepartal care, the first available appointment time may be after the woman's expected delivery date. Consequently, a large number of women from Rosemont deliver at Jefferson Memorial having received no antepartal care. The administrator of the Sunvalley Clinic felt a top service priority to be additional education, support, and monitoring services for the pregnant woman and new mother.

No services have been discontinued in the recent past. With regard to the question of services that are needed, the elderly were identified as a target group. Plans were underway to establish a nursing clinic for the elderly, as well as a wellness program to be offered at daycare for the elderly, and at senior centers. There are presently more than ten such facilities for seniors within the city of Hampton.

Numerous Rosemont residents use the health department services, especially the Sunvalley Clinic. Problems cited include lack of a direct bus connection to the clinic (presently three bus transfers are required) and the impersonal service. Because patients are not assigned to a primary care provider, it is customary for a patient to see a different health provider each visit. Maternity patients have an additional concern. Each woman must make her own delivery arrangements and frequently women that qualify for antepartal care at Sunvalley Clinic do not meet eligibility requirements for delivery at Jefferson Memorial. Consequently the woman must search for a facility that will admit her for labor and delivery. All too often the woman is forced to deliver at home, a situation documented by Sunvalley nurses and confirmed by several Rosemont residents.

Home health agencies

The Visiting Nurses Association (VNA) of Hampton is the largest home health agency in Jefferson County. Services of the VNA include: nursing care, physical and occupational therapy, speech therapy, medical and social services, and home health care. The VNA accepts paying clients and third-party reimbursements. Paying clients are charged on a sliding scale according to income and family size. Patients who are unable to pay a fee can request financial assistance from several community social service agencies such as the United Way.

Numerous other home health agencies are located in Hampton and Jefferson County. Although more limited in scope of service, all offer home health services and require fees or third-party reimbursement for payment.

Long-term, extended care, and continuing care facilities

There are two long-term facilities within eight miles of Rosemont. The Pinewoods Rest Center and the Windsail Nursing Home. Each facility is classified as an intermediate-care facility and licensed by the State Department of Health. A profile of the services, resources, and characteristics of the residents for each facility is presented in Table 6-13. In addition, several hospitals offer extended-care services.

Emergency services

The Poison Control Center provides information to individuals and health providers on harmful substances and methods of assessment and treatment. The center provides educational materials and programs for schools and interested groups.

The Medical Emergency Ambulance Service (MEAS) is financed by Hampton city taxes, public donations, Jefferson County contributions, and organized fund raisers. The MEAS first-aid services are free and available 24 hours a day to all residents of Rosemont. (The MEAS operates in conjunction

TABLE 6-13. SERVICES, RESOURCES, AND RESIDENT
CHARACTERISTICS AT PINEWOODS REST
CENTER AND WINDSAIL NURSING HOME
DURING THE PRECEDING YEAR

	Pinewoods Rest Center	Windsail Nursing Home
Services	Convalescent nursing care, physical, occupational, and speech therapy	Convalescent nursing care
Fulltime personnel	6 RNs, 4 licensed visiting nurses (LVNs), 3 nurse aides, 1 administrator	3 RNs, 2 LVNs, 1 nurse aide, 1 administrator
Licensed bed capacity	96	38
Patient days	33,524	12,965
Occupancy rate	0.96	0.93
Certified bed capacity*	96	38
Median age of residents	79	76
Average duration of stay	Four years	Six years

* Recommended occupancy rate for nursing home beds is 90%.
(Jefferson County Planning Council, Pinewoods Rest Center, and Windsail Nursing record books)

with the local fire stations. See the Safety and Transportation section of this chapter for a description of fire protection services.)

The MEAS closest to Rosemont has two ambulances; one is used daily, the other serves as a back-up. The MEAS averages 90 to 110 calls a month with a response time of less than eight minutes. (Table 6-14 presents specific reasons for ambulance service to persons in Rosemont during the last three-month period.) Calls are received through the central fire department and dispatched by radio to the nearest MEAS team. Each MEAS team consists of 26 persons: 3 paramedics having completed 100 hours of classwork and 200 hours of hospital experience; and 22 emergency medical technicians (EMTs) with basic paramedic training and additional experience in intravenous therapy and intubation. Both paramedics and EMTs are certified. In addition to emergency service, the MEAS team offers CPR and first-aid classes to community groups.

TABLE 6-14.   REASONS FOR MEAS TO PERSONS IN
ROSEMONT DURING THE PRECEDING
THREE-MONTH PERIOD

Reason	Total %
Cardiac-related problems and cerebrovascular accidents	25
Falls and household accidents	19
Respiratory problems	12
Dizziness and weakness	12
Lacerations	11
Fractures and dislocations	9
Abdominal pain	7
Mental–psychiatric disorders	5

(MEAS Paramedics Records)

Special services

Frequently special facilities exist to serve specific groups such as the handicapped or retarded. After surveying the immediate extra-community, no such facilities were located within a 10-mile radius of Rosemont.

Intra-community health facilities

According to the Health Systems Agency (HSA) of Jefferson County, CT 402 is a medically underserved area; CT 403 is not.

The type and number of practitioners offering health services in Rosemont are listed in Table 6-15. A need that was frequently expressed by female residents was for gynecological and obstetric services. Numerous persons cited the need for family practitioners, as well as bilingual health providers. (None of the practitioners listed in Table 6-15 speaks Spanish or Vietnamese.) Rosemont residents with financial resources tend to select from extra-community medical services; indigent residents rely on medical services within the community. All private practitioners require payment when services are rendered, or third-party reimbursement; none uses a sliding scale to calculate fees. In addition to private practitioners, two clinics—the Third Street Clinic and the Rosemont Health Center—are located in Rosemont.

Third Street Clinic was founded in 1968 by concerned citizens and church

TABLE 6-15.   PRACTITIONERS IN ROSEMONT

Type	Number
Dentist	6
General medical	1
Optometrist	2
Orthodontist	1
Osteopath	2
Podiatrist	1
Chiropractor	3

(Windshield Survey, Chamber of Commerce, and Phone Directory)

leaders in Rosemont. The clinic, located in the center of CT 402, was initially financed by public donations and church-sponsored fund raisers. All professional time and supplies were donated. Today the Third Street Clinic serves 30% to 40% of Rosemont residents and has an annual operating budget of $750,000, a reduction of $220,000 from two years ago. The majority of funds are from federal and state grants, as well as client fees and Medicare and Medicaid reimbursements. Although patients are charged according to a sliding scale, no one is denied care. Services provided at Third Street Clinic are summarized in Table 6-16. The clinic provides no acute or trauma care services. One part-time physician, two part-time nurses, one social worker, one administrator, and a clerk form the clinic's staff. Both nurses speak Spanish, none of the staff speaks Vietnamese. Optometry students and supervising faculty provide services one day a week and one nurse midwife provides antepartal care two mornings a week. The clinic is open Monday to Friday, 8 am to 5 pm. On the average 95 people are seen weekly. Medical professionals and citizens form the board of directors. According to the clinic's director, immediate medical needs for the residents of CT 402 include

- Ill infant, child, adolescent and adult assessment, treatment, and follow-up
- Dental assessment and restoration
- Counseling, referral, and, when possible, treatment for drug abuse and alcoholism
- Group health teaching, especially for pregnant women, parents of young children, and adolescents
- Wellness and selfcare classes for all age groups
- Support groups for single parents and senior citizens

TABLE 6-16. SERVICES AND NUMBER OF PEOPLE
SERVED AT THIRD STREET CLINIC

Service	Description	Patient Visits (Weekly Average)
Family planning	Physical exams, education, prescriptions filled	24
Well child examinations	Physical assessment, referral for illness, immunizations, screening	19
Antepartal and postpartum	Physical assessment and monitoring	42
Optometry	Eye exams, prescriptions filled	9
Podiatry	Assessment, treatment	6
Chronic disease counseling and treatment	Treatment and care instructions for hypertension, diabetes, cardiovascular conditions	31

Presently there are no consistent health education or counseling services. Transportation services from area neighborhoods to the clinic, as well as dental and home nursing care were discontinued two years ago following grant reductions. The major problem confronting the clinic is the recruitment of health providers, especially nurses and physicians. Clinic services cannot be expanded (or maintained at the present level) unless additional health providers are recruited and retained.

Most Rosemont residents are aware of the Third Street Clinic, and many use the clinic's services routinely. The major impediment to clinic use is the one to two mile walk to the clinic for many residents (there is no direct bus connection for most people). Rosemont residents feel welcomed at the clinic and low staff turnover has fostered compliance with medical recommendations. Residents did, however, express a need for additional services at the clinic.

The Rosemont Health Center, centrally located in CT 403, is a nonprofit clinic devoted to the diagnosis and treatment of STDs. The clinic is open Monday to Saturday, 6 pm to 10 pm, and Sunday, 2 pm to 10 pm. The center reports 20% of the syphillis cases in Jefferson County and 60% of the gonorrhea cases. Approximately 600 patient visits occur monthly (200 new cases, 200 repeat cases, and 200 followups). All 75 professional staff members are volunteers and donate 4 hours to 10 hours of service a month. The director of the clinic is employed part-time. The state donates penicillin, tetanus cultures, and Venereal Disease Research Laboratory (VDRL) tests. Initially there were no fees for services—presently a fee of $2.00 per visit is assessed to defray costs of equipment, rent, and utilities. (However, no patient is denied care.) Ninety percent of the patients are male homosexuals. Each patient is issued an identification number and card that is used with each visit. Persons in psychologic crises are referred to the City Health Department for counseling. Most patients drive or walk to the clinic.

The director of the health center discussed the immediate need for counseling and support groups, especially for patients with Acquired Immune Deficiency Syndrome (AIDS). A second need is for an orientation program and information update sessions for staff, most of whom are former patients. The majority of patients are from the Rosemont area although an increasing number of patients are commuting to the clinic from Hampton and surrounding Jefferson County. Patients surveyed in the waiting room rated the care as excellent; appointments are rarely cancelled by patients.

Observations made on a visit were: two open trash bags filled with syringes and attached needles, no visible emergency cart, lack of procedure manuals, and no posted protocol for an adverse treatment response (*e.g.,* penicillin reaction).

Social Service Facilities

Because social service agencies are frequently located in office buildings, their location in the community may be difficult to determine during a windshield survey. It is preferable to use a directory such as the type compiled by the Chamber of Commerce or local planning board to begin identifying social service organizations relatively close to the community being assessed. If the community does not have a Chamber of Commerce, use the phone directory.

Extra-community social service facilities

Counseling and support services

The Hampton Comprehensive Counseling Center was founded in 1971 by concerned citizens of Hampton and Jefferson County for the purpose of providing counseling to adolescent drug users. Today the center offers a comprehensive mental health program for all residents of Hampton. The center is located two miles south of Rosemont. Although persons can self-refer to the center, most patients are referred from schools, clinics, and private practitioners. Fees are based on a sliding scale; third-party reimbursements are not accepted. Last year's operating budget was $200,000. The majority of revenues are from clients, although numerous churches and social service agencies sponsor individuals and families. The staff consists of six professionals and two clerks. Services are outlined in Table 6-17. An average of 300 patients are seen monthly. The director describes the patient population as middle to upper class, more males than females, and all patients are white. Most patients use private transportation to arrive at the clinic. No additional services are planned as the center staff feels they are adequately meeting the needs of the population. Rosemont residents queried were unaware of the existence of the counseling center and no one knew of anyone having used the center although all residents interviewed knew of several adolescent drug users.

The YMCA Youth Development Center borders Rosemont and offers a variety of educational and recreational programs. Adjacent to the "Y" is the YMCA Indo-Chinese Refugee Program, an agency that seeks to facilitate the resettlement of asian immigrants. Major services include cultural orientation, job counseling and placement, and courses in English as a second language.

TABLE 6-17. SERVICES OFFERED AT THE HAMPTON COMPREHENSIVE COUNSELING CENTER

Service	Description
Diagnosis	Screening procedure for the mentally handicapped; recommends services required for clients' needs
Information and referral	Liaison teams coordinate services with state schools for the mentally retarded, and state hospitals for the mentally ill
Counseling and therapy	Group and play therapy provided
Alcohol and drug abuse services	Counseling services
Psychiatric evaluation and medical services	Psychiatric department provides evaluations and medications for clients
Emergency service	Handles crisis calls 24 hours/day, 7 days/week
Education and consultation	Center staff works with other community groups, including schools, police, and social service agencies, to solve local problems

(Hampton Comprehensive Counseling Center)

The agency services have experienced a 200% increase in usage during the past three years. Presently, over 100 persons use the facility daily. Although all four staff members are bilingual, they are too small a staff to meet the needs of the Vietnamese community—a large proportion of which lives in Rosemont. Staff feel the immediate need is for counseling and therapy programs for alcohol and drug abuse, as well as teaching basic life-survival skills (*e.g.,* finding a job, housing, and medical care). The staff estimate that 40% to 50% of the asians using their services are from Rosemont. Asian residents in Rosemont agree that the "Y" is responsive to their needs, but they complain about the long waiting period (sometimes weeks) for classes and counseling.

Clothing, food, shelter, and basic welfare services

Most churches and synagogues in the area have a food pantry, and many can arrange emergency shelter and provide clothing and essential transportation services. People are usually helped on a walk-in basis, or the church is referred to a family or individual in need. In Hampton a special organization, The Metropolitan Ministries, serves as an interfaith link between the religious communities of Hampton and community residents in need of social services. The Metropolitan Ministries acts to coordinate services, thereby avoiding duplication, and refers individuals to the program that can best meet their immediate needs.

> NOTE: In most communities, churches must be contacted individually for a listing of services.

In addition to the churches and synagogues, numerous resale clothing shops are located in shopping areas close to Rosemont. Residents are very knowledgeable about available retail stores and actively promote preferred merchants.

The Jefferson County Welfare Department and the Hampton Welfare Department screen and process applicants for food stamps, housing subsidies, and financial aid checks. Each welfare department has a division of child protection that investigates reports of child abuse and neglect. The division provides casework services, foster home placement, emergency shelter for women and children, as well as parenting classes and child therapy groups. Welfare departments are financed by federal, state, and local tax revenues.

Special services

The United Way lists 42 private and public-supported social service agencies located in Hampton or Jefferson County. The United Way directory includes identifying information for each agency, plus services and fees. Agencies on the roster include: the Society to Prevent Blindness, American Lung Association, March of Dimes, Woman's Center, Paralyzed Veterans Association, International Rescue Committee.

> ADVICE: In your community assessment material, this would be an ideal location to append a list of social service agencies, along with identifying information, (*e.g.,* address, phone number, major services, and contact person).

Intra-community

Two churches in Rosemont, South Main Methodist and Westpark Episcopal, have extensive social outreach programs including preschool and daycare services; benevolence funds for food, clothing, and shelter; and numerous support groups (*e.g.,* parents without partners, singles, and solitaires). Westpark has a seniors center open 8 am to 6 pm daily. The seniors enjoy a variety of recreational and educational programs and a hot noon meal. In addition, volunteers are enlisted to complete shopping and errands, minor home repairs, light housekeeping, and meals for fellow seniors who are permanently or temporarily incapacitated. Noticeably absent from Westpark were any support groups or programs directed at the large male homosexual population. When asked about this, staff responded that "that problem does not exist in this community." South Main does offer a coffee-klatch on Friday night and plans to offer additional services to the male homosexual population, although there is strong resistence from the older parishioners.

On the north side of CT 403 is Lambda Alcoholic Anonymous (AA), an Alcoholic Anonymous program specifically for homosexual males, a group originally not allowed to join Alcoholic Anonymous. (Lambda is the Hebrew symbol that Hitler forced the homosexual population to wear as identification in Nazi Germany.) Lambda AA in CT 403 is an active group with the present participation exceeding 120. All socioeconomic groups are represented in the meetings and members take turns leading the support groups.

ECONOMICS

The economic subsystem includes the "wealth" of Rosemont; that is, the goods and services available to the community, as well as the costs and benefits of improving patterns of resource allocation. It should be evident that extra-community factors such as the state of the United States and world economies affect in great measure the local economy. Nevertheless, intra-community economic factors impinge upon all other subsystems so they must be included in the assessment. Table 6-18 lists the suggested areas for study-

---

TABLE 6-18.   ECONOMIC INDICATORS AND SOURCES OF INFORMATION

Indicators	Source
Financial Characteristics	
Households	

Median household income
  % households below poverty level
  % households receiving public assistance
  % households headed by females
Monthly costs for owner-occupied households,
    renter-occupied households
	Census records

Individuals	
Per capital income % of persons who live in poverty	Census records
Labor Force Characteristics	
Employment Status	

General population (age 18+)
  % employed
  % unemployed
  % not participating in employment (retired)
Special groups
  % women with children under age 6 working
	Chamber of Commerce
	Department of Labor
	Census records

Occupational Categories and Number (%) of Persons Employed	
Managerial Technical Service Farming Production Operator/laborer	Census records
Union Activity and Membership	Local union(s) office

ing a community's economy, along with sources of the data. The census data can be used to summarize most of these economic indicators.

Financial Characteristics of Households

The two census tracts that comprise the Rosemont community vary greatly in income characteristics. The 1980 census data show the median income for households in CT 402 to be $4776, while in CT 403 it was $16,019. Table 6-19 lists the household income for the community and Hampton, comparing 1970 and 1980 figures.

Businesses

There are several high-rise office buildings located on the northern boundary of the area along the Audubon Parkway, including the National General Life Insurance complex of three towers; the new National Tower, presently under construction; National Service Corporation; as well as Second Mortgage Corporation's building on Audubon Parkway. Way-on-the-Bayou, a new office complex, is also being constructed at the corner of Way Drive and Buff's Bayou. These buildings all feature spacious landscaped grounds, modern architecture, and covered parking. Some of the residents of the area are em-

TABLE 6-19.   INCOME INDICES FOR THE YEARS 1970
AND 1980 FOR CT 402, CT 403
AND HAMPTON

	CT 402		CT 403		Hampton	
Income Indices	*1970*	*1980*	*1970*	*1980*	*1970*	*1980*
Median household income	$2420	$4776	$6178	$16,019	$9876	$15,321
% of all families with incomes below poverty level	50.2	53.7	11.7	5.4	10.7	7.1
% of all families with public assistance or public welfare income	33.7	36.4	4.4	4.3	3.8	3.4
% of female-headed households	46.3	49.2	14.4	11.1	12.3	15.4

(Data from 1970 Census, Selected Characteristics; 1980 Census, Selected Characteristics)

ployed in these offices; most employees, according to local residents, live in other areas of Hampton.

Other major area businesses include the Rose Milk Company factory at the northern edge of the area on Way Drive, the Sheet Metal Workers Union Local No. 54 at the corner of Way Drive and Jackson, and American Life Insurance Company on Green.

All of the main thoroughfares in the area are lined with neighborhood-type businesses such as grocery stores, craft stores, antique shops, cleaners, and small restaurants (see the Physical Description section). In addition, these kinds of businesses are also dispersed throughout the area within the residential districts. The Hampton Lighting and Power Service Center is located near the northern edge of the area. Hampton's Vehicle Maintenance Department and its Street Repair Department are also located on West Pleasant in the northern part of the Rosemont area. There is also a considerable number of printing houses (probably the largest concentration in Hampton) on the northern edge of the area, as well as the broadcast studios of Channel 11 (KHAM TV).

According to local residents, the economic impact of these businesses on the Rosemont area is minimal because most residents are employed outside of Rosemont and, other than the minimal shopping done in neighborhood convenience stores, they tend to shop for major purchases in other areas of the city. The residents also indicated that the vast majority of the businesses do not directly participate in the life of the community. Selected industries of the area are listed in Table 6-20.

When there are major businesses within a community that employ a substantial number of community residents a thorough assessment is required. An excellent guide for assessing an occupational setting is included as Table 6-21.

(*Text continues on page 206*)

TABLE 6-20.   SELECTED INDUSTRIES IN ROSEMONT

	CT 402		CT 403	
	Number	*Total %*	*Number*	*Total %*
Manufacturing	92	10	430	15
Wholesale and retail trade	450	48	1084	37
Professional and related services	387	42	1423	48
Total	929	100	2937	100

(Data from 1980 Census, Selected Characteristics)

TABLE 6-21. A MODEL ASSESSMENT GUIDE
FOR NURSING IN INDUSTRY

Components	Questions to Ask
The Company	
Historical development	How, why, and by whom was the company founded?
Organizational chart	What is the formal order of the system and to whom are the health providers responsible?
Company Policies	Is there a policy manual? Are the workers aware of existence of the manual?
Length of the work week	How many days a week does the industry operate?
Length of the work time	Are there several shifts? How many breaks? Is there paid vacation?
Sick leave	Is there a clear policy and do the workers know it?
Safety and fire provisions	Is management aware of situations or substances in the plant that represent a potential danger? Are there organized fire drills? (The *Federal Register* is the source of information for federal standards and serves as a helpful guide)
Support services (benefits)	
Insurance programs	Is there a system for health insurance and life insurance and is it compulsory? Does the company pay all or part? Who fills out the necessary forms?
Retirement program	Are the benefits realistic?
Educational support	Can the workers further their education? Will the company help financially?
Safety committee	If there is no committee, do certain people routinely handle emergencies? The Red Cross First Aid Course through programmed instruction is excellent (for information consult your local Red Cross).
Recreation committee	Do the workers have any communication with or interest in each other outside the work setting?
Employee relations	Are there problems in employee relations? (This is difficult information to get, but it is important to get a sense of how employees feel generally about management, and vice versa.)
The Plant	
General physical setting	What is the overall appearance?
The construction	What is the size and general condition of buildings and grounds?

(continued)

TABLE 6-21. (Continued)

Components	Questions to Ask
Parking facilities and public transportation stops	How far does the worker have to walk to get inside?
Entrances and exits	How many people must use them? How accessible are they?
Physical environment	What conditions exist in the physical environment? (Comment on heating, air-conditioning, lighting, glare, drafts, etc.)
Communication facilities	Are there bulletin boards, newsletters?
Housekeeping	Is the physical setting maintained adequately?
Interior decoration	Are the surroundings conducive to work? Are they pleasing?
Work areas	
Space	Are workers isolated or crowded?
Heights: workplace and supply areas	Is there a chance of workers falling or being injured by falling objects? (Falls and falling objects are dangerous and costly to industry.)
Stimulation	Is the worker too bored to pay attention?
Safety signs and markings	Are dangerous areas well marked?
Standing and sitting facilities	Are chairs safe and comfortable? Are there platforms to stand on, especially for wet processes?
Safety equipment	Do the workers make use of hard hats, safety glasses, face masks, radiation badges, etc.? Do they know the safety devices the OSHA regulations require?
Nonwork areas	
Lockers	If the work is dirty, workers should be able to change clothes. Are they accidentally carrying toxic substances home on their clothes?
Hand-washing facilities	If facilities and supplies are available, do workers know how and when to wash their hands?
Rest rooms	How accessible are they and what condition are they in?
Drinking water	Can workers leave their jobs long enough to get a drink of water when they want to?
Recreation and rest facilities	Can a worker who is not feeling well lie down? Do workers feel free to use the facilities?
Telephones	Can a worker receive or make a call? Does a working mother have to stay home for a call because she can't be reached at work?
Ashtrays	Are people allowed to smoke in designated areas? Are they safe areas?

(continued)

TABLE 6-21.   (*Continued*)

Components	Questions to Ask
The Working Population: Include worker and management, but separate data for comparison.	
General characteristics	(Be as accurate as possible, but estimate when necessary.)
Total number of employees	(Usually, if an industry has 500 or more employees, full-time nursing services are necessary.)
General appearance	Are there records of heights, weights, cleanliness, and so forth? Ask to see them.
Age and sex distribution	What are the proportions of the different groups? (Certain screening programs are specific for young adults, while others are more for the elderly. Some programs are more for women; others are more for men.) Is there any difference between day and evening shift populations? Are the problems of the minority sex unattended?
Race distribution	Does one race predominate? How does this compare with the general community?
Socioeconomic distribution	Are there great differences in worker salaries? (This can sometimes cause problems.)
Religious distribution	Does one religion predominate? Are religious holidays observed?
Ethnic distribution	Is there a language barrier?
Marital status	What proportion of the workers are widowed, singles, or divorced? (These groups often have different needs.)
Educational backgrounds	Can all teaching be done at approximately the same level?
Lifestyles practiced	Is there disapproval of certain lifestyles?
Types of employment offered	
Background necessary	What educational level is required? Skilled versus unskilled?
Work demands on physical condition	What level of strength is needed? Is the work sedentary or active?
Work status	How many employees work full-time? Part-time? Is there overtime?
Absenteeism	Is there a record kept? By whom? Why?
Causes	What are the five most common reasons for absence?

(*continued*)

TABLE 6-21. *(Continued)*

Components	Questions to Ask
Length	What are the patterns of absences? (Absenteeism is costly to the employer. There is some difference between one ten-day absence and ten one-day absences by the same person.)
Physically handicapped	Does the company have a policy about hiring the handicapped?
Number employed	Where do they work? What do they do?
Extent of handicaps	Are they specially trained? Are they in a special program? Do they use prosthetic devices?
Personnel on medication	What medication does each of these employees take? Where does each person work?
Personnel with chronic illness	At what stage of illness is the employee? Where does the employee work? Will he or she be able to continue at this job?

The Industrial Process: What does the company produce and how?

Equipment used	Is the equipment portable or fixed? light or heavy?
General description of placement	Ask to have each piece of large equipment marked on a scale map.
Type of equipment	Fans, blowers, fast moving, wet or dry?
Nature of the operation	Ask for a brief description of each stage of the process so you can compare the needs and abilities of the worker with the needs of the job.
Raw materials used	What are they and how dangerous are they? Are they properly stored? Check the *Federal Register* for guidelines on storage.
Nature of the final product	Can the workers take pride in the final product or do they make parts?
Description of the jobs	Who does what? Where? (Label the map.)
Waste products produced	What is the system for waste disposal? Are the pollution-control devices in place and functioning?
Exposure to toxic substances	To which toxins are the workers exposed? What is the extent of exposure? (Include physical and emotional hazards. Remember that chronic effects of industrial exposure are subtle; a person often gets used to having mild symptoms and won't report them. The *Federal Register* contains specifications for exposure to toxins and some states issue state standards.)

(continued)

TABLE 6-21.   (*Continued*)

Components	Questions to Ask

The Health Program: Outline what is actually in existence as well as what employees perceive to be in existence.

Existing Policies	Are there informal, unwritten policies?
Objectives of the program	Are they clear?
Pre-employment physicals	Are they required? Are they paid for by the company? Is the information used to select?
First aid facilities	What is available? What is not available?
Standing orders	Is there a company physician who is responsible for first aid or emergency policy? (If so, work closely with him in planning nursing services.)
Job descriptions for health personnel	Are they in writing? (If there are no guidelines to be followed, write some.)
Existing Facilities and Resources:	Sometimes an industry that denies having a health program has more of a system than they realize.
Trained personnel	Who responds in an emergency?
Space	Where is the sick worker taken? Where is the emergency equipment kept?
Supplies	What are they? Where are they kept? (Make a list and describe the condition of each item.)
Records and reports	What exists? (The OSHA requires that employers keep three types of records: a log of occupational injuries and illnesses, a supplemental record of certain illnesses or injuries, and an annual summary [forms 100, 101, and 102 are provided under the Act]. Good records provide data for good planning.)
Services rendered in the past year:	Describe as specifically as possible.
Care needed	Chronic or acute? Why?
Screening done	Where? By whom? Why?
Referrals made	By whom? To whom? Why?
Counseling done	Formal or informal? (Often informal counseling goes unnoticed.)
Health education	What individual or group education was offered by the company?
Accidents in the past year	During working hours? After hours? (Include those that occur after work hours, some may be directly or indirectly work related.)
Reasons employees sought health care	What are the five major reasons?

(*continued*)

TABLE 6-21. (*Continued*)

Components	Questions to Ask
Stressors	
As identified by employees	What pressures are felt on the job?
As identified by health providers	What problems do they perceive?

(Adapted from: Serafini P: Nursing assessment in industry: A model. Amer J Public Health 66(8):755–760, 1976)

This guide may be used by either the community nurse who needs more information about a major economic factor in the community or by the occupational health nurse employed by the business. A complete industry assessment using the guide is presented in Table 6-22.

Labor Force

Employment status

The labor force of a community is comprised of persons 16 years of age and over. Table 6-23 summarizes key data relating to the workforce of the Rosemont community. The majority of workers are classed as "private wage and salary," as shown in Table 6-24.

Occupation

General occupational categories are included in the census. Table 6-25 lists the occupations of the citizens of Rosemont.

NOTE: Census occupational categories are quite general. To determine more precisely what sort of work is incorporated in a category it is necessary to ask those who do the job or to look up the category in the Department of Labor publications.

Differences between the two census tracts that comprise Rosemont are clearly seen in the occupational makeup of the community. Whereas almost half of the workers in CT 402 are categorized under "Service Occupations," a similar percentage of workers in CT 403 are classified under "Managerial and Professional."

(*Text continues on page 213*)

TABLE 6-22.   ASSESSMENT OF AN INDUSTRY

Components	Description

The Company	The AAB Chemical Company
	   Hampton Industrial Complex
	   Located west of State Highway 519 and Loop 177

Historical development	The AAB Chemical Company separated from the AAB Refinery in 1957 and the present plant was completed in 1961. The parent company is a major oil company with headquarters in Chicago. The plant is today the most complex and versatile in the AAB system.
Organizational chart	A formal organizational chart was not available. However, by observation and interview, a structure consisting of a Plant Manager, with supervisor for each production area, safety, and maintenance was noted. There are foremen for each area of operation for each shift. The medical staff, which consists of one doctor and one nurse, are not hired by the plant personnel department, but by the parent company in Chicago.
Company policies	The plant operations are never shut down. There are shifts around the clock for operators and craftspeople. Employees such as clerical staff, administrative, and medical work 8-hour days, 40-hour weeks. Breaks are provided during the work period. Employees are eligible for 2 weeks of paid vacation per year after working 1 year. This increases in 5-year increments. A 20-year employee is eligible for 5 weeks of vacation. Employees are eligible for sick leave after 6 months of service. Benefits vary with length of service. All benefits are published in an employee handbook, distributed to all employees. Management is well aware of situations and substances that pose danger to the workers. The safety program, run by a safety supervisor and a safety engineer, is extensive. Organized fire drills are held frequently. Procedures for dealing with spills and other hazards are also well organized. Fire-fighting equipment and an ambulance are available on the plant site at all times. Certain employees are trained as fire fighters. There are EMTs available inside the plant in addition to the nurse. Fire extinguishers are placed throughout the plant in strategic locations.
Support services	A comprehensive medical expense plan is compulsory for all employees. In addition, disability up to 40 weeks owing to occupational illness or injury is provided to all employees regardless of length of service. Term life insurance under

(continued)

TABLE 6-22.   (*Continued*)

Components	Description
	a group plan is available at a low rate. A long-term disability plan is available to employees covered under the basic life insurance plan. A retirement plan is provided at complete cost to the company. A savings plan in which employees may invest in company stock and U.S. Savings Bonds is also available.
	Employees are offered an educational assistance program and are encouraged to advance their careers. On the job training is provided to help employees advance.
Employee relations	The workers are affiliated with the Oil, Chemical and Atomic Workers International Union, a part of the AFL–CIO. It was difficult to perceive how management and labor relate to each other. However, several workers mentioned the familylike atmosphere among employees, and hopefully, this bridges the gap between labor and management. The last strike occurred approximately two years ago.

The Plant

General physical setting	The appearance of the plant is best described as an intimidating maze of pipes, towers, and vessels. The main building, in which the clinic is located, is modern and attractive with well-tended grounds. Ample parking is available, with areas provided for the handicapped. The building is air conditioned, spacious, and clean, with a pleasing interior.
	The grounds and buildings inside the plant are also neat and well maintained. Scattered through the plant in strategic locations are eye-bubbling devices for flushing the eyes and showers for removing irritants from the skin. Danger areas are clearly marked with yellow paint and warning signs. Employees working in areas where hydrofluoric acid is used are provided with complete protective covering, and they shower immediately upon leaving the area. Ear plugs and ear muffs are required in high-noise areas. Compliance in use of safety devices is good, and workers are aware of Occupational Safety and Health Association (OSHA) regulations.
Work areas	Some work areas, especially where craftpeople are involved, are cramped and close, owing to the physical structure of the myriad pipes and lines. Some areas are also elevated

(continued)

TABLE 6-22.   (*Continued*)

Components	Description
	in height. One problem noted by the plant nurse is occasional heat stress during summer months when employees are working in these areas upon equipment that reflects heat. Another problem noted was the stress, manifested in muscle and joint discomfort, of working in cramped quarters, especially when employees work a lot of overtime. Occasionally employees are injured by falling objects such as heavy wrenches. Burns are the most common type of injuries. Operators who work in the processing units and monitor the gauges and flow rates are in stressful jobs because a mistake could be costly and dangerous.
Nonwork areas	Each work area has a kitchen area, restrooms, and water fountains that are easily accessible. Lockers and showers are also available. Communication by phone is possible in all areas of the plant. Facilities are available in the clinic so that workers who are ill may lie down. However, in some areas, repeated visits to the clinic are discouraged. Employees are instructed regarding handwashing and prompt attention to small wounds by the nurse as part of new employee orientation. Smoking is permitted only in specifically designated parts of the fenced area of the plant, the docks, and warehouses.

The Working Population

General characteristics	AAB Chemicals employs approximately 500 people. Age and sex distribution data were not available. However, the plant nurse stated that employees range in age from age 18 to retirement at age 65, and that male employees outnumber female employees. The nurse also stated that some women were moving into previously male-dominated jobs. Race distribution data were not available. By observation, the distribution appeared to be predominantly white, followed by black and then hispanic employees, which is in line with the population distribution in the community. Data regarding religious and marital status were not available. Wages and salaries are commensurate with education, qualifications, and years of service. Educational backgrounds range from high school graduates to advanced degrees in engineering and the sciences. Therefore health teaching must be geared to match the educational level of the group being instructed.

(continued)

TABLE 6-22.   (*Continued*)

Components	Description
Type of employment offered	Types of employment include skilled craftspeople, operators, lab analysts, chemists, engineers, clerical and administrative personnel, and a nurse and a physician. The background required for each area varies with the complexity and nature of the job. Most employees are full-time and work overtime as required.
Absenteeism	Records of absences are kept in the employee's work unit. The nurse keeps records on illness- or injury-related absences. An employee who has been absent for an extended or serious illness, an injury, or for surgery must report to the medical department before returning to work and must supply a statement from a doctor regarding the nature of his disability, and the limitations, if any, on permissible work. The medical department then determines the physical condition of the employee and notifies his or her supervisor regarding the employee's return to work. Strict record keeping also is done for OSHA requirements. According to the nurse, the most common reasons for absence are not occupationally related. They are most often for upper respiratory infections and other common health problems, or for accidents that occurred away from the plant.
Physically handicapped:	The AAB Company is an equal opportunity employer. Information regarding handicapped employees, the nature of their handicaps, and the jobs they fill was not available.
Personnel on medication Personnel with chronic illness	The nurse keeps records of employees on medication. This information is confidential. The confidentiality of employees' medical records is strictly enforced.

The Industrial Process

Equipment used Nature of the plant operation	The basic job of the plant is to produce specialty chemicals and petrochemical intermediates for manufacture of products that range from boats and surfboards, to carpets and furniture. Production of these chemicals involves moving raw materials (called "feedstock") from AAB's Hampton Refinery and another chemical plant and mixing them with xylenes and benzenes. Some of the chemicals produced are propylene, styrene, paraxylene, metazylene, aromatic solvents, oil-recovering chemicals, oil-producing chemicals, and polybutenes. The equipment used involves

(*continued*)

TABLE 6-22. *(Continued)*

Components	Description
	miles of pipes and many towers and vessels. Process units are designed to be energy efficient, and in many instances energy-producing hydrocarbons are a by-product of a process. These are then recovered and used as fuel in other operations.
	Flammability and danger of explosion are major concerns when dealing with the above-named chemicals. Proper storage is essential and is carried out with care in this plant.
	The final product of the production process are barrels of chemicals. Workers take pride in turning out a certain number of barrels in a time period, and in keeping the plant operating efficiently.
	The treatment of waste-water is through an effluent water-control system that is one of the most sophisticated in the industry. The facility handles waste-water not only from AAB Chemicals, but also from the AAB Refinery and another chemical plant in the area. Air-pollution control is done in two steps, first by eliminating potential contaminants whenever possible, and then through the use of devices such as scrubbers, filters, cyclone separators, and a flare system to burn up the waste hydrocarbons.
Exposure to toxic substances	The major substances of concern are benzene and xylene. Benzene is a colorless, flammable, volatile liquid. The major hazard with this chemical is chronic poisoning by inhalation of small amounts over a long time. It is one of the most dangerous organic solvents in common use. Benzene acts primarily on the blood-forming organs. Skin contact also is to be avoided. Benzene is suspected of being carcinogenic. Xylene resembles benzene in many chemical and physical properties, but is not involved in causing chronic blood diseases. It has a narcotic effect and can cause dermatitis with repeated contact. Benzene screening is done on all employees on a yearly basis.

The Health Program

Existing policies	The objectives of the program are to monitor the status of each employee's health in order to pinpoint problems at an early stage, and to provide prompt attention to accidents or emergencies as they occur at the worksite.

(continued)

TABLE 6-22.   (*Continued*)

Components	Description
	The employees perceive the second objective more readily than the first. Many of them perceive the yearly physicals as a low priority.
	Pre-employment physicals are done by the nurse and company doctor at no charge to the client and are used as a baseline for future reference.
	The ambulance kept at the plant is equipped for all emergencies. Injured or ill employees requiring more than initial first aid are taken immediately to Jefferson Memorial Hospital.
	There is a set of comprehensive standing orders, written through collaborative effort by the nurse and doctor. Yearly physicals include chest x-ray, blood work that includes benzene screening, urinalysis, vision and hearing assessments, and physical exams by the physician. Pregnant women are seen each month by the doctor in addition to their own private doctors. No screening programs alone are done, but they are incorporated into the yearly physical. Health teaching and informal counseling are done on an individual basis by the nurse and doctor.
	CPR is taught to selected personnel throughout the plant by the nurse.
Existing facilities and resources	The medical department consists of one full-time nurse and a physician who cover this plant and AAB's larger plant near Avina, as well as a part-time secretary. The facilities include the nurse's office, where all medical records are kept and where employees check in when visiting the clinic; a treatment room; a small lab and dispensary; an x-ray room; an exam room; and the physician's office. First aid facilities are extensive and well supplied. EKG equipment also is available.
	The nurse sees between 12 and 15 clients per day in the clinic. The major reasons employees seek health care are nonoccupationally related sicknesses or accidents, stress-related complaints, and minor accidents on the job.
Stressors	
Employees	Job pressure, as with operators who control the process units
	Over-time hours, when worked frequently

(*continued*)

TABLE 6-22. *(Continued)*

Components	Description
Health providers	Knowledge of potential fire or explosion
	Shift work that may not be in sync with normal body rhythms
	Strikes or lay-offs
	Problems with role definition. Nurse wishes to do more health teaching, but feels Safety Department has taken over many of her functions. Feels powerless to change the situation. Feels that physician also perceives her role as limited to specific, traditional areas.

(*Text continued from page 206*)

SAFETY AND TRANSPORTATION

Table 6-26 lists the major components of safety and transportation that affect the community.

Protection Services

Fire, police, and sanitation services are provided by the city of Hampton. Rosemont residents pay for these services through their city taxes. Therefore, these services are extra-community, located outside the community of Rosemont.

TABLE 6-23.   ROSEMONT LABOR FORCE, 1980

	CT 402	CT 403	Hampton
Persons 16 and over	4580	6470	1,189,136
Labor force	1825	5472	850,389
Percent of persons 16 and over	39.8	85.4	71.5

(Data from 1980 Census of Population and Housing)

TABLE 6-24.   CLASS OF WORKER, ROSEMONT, 1980

	CT 402		CT 403	
	Number	*Total %*	*Number*	*Total %*
Private wage and salary	1219	67	4168	76
Government	326	18	664	12
Local government	238	13	307	6
Self employed	42	2	333	6
Total	ˉ825	100	5472	100

(Data from 1980 Census of Population and Housing)

Fire protection

The fire department and MEAS are combined in Hampton. (For a description of the MEAS, see the Health and Social Services section.)

   The fire station serving Rosemont maintains two fire trucks, one air boat (for evacuations during flooding), and 20 personnel. Firemen must complete 335 hours of basic certification courses. The fire captain reports a response

TABLE 6-25.   OCCUPATIONS, ROSEMONT, 1980

	CT 402		CT 403	
	Number	*Total %*	*Number*	*Total %*
Managerial and professional specialty	117	7.1	2238	42.1
Technical, sales, administrative support	198	12.1	1813	34.1
Service	724	44.2	560	10.5
Farming	28	1.7	11	0.2
Precision production	186	11.3	463	8.7
Operators, fabricators, laborers	387	23.6	230	4.3
Total	1640	100	5315	100

(Data from 1980 Census of Population and Housing)

TABLE 6-26.   SAFETY AND TRANSPORTATION

	Sources of Information
Safety	
Protection services	Planning office (city, county, state)
Fire	Fire department (local)
Police	Police Department (city, county)
Sanitation	
Waste Sources and Treatment	Waste and water treatment plants
Solid Waste	
Air quality	Air control board (state, regional, and local offices)
Transportation	
Private	
Transportation sources	Census data. Population and Housing Characteristics
Number of Persons with a Transportation Disability	
Public	
Bus Service (routes, schedules, fares)	Local and city transportation authorities
Roads (number and condition; primary, secondary and farm-to-market roads)	State Highway department
Interstate Highways	
Freeway System	
Air Service (Private and Public-Owned)	Local airports (Note: Local airports are frequently owned and operated by city government)
Rail Service	In the United States, AMTRAK is the primary source of intercity rail transportation.

time of less than 10 minutes. During the past 90 days previous to the analysis, the station responded to 45 fires. This compares to 39 responses during the same period one year ago. Forty responses were to homes—the major culprit being grease fires that started in the kitchen. Other leading causes of fires include children playing with matches, and lighted cigarettes. In addition to responding to fires, personnel perform safety checks of homes, teach fire prevention classes to school and community groups, and distribute window stickers that specify the location of children, elderly citizens and pets for emergency alert during a fire.

Police protection

The police department serving Rosemont has a staff of 27 full-time employees, including 21 police officers and 6 civilians (4 dispatchers and 2 record clerks). Equipment includes five marked and four unmarked patrol cars, two motorcycles, and a complete computerized data storage and retrieval system. This station has one holding cell where persons are detained until they can be transported to the Hampton Jail.

According to the dispatcher, response time to Rosemont is four to six minutes. Crime statistics for CT 402 and CT 403 are presented in Table 6-27.

The most frequent crimes are burglaries and thefts, which the police captain feels are committed mainly by nonresidents of Rosemont. Speeding, and driving while intoxicated (DWI) are also frequent crimes in Rosemont, although following the addition of two motorcycle policemen two years ago, the number of traffic accidents has decreased by 38%. The police department offers the following services to Rosemont residents

- Housewatch—When residents are out of town, the police will check their house three times a day for up to 30 days.
- Identification—The police department loans an engraver to citizens who wish to engrave personal belongings. The department also provides household possessions registration and pamphlets on how to protect one's home from burglary.

TABLE 6-27. CRIME STATISTICS FOR CT 402 AND CT 403

	1980		1981		1982		1983	
	CT 402	*CT 403*	*CT 402*	*CT 403*	*CT 402*	*CT 403*	*CT 402*	*CT 403*
Murder	5	3	7	7	8	6	10	3
Rape	24	19	22	18	27	11	34	17
Robbery	196	100	204	104	252	165	328	186
Aggravated assault	40	17	47	27	58	27	94	29
Burglary	263	288	274	279	295	321	345	339
Theft	403	462	423	371	397	384	384	363
Vehicle theft	103	144	113	214	112	232	109	327
Total	1034	1033	1090	1020	1149	1146	1304	1264

(Data from City of Hampton Police Department)

- Fingerprinting—Fingerprinting is done and a record provided to the person for personal identification, as well as immigration requirements. The police department is presently pursuing a special project, a citywide campaign to fingerprint all children and adolescents. A copy of the fingerprint record is given to parents and a copy remains with the police. Following several weeks of radio and TV announcements, police personnel are now present at local shopping centers every weekend to explain and complete the fingerprinting process. This special project is in response to citizen concern and requests for police assistance in locating an increasing number of missing children.
- Animal Protection Officer—The city of Hampton has a leash and fence law for dogs. The animal protection officer picks up stray animals and detains them in the city kennel until the owner or an adopter can be found.
- Public Education—Crime prevention programs are offered to community and school groups.

Residents of Rosemont repeatedly voiced concern about their personal safety. Elderly citizens expressed fear of being mugged and related stories of friends who have been harassed and robbed during the day as they walked to and from local stores. (One area grocery store owner reported that he has stopped cashing social security checks because so many patrons had been mugged after leaving his store.) The feeling of being a prisoner in one's own home was repeatedly expressed, as were questions regarding what people could do to protect themselves.

Homosexual males described experiences of perceived harassment by police, as well as incidences of marked delay (up to 30 minutes) in police response time to requests for help. Residents reported that brawls, quarrels, and physical violence are becoming commonplace in Rosemont. The citizens are concerned for themselves and others; they want a safe place to live.

Sanitation

Water sources and treatment

The terrain of Rosemont is flat with minimal changes in elevation. Stagnant pools of water are common—a situation that promotes mosquito populations during the warm months. Drainage is toward the northeast and into Buff's Bayou, the only open stream in Rosemont. All storm water and sewage is gathered into Hampton's sewage system. There is no separate system for storm water disposal. As a result, during a heavy rain raw sewage backs up and residents complain of the smell and problems associated with toilets that cannot be flushed.

Sewage from Rosemont is treated at the 5th Street Plant. Presently a sewage moratorium exists for Rosemont owing to overcapacity at the 5th Street Plant. Consequently, only single-family dwellings can be built on plotted lots. Builders requesting permits for multifamily dwellings are given the option of delaying building indefinitely *or* being assessed a fee based on projected occupancy of their building and the associated gallons of sewage that will be produced. The assessed fee is used to increase the capacity of the treatment plant. However, even if the assessed fee option is chosen, it may be three to four years before the permit is issued.

Potable (drinking) water for Rosemont comes from Lake Hampton located 20 miles north of the city. Residents are concerned about possible contamination of the drinking water with arsenic and heavy metals. Presently there is no routine testing of the drinking water except to meet state health requirements for chlorine content. Fluoride is not added to the Rosemont's drinking water, nor does it occur naturally.

Solid waste

Garbage is collected twice weekly; residents state the service and frequency is adequate. The major complaint is that illegal dumping of large items, such as refrigerators, stoves, and so forth, has increased and despite numerous calls to proper authorities, the trash is not cleaned up with any regularity. Parents are concerned that children, attracted by abandoned machinery and appliances, may be hurt as they explore. In addition, inoperable automobiles are abandoned in parking spaces on the streets and months can pass before the cars are removed by the city.

Air quality

The Federal Air Quality Act of 1967 provided for the establishment of air-quality control regions. Regional offices maintain an inventory of air-pollution sources and monitor air status. In similar fashion, individual states formed air-quality boards that developed air-quality standards and long-range air-quality programs. Local air-monitoring stations sample and record information levels on such pollutants as ozone, carbon monoxide, sulfur dioxide, and nitrogen dioxide. In addition, some 30 to 40 suspended particles in the air (solids) are measured and recorded, as are certain gaseous substances (*e.g.*, ammonia).

To assess the air quality of Rosemont, the local air control office was contacted. Recent reports of the air control board document a rise in air pollution. Area pollution is attributed to an increase in industrial growth and a high population density. Some 25 miles east of Rosemont is a large industrial complex and although the daily emissions from the industries are within acceptable limits, certain wind and temperature patterns act to compound emissions. This causes a visible yellow haze to form that shrouds Rosemont and surrounding communities many days of the year. Area residents complain of eye irritation and increased frequency of respiratory conditions. The chemical reactions that lead to the haze and the contribution of automotive and industrial emissions, as well as potential health effects associated with the haze are unknowns presently being researched.

NOTE: Air pollution is a frequently-used term; it means the presence of one or more contaminants in such concentration and of such duration that they may adversely affect human health, animal life, vegetation, or property.

Despite the pollution increase and industrial growth there has been no significant increase in the amount of pollutants introduced into the atmosphere surrounding Rosemont. This is attributed to compliance of industries with the Air Control Board regulations and permit system for new industries. Citizens can contest industry construction permits; and through this process provide a forum for public opinion and objections that regulation boards take into consideration during the permit decision-making process. Citizens also are entitled to complain to the Board regarding a specific industry's emissions; the Board will then investigate and file a report.

During the past year, Rosemont has experienced three air stagnation advisories. Because the pollution concentration is greater than usual, persons with respiratory conditions such as bronchitis and emphysema are advised to remain indoors and limit outside activities until the air stagnation clears.

NOTE: Air stagnation occurs when a layer of cool air is trapped by a layer of warmer air above it; the bottom air cannot rise and pollutants cannot be dispersed.

The Board feels citizens are ill-informed regarding the meaning of and the appropriate actions that should be taken during air stagnation advisories, as well as each citizen's responsibility in minimizing pollution. For example, citizens seem unaware that transportation sources, not industry, are the major contributors of air-pollution problems; and that a citizen who burns leaves or trash is releasing tiny particles of matter into the air that can irritate eyes, nose, and lungs. To promote public awareness and understanding, the local office makes presentations to organizations, schools, and citizen groups. Numerous public television and radio programs were planned for the year following the assessment.

Transportation

Private

The primary means of transportation in Rosemont include: walking, bicycle riding, private automobiles, Hampton city buses, Hampton city vans (special transportation for the elderly and handicapped), and school buses.

The major source of private transportation is the automobile. Table 6-28 presents the types of transportation used to commute to work and Table 6-29 indicates the number of persons 16 years of age or older that have a transportation disability. According to the 1980 census data, mean travel time to work for Rosemont residents is 17.7 minutes as compared to 26.6 minutes for Hampton residents.

TABLE 6-28. TRANSPORTATION SOURCES TO WORK THAT ARE USED BY RESIDENTS OF CT 402 AND CT 403

	CT 402		CT 403	
	Number	*Total %*	*Number*	*Total %*
Drive alone	1351	42.8	3279	63.8
Carpool	749	23.7	808	15.7
Public transportation	721	22.8	567	11
Walk	231	7.3	300	5.8
Other means	79	2.5	130	2.5
Work at home	27	0.9	58	1.2
Total	3158	100	5142	100

(Data from 1980 Census of Population and Housing.)

TABLE 6-29. NONINSTITUTIONALIZED PERSONS
16 YEARS OF AGE OR OLDER BY
TRANSPORTATION DISABILITY STATUS
FOR CT 402 AND CT 403

	With Disability		Without Disability		Total	
	Number	*Total %*	*Number*	*Total %*	*Number*	*Total %*
Age 16–64						
CT 402	221	5.9	3495	94.1	3716	100
CT 403	15	0.3	5908	99.7	5923	100
Age 65 and Over						
CT 402	197	21.3	728	78.7	925	100
CT 403	55	10.5	469	89.5	524	100

(Data from 1980 Census of Population and Housing.)

Public

The major source of public transportation within Rosemont and surrounding communities is the Hampton bus system. The city provides east–west bus service at half-hour intervals throughout the days on Pecan Drive and Live Oak Boulevard. The same service is provided on north–south routes for Way Drive, Rosemont Boulevard and Hampton Street. For persons that qualify (*e.g.,* the elderly and/or handicapped), the bus company provides door-to-door service from the individual's home to essential services such as food shopping or medical-care visits. The cost of this service varies from $0.50 to $1.00 per trip according to geographic area. Although all users agree the service is reliable, it is only available Monday through Friday, 8:30 am to 5:00 pm, and reservations are required several days in advance—a requirement that is impossible to meet in situations such as during acute illnesses.

Roads

Jefferson County has adequate primary, secondary, and farm-to-market roads. In addition, several miles of a freeway system circle of Hampton. Two major interstate highways transect Hampton and the State Highway Department has budgeted two billion dollars for highway construction and maintenance for Jefferson County over the next 20 years. Recently, the residents of Jefferson County (of which Rosemont is a part) voted for an additional tax devoted entirely to improving intra-county transportation. Rosemont residents complain of congested freeways and damaged roads that go without repair for months. The need was expressed for a road system that efficiently handles local traffic.

Air service

Jefferson County has four small, privately owned airports. The city of Hampton owns and operates two airports; both provide national and international service.

Rail service

Amtrak connects Hampton to other major cities in the state, as well as other states. There are no private or public commuter rail services within Jefferson County or Hampton.

POLITICS AND GOVERNMENT

Rosemont falls within the city limits of Hampton, which has a mayor–council form of government. There are 14 council members (five at-large), one of whom represents Rosemont and nearby communities. Each serves a two-year term. The City Council meets at City Hall on the first Tuesday of each month. The meetings are open to the public and Rosemont residents often attend.

The city council and mayor comprise the policy-making body, as well as the administrative head of Hampton. Their duties include the following: maintaining competent staff to operate all city services (the health department and police, for instance), passing ordinances, and appropriating funds to carry out policies.

The councilman for District Three, which includes Rosemont, is James Browning. Councilman Browning was elected by a wide margin of votes and has been popular with the Rosemont community because he has spearheaded the fight against sexually-oriented businesses (the ''SOB Fight'' as it popularly is called). This issue has not been settled and the citizens are supporting Councilman Browning's re-election so that he may continue the fight.

The active participation in the Hampton council of Councilman Browning is only one indicator of Rosemont's politics. There are several politically oriented organizations and civic clubs in the area, all of which seek to improve the quality of life in Rosemont and help to support inter-community activities.

A brief synopsis of several organizations that are politically active in Rosemont is presented in Table 6-30. (Contact person, address and phone number should be included in such lists, but have been omitted from this description.)

TABLE 6-30. ORGANIZATIONS POLITICALLY ACTIVE IN ROSEMONT

	Description
Neartown Business Alliance (Founded: 1949)	Owners of businesses in the area meet monthly and work to promote the area and its businesses. The alliance contributes to campaigns of supporters of Rosemont.
Gay Political Caucus (Founded: 1964)	This is a very active and visible group. It works to influence elections through voter registration, campaign work, and education. It has been credited with the election or defeat of certain candidates. Membership is open to all interested in community improvement. It meets on third Tuesday, 7:00 pm.
Rosemont Firehouse (Founded: 1973)	This is a coordination and referral group; it operates a 24-hour crisis hotline. It is sponsored by donations from most of the area's churches as well as the civic groups, and most of the workers are community volunteers.
Rosemont Watch (Founded: 1978)	The Watch works to prevent crime in the area through education and visible activities such as "Block Awareness Week." It coordinates activities with the Hampton City Police. All citizens are encouraged to become involved. It meets monthly.
Seniors for a Safe Community (Founded: 1980)	Comprised primarily of retired persons (but open to all interested residents), this group was formed to address the problem of the mugging or robbing of senior citizens, especially on the days in which social security checks arrived. The original small group has expanded, as have their goals, so that now they are actively involved in promoting a better quality of life for all in the community (with a special emphasis on the elderly). This group is active in the "SOB Fight" and also works closely with Rosemont Watch.

A number of other groups in the community are less visible and active unless an issue of particular interest becomes "hot." For instance, many voluntary agencies such as the American Lung Association—Hampton Chapter are located in the community and can be called upon to assist specific campaigns (*e.g.,* smoking-prevention programs in the schools or antipollution campaigns aimed toward extra-community sources). The Community Services Directory lists all such organizations both by interest (*e.g.,* heart, lung, crime, etc.) and general area (Rosemont groups can usually be found under, "Southwest, near downtown").

Political activism is evident throughout Rosemont: during election years there are campaign posters everywhere; talk at gathering places (barbershops, grocery stores, bars) inevitably turns to politics; and numerous rallies are held in support of candidates or issues. In Rosemont there appear to be two major political factions. Voting records show CT 403 residents to be more liberal than residents in CT 402. This may reflect the fact that CT 403 is comprised of more affluent, younger, and professional residents than is CT 402.

COMMUNICATION

Communication may be formal or informal. Formal communication usually originates outside the community (extra-community) as opposed to informal communication, which almost always originates and is disseminated within the community. Salient components of formal and informal communication, as well as sources of data are presented in Table 6-31.

Formal Communication

Hampton has one major newspaper, *The Hampton Herald*. Additional daily newspapers include a business journal, *Current Issues;* a black-oriented paper, *Progress;* one Spanish-language paper, *La Prensa;* and a Vietnamese tabloid. Hampton has 12 AM stations and 10 FM stations, six commercial TV stations and one educational network. Cable television is available to Rosemont residents on a monthly subscription basis. Residents receive home mail delivery.

Informal Communication

Bulletin boards and posters dot community and municipal buildings in Rosemont. Posters are placed on trees and tacked to buildings throughout the

TABLE 6-31.   COMMUNICATIONS

Components	Sources of Information
Formal	Chamber of Commerce
	Newspaper office
Newspaper (number, circulation, frequency, scope of news)	Telephone Company
	Yellow Pages
Radio and television (number of stations, commercial versus educational, audience)	Telephone book
	Census data on phone use
Postal service	
Telephone status (number of residents with service)	
Informal	
Sources: bulletin boards; posters; hand-delivered fliers; church, civic, school newsletters	Windshield survey
	Talking to residents
Dissemination (How do people receive information?)	Survey
Word of mouth	
Mail	
Radio, television	

community and a rainbow of handfliers can be seen tucked into fence and door crevices. Radio and television announcements herald forthcoming events, and offer open forums on community issues. The Rosemont Civic Association publishes a four-page newsletter bi-monthly to notify residents of upcoming meetings and social activities. Polls and surveys are a regular feature of the newsletter that is distributed free to all residents.

Key informants within Rosemont include the civic association secretary, local ministers, fire and police personnel, as well as community civic board members. People can be seen "chatting" throughout Rosemont and when asked how information is received, all of the above formal and informal sources were mentioned.

EDUCATION

The general educational status of a community can be summarized using census data. Census information lists the number of residents attending schools, years of schooling completed, and percentage of residents who speak English. To supplement this broad assessment, information is needed about major educational sources (*e.g.,* schools, colleges, and libraries) located inside the community. Table 6-32 is a suggested guide for assessing a community's educational sources.

> NOTE: It is sometimes difficult to decide which educational sources to include in the assessment. Community usage is probably the single most important indicator. Primary and secondary schools attended by the majority of youngsters in a community, regardless of intra- or extra-community location, are major educational sources and require a thorough assessment, whereas schools composed primarily of students from outside the community do not require such an extensive appraisal.

Educational Status

Table 6-33 presents the years of schooling completed by adults in CT 402 and CT 403. In a similar format, Table 6-34 lists school enrollment by type of

---

TABLE 6-32.   EDUCATION

Components	Sources of Information
Educational Status	
Years of school completed	Census data—Social characteristics section
School enrollment by type of school	Census data—Social characteristics section
Language spoken	Census data—Social characteristics section
Educational Sources	
Intra-community *or* Extra-community (collect data for each facility)	Local Board of Education
Services (educational, recreational, communication, health)	School administrator (*e.g.,* principal, director), school nurse
Resources (personnel, space, budget, record system)	School administrator
Characteristics of users (geographic distribution, demographic profile)	Teachers and staff
Adequacy, accessibility, and acceptability of education to students and staff	Students and staff

TABLE 6-33.   YEARS OF SCHOOL COMPLETED
FOR CT 402, CT 403, AND HAMPTON

	CT 402	CT 403	Hampton
Persons 25 years and over	3459	4948	888,269
Elementary			
0 to 4 years	611	26	41,695
5 to 7 years	665	164	66,775
8 years	409	101	37,373
High School			
1 to 3 years	800	278	136,179
4 years	661	914	240,320
College			
1 to 3 years	181	1173	160,999
4 or more years	132	2292	204,928
% High school graduates	28.2	88.5	68.3

TABLE 6-34.   SCHOOL ENROLLMENT AND TYPE
OF SCHOOL FOR CT 402, CT 403,
AND HAMPTON

	CT 402	CT 403	Hampton
Type of School			
Public nursery school	94	44	20,735
Private nursery school	77	44	15,427
Public kindergarten	194	14	21,863
Private kindergarten	25	14	4,833
Public elementary (1 to 8 yr)	1258	186	198,367
Private elementary (1 to 8 yr)	10	136	18,440
Public high school (1 to 4 yr)	482	92	94,099
Private high school (1 to 4 yr)	12	25	7,154
College	92	922	78,472
Total enrolled in schools (age 3 years and over)	2120	1258	413,536

(Data from 1980 Census of Population and Housing.)

school and Table 6-35 presents the number and percentage of community residents who speak English.

Educational Sources

Intra-community

Temple Elementary School is located on the corner of Pecan Drive and Magnolia Drive, close to the center of CT 402. Asphalt lots bound three sides of Temple, two are used for vehicle parking and one is for play. A small patch of grass persists on the remaining side, a fenced-in area that contains several large trees, a swing set, and three teeter-totters. Several broken windows were seen, and no graffiti was noted.

Temple is in its 54th year of continuous operation; teaching grades kindergarten to eighth. Present enrollment is 924: 42% of the students are black; 33%, Asian; 18%, hispanic; and 5%, white. Most of the children live in Rosemont and either walk to school or ride the school bus (provided for children living further than two miles from Temple). As part of the Hampton School District (HSD), Temple receives funding from the district revenues obtained from local property taxes, state coffers, and the federal budget. State monies to HSD are based upon average daily attendance of students at each school. Most policies affecting Temple are formed and enforced by the HSD Board. The Board is composed of eight nonsalaried persons, each elected from one of eight regions in the school district. Each term of office is four years. Board member Jane Roberts represents Rosemont; at the time of assessment, she was in the second year of her four-year term. Responsibilities of the HSD board

TABLE 6-35. ABILITY TO SPEAK ENGLISH FOR CT 402, CT 403, AND HAMPTON

| | Percentage Who Speak English Poorly or Not at All | |
	Age 5–17 Yrs	Age 18 Yrs and Over
CT 402	75.9	73.8
CT 403	11	19.3
Hampton	21.4	26.2

(Data from 1980 Census of Population and Housing.)

include: prescribing qualifications of employees, establishing salary schedules, setting goals and objectives for the district, establishing the policies to implement the goals and objectives, and evaluating the performance of the district in relationship to adopted goals and objectives. The General Superintendent is the administrative head of the Board. The superintendent is salaried and actively recruited by the Board.

Temples' principal cited truancy and the related problem of academic failure as the school's major problems. According to office records, some 6% to 8% of the student body is absent each day and most are not ill. Compounding the problem is the fact that many parents do not have phones. As a result it is not uncommon for a youngster to be absent two or three days before parental contact is made. (Almost always it is found that the parent assumed the child was in school.) The principal believed that truancy is most common among seventh and eighth graders, especially among hispanic boys. Regarding bilingual education for non-English speaking students, the principal felt that all classes should be in English and the presence of bilingual education at Temple only slows the progress of the children who are learning English. Presently there are two bilingual teachers at Temple; they reported that they have a list of over 100 youngsters who have requested and have been assessed as needing the bilingual program.

Teachers repeatedly stated the need for improved communication with parents. Teachers felt that parents need to have current information about their child's learning needs and school performance, as well as a knowledge of specific techniques for fostering academic achievement. (Presently school policy allows for two, 20-minute, parent–teacher conferences yearly—a time allotment that was rated as extremely inadequate by the teachers.) The teachers reported that 22% of the student body at Temple failed last year. Major impediments to learning were listed as: poor English-speaking skills and understanding of English, stressful home environments, and inadequate adult supervision at home. Teachers felt overwhelmed and frustrated; the average employment stay at Temple is two years.

The school nurse at Temple is present two days a week; she is at West Hampton High the remaining three days. A review of the daily clinic register for the preceding six weeks noted a clinic attendance of 141; the majority (72%) were complaints of a stomach or headache. Although none of the stomach ailments required early dismissal, 60% of the headaches were associated with fever and necessitated early dismissal from school. Remaining complaints were sore throats and minor cuts or falls. All children were screened biannually for vision and hearing problems. The nurse recognized the need for yearly screening but said she lacked the necessary time. She stated that if school policy would permit the recruitment and training of a parent volunteer(s), then yearly screening would be feasible. In addition to vision and hearing testing, all children are screened for head lice twice a year; children found to be infected are dismissed from school and are not readmitted until they have been successfully treated. Some 62% of the youngsters participate in the free lunch program. The nurse expressed concern that several children who appear undernourished (*i.e.,* low weight for height, and small arm circumference for age) do not qualify for the lunch program, whereas others who appear to be well-nourished do qualify. Eligibility is based on family size and income.

Major health problems as described by the nurse include: lack of hygiene (children frequently come to school dirty and inadequately clothed for cold weather), dental caries, high (30%–40%) annual incidence of youngsters with head lice, especially in primary grades (kindergarten, 1st, and 2nd), incomplete immunization status (92% of the youngsters have up-to-date immunizations), and lack of parent follow-through for needed medical care and treatment during illnesses. To assess dental status the nurse performed oral assessment of children who came to the clinic during one four-week period. She found 62% of the children to have discolored areas or cavitations in the pits of their teeth or between teeth. Most of the youngsters stated they had never been to a dentist and many reported frequent tooth pain and difficulty chewing.

Presently the nurse does not do any health teaching in the classroom because school policy mandates that the nurse be present in the clinic at all times. The ruling causes considerable frustration as the nurse's participation in the teaching and promotion of health habits is restricted to one-to-one clinic encounters (a time when the child is ill and not receptive to learning). When asked about staff and teacher usage of the clinic, the nurse discussed at length the need for health information expressed by both teachers and staff. Questions regarding exercise, stress, and diet modifications are common. The nurse would like to assess and identify specific health needs of staff and teachers.

As a community service, Temple sponsors scout troops, a basketball and softball team, and provides a meeting place for several newly formed church and community-action groups. In addition, Monday through Thursday nights, Temple houses extension courses from Hampton Community College. A full range of subjects is offered, including academic, vocational, and enrichment courses. Present enrollment exceeds 1200, an increase of 22% from the previous year.

All Rosemont residents were familiar with Temple Elementary and most had children that attended Temple or they themselves attended Temple as youngsters. Residents felt Temple was a community landmark and symbol of unity that links one generation to the next. The primary complaint, repeated by several families, was a perceived insensitivity of Temples' staff and teachers to ethnic and racial differences and needs. For example, all school notices are written in English, and all programs offered by the Parent Teachers Organization (PTO) are presented in English. Both asian and hispanic parents have brought specific concerns and needs to the staff and teachers at Temple, but have repeatedly been told that all parental requests must come from appropriate PTO committees–an organization that seems alien to many asian and hispanic parents.

One daycare center is located in CT 402—the Busybee Nursery. There are no daycare facilities in CT 403. Housed in a renovated building, the Busybee accepts children aged two to five years. Some 60 youngsters are cared for by five staff and 43 children (primarily toddlers) are on the waiting list. The center is licensed by the state. Rosemont residents repeatedly lamented the lack of daycare facilities. Many parents felt forced to leave their young children with other mothers or teenagers who have dropped out of school. Several mothers reported leaving their children daily with a babysitter who cares for from eight to ten youngsters.

The Rosemont library is conveniently located adjacent to the main shopping district and offers a variety of adult, teen, and youth book programs, films, and special educational activities. Notices of all programs are published in the Rosemont civic association newsletter and posted on local bulletin boards.

Extra-community

High school students from Rosemont attend Central Hampton High, a complex that houses 4800 students and is located eight miles from Rosemont. Concerned about truancy and grade failure, Central Hampton began a "Failproof" program two years ago. Some 82% of students and their parents have participated. As a result, school scores on state and national proficiency tests have improved and truancy has decreased. The principal described numerous community outreach services offered by the school, including recreational programs in the evening and on the weekends, as well as a full compliment of adult education courses.

The nurse at Central Hampton is present five days a week. The majority of visits to the clinic (an average of 30 daily) are allergy-related complaints, gastrointestinal upsets, and minor sprains or strains that occur during physical exercise class. Because of HSD policies, the high school nurse also is prohibited from offering health education in the classroom.

The nurse's major concern is the increased number of teenage pregnancies and the HSD Board's decision of two years ago not to permit sex education information in the classroom. Classes in sexuality, sexually transmitted disease, contraception, and decision-making in the area of sexual activity had been offered at all high schools in Hampton prior to the new ruling. The nurse does not know the sequence of events that resulted in the sex-education decision. A second major concern is the increased use of alcohol among students. A drug-awareness curriculum was prepared by the State Board of Education and will be implemented during the next semester as part of the biology courses' content.

Numerous private preschool and grade schools are available in Hampton and some are used by the residents of Rosemont, especially persons in CT 403. Some 20 colleges and universities are located in Hampton and Jefferson County; most offer a variety of general-education and specialty-training programs. One unique aspect of the educational resources is Hampton Community College, a junior college that provides classes in 21 public schools in Hampton and Jefferson County. (Temple Elementary is one of these campuses.) Numerous residents state that they prefer Hampton Community College to other area resources because of its convenient locations, low tuition, and employment-oriented approach to education.

RECREATION

The recreation facilities within and adjacent to Rosemont are listed in Table 6-36 and pictured in Figure 6-3. With the exception of the schoolyards, there is very little recreation area for children, and almost none for adults and teenagers. Although there are funds in the budget of the Hampton Parks and Recreation Department for the acquisition of parks, there are no plans for any development in the Rosemont area. However, the city has recently begun an improvement program along the banks of Buff's Bayou in order to create a "River Walk" similar to those in other cities with rivers. It will be several years before the project is completed.

The Rosemont Sports Association, according to its president, provides "quality organized recreation opportunities" for the Rosemont people. Pro-

TABLE 6-36.   RECREATIONAL FACILITIES IN ROSEMONT
AND ADJACENT AREAS

	Acreage	Location	Facilities
San Juan	2.6	1650 Pleasant	Shelter building, playground equipment, softball field, baseball field
Richards	1	1414 Redbud	Shelter building, playground equipment, picnic area, basketball court (swimming pool recently filled in)
Applehurst	1.9	600 Water Oak	Recreation center, rest room, playground equipment, picnic area, tennis, basketball, and volleyball courts
Jeckle Park	0.08	1500 Maple	None
Buff's Bayou	?	"Greens" along the bayou	Park benches, jogging–bicycle trail

(City of Hampton, Parks and Recreation Department, interview with JB, (Director), May, 1984)

grams consist of teams for winter bowling, spring bowling, summer bowling, softball, flag football, tennis, and so forth. The Rosemont Sports Association, however, is open only to members who pay a fee of $20 per year.

Churches of Rosemont (two were visited, see the Social Services section) offer a wide variety of activities for all ages. Exercise classes, craft classes, Mother's Day Out, preschool classes, senior citizens' groups, and many other programs are available to church members. Although other community residents are welcome to take advantage of these activities, the persons interviewed at the churches reported that their participants are almost all church members.

Several residents spoke of an area along the northern bank of Buff's Bayou (just east of Way Drive) that is used as a gathering place by residents who live nearby. Families take their children there on summer evenings so that parents can visit while the children play. The only facilities at this area are benches that have been placed along the grassy area.

A bicycle/jogging trail follows the bayou for several miles and is popular with the "health conscious" residents who use it frequently, especially in the early morning and late evening hours. Some people have expressed fear of being mugged while using this trail, but there have been no official reports of crime in this area over the past year. The trail and all the land along the bayou are maintained by the city of Hampton.

The area residents of the east side tend to congregate for recreation on sidewalks and in neighborhood bars. The one playground in the area, other than the one at Temple Elementary, is located adjacent to the Audubon Parkway Village (the low-rent housing complex), but it is used exclusively by the residents of that complex. The playground equipment is very poor and there is virtually no grass left in the area. The Parks and Recreation Department has no plans to upgrade or replace the equipment or to replant the grass.

There is one movie theater and one theater for stage production in the Rosemont Community, but movie theaters are accessible and near almost all areas. Other forms of evening entertainment are reflected in the numerous bars and restaurants that feature live music (as was mentioned in the physical examination of the community).

Extra-community recreational facilities abound. A large city park that includes museums, a zoo, a bandshell, and picnic areas is less than a mile to the south of Rosemont. Another city park in downtown Hampton, called Serenity Park, is less than a mile to the northeast.

Virtually every major league sport has a team in Hampton. The sports arenas are some distance from the area but there is adequate bus service to them.

There is an abundance of music and theater available to those who can afford it. Hampton has a symphony orchestra, a ballet, both grand and light opera, and legitimate stage company, to name a few options.

In addition, water activities such as boating and fishing are as close as 30 miles away. According to several residents of Audubon Parkway Village, a special day out includes crabbing along the bay—which is often a successful endeavor to fill the dinner pot, as well as a fun day for the whole family.

SUMMARY

The community assessment is complete. A description of each community subsystem has been recorded. The next step is *analysis,* a process that synthesizes the assessment information and derives from it nursing diagnoses specific to the community. Crucial to community assessment is a model, or map, to direct and guide the assessment process. The model shown in Figure 6-1 was used to guide the assessment of Rosemont. In the Suggested Reading list several other approaches to community assessment have been presented. Consider these sources as you continue your practice of community health assessment.

SUGGESTED READINGS

Aneshensel CS, Frerichs RR, Clark VA, Yokopenic MA: Telephone versus in-person surveys of community health status. Amer J Public Health 72(9):1017–1021, 1982

Braden CJ: Herban NL: Assessment. In Braden CJ, Herban NL (eds): Community health: A systems approach, New York, Appleton-Century-Crofts, 1976

Cordes SM: Assessing health care needs: Elements and processes. Family & Health Care 1(2):1–16, 1978

Griffith JW, Christensen PJ: Nursing assessment: Data collection of the community client. In: Nursing process: Application of theories, frameworks, and models, p. 66. St. Louis, CV Mosby, 1982

Knight JH: Applying nursing process in the community. Nurs Outlook 22(11):708–711, 1974

Luce BR, Stamps PL: An approach to accessibility analysis. Amer J Public Health 66(6):581–582, 1976

Ruybal SE, Bauwens E, Fasla MJ: Community assessment: An epidemiologic approach. Nurs outlook 23(6):365–368, 1975

Serafini P: Nursing assessment in industry. Amer J Public Health 66(8):755–760, 1976

Sheahan SL, Aaron PR: Community assessment: An essential component of practice. Health Values 7(5):September–October, 1982

Stewart M: Community health assessment: A systematic approach. Nursing Papers 14(1):30–47, 1982

7

Analysis and Nursing Diagnosis

OBJECTIVES

This chapter is focused on the second phase of the nursing process, *analysis,* and the associated task of forming community nursing diagnoses. After studying the chapter, you will be able to

- Critically analyze community-assessment data
- Formulate community-nursing diagnoses

INTRODUCTION

Analysis is the study and examination of data. Analysis is necessary to determine community health needs and community strengths, as well as to identify patterns of health responses and trends in health care use. During analysis, any need for further data collection is revealed as gaps and incongruencies in community assessment data surface.

COMMUNITY ANALYSIS

To analyze community assessment data, it is helpful to first *categorize the data.* Data can be categorized in a variety of ways. Traditional categories of community-assessment data include

1. Demographic characteristics (*e.g.,* family size, age, sex, ethnic, and racial groupings)
2. Geographic characteristics (*e.g.,* area boundaries, number and size of neighborhoods, public spaces, and roads)
3. Socioeconomic characteristics (*e.g.,* occupation and income categories, educational attainment, and rental or home-ownership patterns)
4. Health resources and services (*e.g.,* hospitals, clinics, mental health centers, and so forth)

However, models are being used increasingly in the organization and analysis of community health data because they provide a framework for data collection and a map to guide analysis. Because the Community Assessment Wheel (see Figure 6-1) was used to direct the community assessment process in the Rosemont sample study, the same model can be used to guide analysis. Each of the community subsystems will be analyzed and components within each subsystem specify the categories to be evaluated.

Once a categorization method has been selected, the next task is to *summarize the data* within each category. Both summary statements and summary measures such as rates, charts, and graphs are required.

> NOTE: Many health care agencies and educational institutions have access to computerized information systems—a system through which formated data can be retrieved in a variety of forms—including summary health statistics. For example, data entered into a computer system as census figures can be configured into population pyramids, and census and vital statistics information can be programmed to calculate birth, death, and fertility rates. Calculations that previously required hours to complete are now computed in seconds. In your practice, make it a point to inquire as to the availability of computer systems and, if possible, use computer processes to complete data analysis.

Additional tasks of data analysis include the *identification of data gaps, incongruencies, and omissions.* Frequently, comparative data are needed to determine if a pattern or trend exists, or data do not seem correct and the need for revalidation of original information is required. Data gaps are inevitable, as are mistakes in recording data; the important task is to analyze data critically and be aware of the potential for gaps and omissions. To have professional colleagues review the analysis is helpful. Every person has a unique perspective; it is only through the sharing of views that a whole and comprehensive picture of community assessment data can evolve.

The final stage of analysis is *inference*—the process of deriving logical conclusions from evidence. It is from inferences that nursing diagnoses are formed.

ROSEMONT SAMPLE COMMUNITY ANALYSIS

Following the analysis examples given below, information on how to form community nursing diagnoses is presented (see Community Nursing Diagnosis). The analysis of the Rosemont assessment data, as in the assessment process, begins with the community core, and then proceed to analyzes each subsystem.

COMMUNITY CORE

An analysis of Rosemont's core is presented in Table 7-1. Community core data include many demographic measures, a type of data that is especially amenable to graphs and charts. The adage, "one picture is worth a thousand words," is particularly meaningful for demographic characteristics.

Perhaps the most representative illustration of the age and sex composition of a population is the *population pyramid.* Population pyramids for census tracts (CTs) 402 and 403 appear in Figure 7-1.

> NOTE: The population pyramid is formed of bars; each bar represents an age group. Usually 5- or 10-year age groups are used although adaptations can be made for smaller or larger age ranges. Bars are stacked horizontally, one on another, with bars for men on the left of a central axis and those for women on the right. The percentage of men and women in a particular age group is indicated by the length of the bars, as measured from the central axis. All age groups in a pyramid should be the same interval.

To construct a population pyramid, use Table 7-2 to calculate the percentage contribution of each age and sex class and Table 7-3 for actual pyramid construction. Note that parts of the population pyramids in Figure 7-1, those age

(*Text continues on page 246*)

TABLE 7-1.   ANALYSIS OF ROSEMONT'S CORE

Categories of Data	Summary Statements/ Measures	Inferences
History		
	Cultural and ethnic diversity	Community revitalization
	Renovation of businesses and homes	Community pride
	Pride and concern evident	
Demographics		
Age		
CT 402	42.5% of population ≤19 years	Large % of children and adolescents
	53% of population ≤19 years or ≥65 years	High dependency ratio*
	10% of population ≥65 years	Large % of elderly compared to Hampton and Jefferson County
Data Gap: Need census data from 1970 to determine if demographics are consistent or changing		
CT 403	7.5% of population ≤19 years	Small % of children and adolescents
	15.2% of population ≤19 years or ≥65 years	Low dependency ratio
	7.7% of population ≥65 years	
Data gap: Need census data in 5-year increments to construct population pyramids		
Sex		
CT 402	48% of population is male	Equal % of males and females
	45% of population aged 20–64 is male	
CT 403	65% of population is male	High % of males
	69% of population aged 20–64 is male	
Data gap: Need census data from 1970 to determine if demographics are consistent or changing		
Racial/ethnic		
CT 402	Diversity: black 54%, asian 19%, white 12%, hispanic 9%	Racial and ethnic diversity
CT 403	Homogeneity: white 89%	Racial and ethnic homogeneity
Data gap: Need census data from 1970 to determine if demographics are consistent or changing		

(*continued*)

TABLE 7-1.   (Continued)

Categories of Data	Summary Statements/ Measures	Inferences
Household types		
CT 402	83% of households are family	Family households dominate
CT 403	36% of households are family	Nonfamily households dominate
Marital status		
CT 402	15% single, 60% married, 14% divorced	Small % of single adults Majority of adults married
CT 403	53% single, 24% married, 15% divorced	Large % of single adults Small % married

Data gap: Need census data from 1970 to determine if demographics are consistent or changing

Vital statistics

(Refer to Chapter 2 for rate calculation)

Births	*Rate per 1000*	*(When compared to Hampton and Jefferson County)*
CT 402	30.5	A higher birth rate
CT 403	17.3	A lower birth rate
Hampton	19.4	
Jefferson County	25.2	

Data gap: Need general fertility rate and age-specific birth rate

Deaths	*Rate per 1000*	*(When compared to Hampton and Jefferson County)*
CT 402		
Infant	33.3	A higher death rate for all ages
Neonatal	23.8	
Fetal	76.2	
Crude	10.4	
CT 403		
Infant	17.1	A higher infant and neonatal
Neonatal	17.1	rate
Fetal	8.5	
Crude	6.2	

(continued)

TABLE 7-1.   (Continued)

Categories of Data	Summary Statements/ Measures	Inferences
Data gap: Need vital statistics from previous 3–5 years to determine if rates are consistent or changing		
Hampton		
Infant	12.1	
Neonatal	7.9	
Fetal	12.6	
Crude	6	
Jefferson County		
Infant	12.3	
Neonatal	8.3	
Fetal	15.3	
Crude	7.3	
Causes of death	*Rate per 1000*	*(When compared to Hampton and Jefferson County data)*
CT 402	Heart disease 22.2%; malignant neoplasms 23.6%; cerebrovascular 8.3%; accidents 5.6%; diseases of early infancy 9.7%; homicides 8.3%; pneumonia 2.8%; suicides 4.2%; tuberculosis 1.4%; all other causes 13.9%	A much higher % of deaths owing to Diseases of infancy Homicides Suicides Tuberculosis A higher % of deaths owing to cerebrovascular disease A lower % of deaths owing to heart disease
CT 403	Heart disease 23.8%; malignant neoplasms 26.1%; cerebrovascular 4.7%; accidents 9.5%; diseases of early infancy 2.4%; homicides 2.4%; cirrhosis of liver 2.4%; pneumonia 2.4%; suicides 2.4%; diabetes mellitus 4.8%; congenital anomalies 4.8%; all other causes 14.3%	A higher % of deaths owing to Accidents Diabetes mellitus Congenital anomalies A lower % of deaths due to heart disease

(continued)

TABLE 7-1. (Continued)

Categories of Data	Summary Statements/ Measures	Inferences
Data gap: Need comparative data for past 3–5 years		
Hampton	Disease of heart 33.4%; malignant neoplasms 21.8%; cerebrovascular 7.3%; accidents 6.2%; emphysema, asthma, bronchitis 0.8%; diseases of early infancy 2.6%; homicides 6.2%; cirrhosis of liver 1.7%; pneumonia 2.2%; suicides 2%; diabetes mellitus 1.4%; congenital anomalies 1%; nephritis and nephrosis 0.1%; tuberculosis 0.2%; all other causes 13%	
Jefferson County	Disease of heart 36%; malignant neoplasms 24.2%; cerebrovascular 7.4%; accidents 5.7%; emphysema, asthma, bronchitis 0.7%; diseases of early infancy 3%; homicides 1.5%; pneumonia 2.2%; suicides 1.4%; diabetes mellitus 1.8%; congenital anomalies 1.5%; nephritis and nephrosis 0.2%; tuberculosis 0.2%; all other causes 9.1%	

* *Dependency ratio* describes the potentially self-supporting portion of the population and the dependent portions at the extremes of age. The dependency ratio is usually computed as follows:

$$\frac{\text{population under 20 + population 65 and over}}{\text{population 20 to 64 years of age}} \times 100$$

The dependency ratio for CT 402 is 91, meaning for every 100 persons age 20 to 65 (supposedly self-supporting because of age) there are 91 persons under age 20 or over age 65 needing support (because of age). In contrast, the dependency ratio for CT 403 is 19.

TABLE 7-2.   CALCULATIONS FOR A POPULATION PYRAMID

COMMUNITY NAME, CENSUS TRACT, OR
   GEOGRAPHIC BOUNDARIES: _____
TOTAL POPULATION: _____

Ages (Years)	Males		Females	
	Number	% of Total Population	Number	% of Total Population
Total				
Under 5				
5–9				
10–14				
15–19				
20–24				
25–29				
30–34				
35–39				
40–44				
45–49				
50–54				
55–59				
60–64				
65–69				
70–74				
75 and over				

TABLE 7-3. CONSTRUCTING A POPULATION PYRAMID

POPULATION PYRAMID FOR _____ :   19____

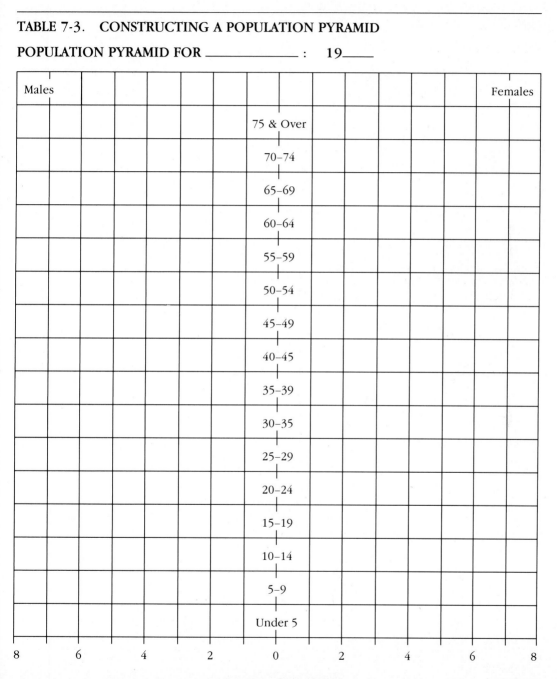

Percentage of Population

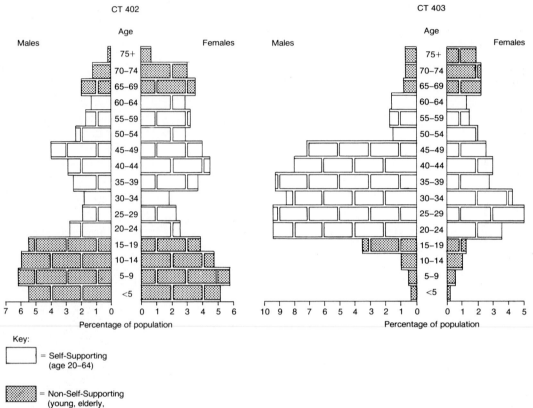

Figure 7-1. Population Pyramid: Age and sex structure of CT 402 and CT 403.

groups less-than-20-years and older-than-65, are shaded; this was done to denote the dependent portions of the population.

Studying the population pyramids for CT 402 and CT 403, striking age and sex differences are evident; and this illustrates an important lesson. If the demographics of Rosemont had been presented as one population pyramid (Figure 7-2), important age and sex differences might have been minimized or have gone unrecognized, and their associated age- and sex-related health needs would be left unmet. This hazard in data analysis is referred to as *aggregating* or *pooling the data.* It is important to divide data along all possibly meaningful lines so that important information is not overlooked. Be alert to this problem as you proceed with your analysis.

Studying the inferences presented in Table 7-1, in conjunction with the population pyramids, Figure 7-1, the following statements can be made about Rosemont's core.

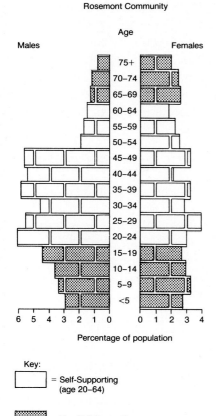

Figure 7-2. Population Pyramid of Rosemont Community: Age and sex structure.

In CT 402 there exists the following

- A large percentage (42.5%) of children and adolescents
- A high dependency ratio
- An equal percentage of adult men and women aged 20–64 years
- A larger percentage (10%) of elderly than Hampton or Jefferson County
- A small percentage (15.2%) of single adults
- A moderate percentage (60.7%) of married adults
- A predominance (83%) of family households
- A mixed racial/ethnic composition with 54% black, 19% asian, 12% white, and 9% hispanic
- An extremely high infant and fetal death rate
    Infant mortality rate (33 per 1000 live births),
    Neonatal mortality rate (24 per 1000 live births),
    Fetal mortality rate (76 per 1000 live births)

- A higher birth rate (31 per 1000 population) than Hampton (19 per 1000 population), or Jefferson County (25 per 1000 population)
- A higher crude death rate (10 per 1000 population) than Hampton (6 per 1000 population) or Jefferson County (7 per 1000 population);
- A much higher percentage of deaths owing to diseases of early infancy, homicides, suicides, and tuberculosis than Hampton or Jefferson County
- A slightly higher percentage of deaths owing to cerebrovascular disorders than Hampton or Jefferson County

In contrast, it can be seen that CT 403 has the following factors.

- A small percentage (7.5%) of children and adolescents
- A low dependency ratio
- A larger percentage (7.7%) of elderly than Hampton or Jefferson County
- A high percentage (69%) of adult males ages 20–64 years
- Racial and ethnic homogeneity with 89% of the population white
- A predominance (64%) of nonfamily households
- A large percentage (53%) of single adults
- A small percentage (24%) of married adults
- A lower birth rate (17 per 1000 population) than Hampton or Jefferson County
- A higher infant mortality (17 per 1000 live births) and a higher neonatal mortality (17 per 1000 live births) than Hampton or Jefferson County
- A lower crude death rate (6.2 per 1000 population) than Hampton or Jefferson County
- A higher percentage of deaths owing to accidents, diabetes mellitus, and congenital anomalies than Hampton or Jefferson County
- A lower percentage of deaths due to heart disease than Hampton or Jefferson County

Having analyzed the core characteristics of Rosemont, it is evident that major differences exist between CT 402 and CT 403, although both are part of Rosemont. In the following sections, this finding will be given more detail as each subsystem in our Community Assessment Wheel model is analyzed.

PHYSICAL ENVIRONMENT

To study the physical components of Rosemont, data were collected that began with community inspection (*i.e.,* the windshield survey) and concluded with a systems review and laboratory studies (*i.e.,* census and Chamber of Commerce data). Table 7-4 presents an analysis of the *physical examination data.*

Studying the inferences in Table 7-4, the following statements about Rosemont's physical components can be made

- Rosemont is a community of contrasts and diversity
- Densely populated residential areas, composed mainly of older homes, abut businesses of various types.
- Industry is minimal and it is concentrated entirely in CT 402.
- Housing values and rents have skyrocketed in CT 403; in CT 402 only rents have increased dramatically.

HEALTH AND SOCIAL SERVICES

An analysis of the health and social services in Rosemont is presented in Table 7-5. Because the data were categorized initially as extra- and intra-community health and social services, the same format has been used in the analysis. Notice that statements from health care providers have been reported separately from those of health care recipients. This is because health care providers frequently have a different concept of the adequacy, accessibility, and acceptability of health services compared to that held by health care recipients. Be sure to collect and analyze data from both perspectives.

After reviewing Table 7-5, the following statements can be deduced about Rosemont's health services

- A variety of private hospitals, home health care agencies, and continuing-care facilities are located outside Rosemont; however most require fee-for-service or third-party reimbursement.
- There is only one full-service public hospital in the area, Jefferson Memorial, is located five miles from Rosemont; users of Jefferson Memorial complain of lengthy waits for outpatient care and fragmented service.
- The Sunvalley Clinic, operated by the city health department, has inadequate antepartal services for Rosemont women; this results in
    Many women delivering at Jefferson Memorial with no antepartal care
    Women forced to self-deliver at home because they do not meet eligibility requirements at Jefferson Memorial
- There are no practicing private obstetric, gynecologic, or family practitioners in Rosemont.

TABLE 7-4. ANALYSIS OF ROSEMONT'S PHYSICAL EXAMINATION DATA

Categories of Data	Summary Statements/ Measures	Inferences
Inspection		
Windshield survey	A community of contrast; bustling business areas and quiet neighborhoods Ethnic diversity evident in foods	Ethnic and business diversity Congested streets lined with homes or businesses Minimal industry Little "open" space
Vital signs		
	Flat terrain and mild climate Densely populated (14 persons per acre) Posters abound sharing information and heralding forthcoming events	Mild climate, abundant flora Densely populated (14 persons per acre) Note: In CT 402 there are 221 persons per acre at one housing development
Systems review		
Land usage		
CT 402	37% of land in commercial usage, 28% single family, 8% multifamily and 9% open	CT 402 has almost twice the commercial usage of land (37%) compared to CT 403 (20%)
CT 403	20% of land in commercial usage, 32% single family, 15% multifamily and 18% open	CT 403 has twice the percentage of open space (18%) compared to CT 402 (9%)
Housing values		
CT 402	From 1970 to 1980 average home values increased 50%; average rents increased 200%	Sharp contrast between average home values; in CT 402 average home value is $26,000 compared to $58,000 in CT 403
CT 403	From 1970 to 1980 average home values increased 350% and average rents increased 500%	Average rent is similar for both census tracts and comparable to Hampton

(Note: No data gaps identified; data for this area is complete.)

- The Third Street Clinic has inadequate health services, specifically a lack of
    Assessment and treatment of persons who are ill
    Dental assessment and restoration
    Counseling and treatment programs for substance abuse
    Health-education programs responsive to residents' needs
    Support and self-help groups as needed and requested by residents
- The Rosemont Health Center offers acceptable, accessible, and affordable services for sexually transmitted diseases (STD); however, there is a lack of
    Orientation and education for the staff
    Procedure manuals and posted protocols for emergency care
    Safe disposal methods for syringes
    A visible emergency cart

    The following deductions can be made about Rosemont's social services

- Hampton Community Counseling Center (HCCC) is located close to Rosemont, but is not used by Rosemont residents, although resident repeatedly expressed a wish for substance-abuse counseling programs.
- The YMCA Indo-Chinese Refugee Program is heavily used by asians in Rosemont; however, present programs of cultural orientation are inadequate to meet demand. Both the YMCA staff and Rosemont residents see a need for additional programs.
- South Main and Westpark churches offer numerous social service programs; however only South Main offers a social program especially for the male homosexual population—a program that is resisted by older parishioners.
- An active chapter of Lamda AA is located in Rosemont.

ECONOMICS

An analysis of the economic and financial characteristics of Rosemont is presented in Table 7-6. The analysis begins with individual wealth indices (*e.g.,* income), proceeds to indicators of business and industrial wealth, and concludes with employment status of community residents. As with other subsystems, the categories for data assessment have become categories for data analysis.

After studying Table 7-6, the following statements can be made about the economic status of Rosemont. Striking differences exist between the financial characteristics of households in CT 402 and CT 403.

(*Text continues on page 255*)

TABLE 7-5. ANALYSIS OF HEALTH AND SOCIAL SERVICES IN ROSEMONT

Categories of Data	Summary Statements/ Measures	Inferences
Health facilities		
Extra-community		
Hospitals	Most are referral or private One public hospital, Jefferson Memorial, has problems of Long waits ($\geq$8 hr) Fragmented care Inaccessibility	Only one public hospital; users complain of lengthy waits and fragmented care
Private care	Numerous options including HMOs	Variety of private care options
Health department (Sunvalley Clinic)	Health providers feel Sunvalley Clinic has Inadequate antepartal services; women wait 8–10 weeks for an initial appointment that is often after their expected date of confinement (EDC) Inadequate nursing services to meet elderly's needs Rosemont residents feel the clinic is: • inaccessible (no direct bus connection) • impersonal (no primary care providers)	Inadequate antepartal services. Many women deliver at Jefferson Memorial with no antepartal care. Many women are forced to self-deliver at home because they do not meet eligibility requirements at Jefferson Memorial. Inaccessibility and unacceptability of Sunvalley services.

Data gap:
  Number of Rosemont residents using
    Well and ill infant, child, adolescent, adult services
    Mental health counseling and referral services
  User's perception of adequacy, accessibility, and acceptability of the above services

| Home health | One large Visiting Nurse Association (VNA) Numerous home health agencies; most require fee-for-service or third-party reimbursement | Numerous options for home health care |

Data gap: Frequency and type of VNA services used by Rosemont residents

(continued)

TABLE 7-5.   (Continued)

Categories of Data	Summary Statements/ Measures	Inferences
Continuing care	Two long-term licensed facilities close (8 miles) from Rosemont	Two long-term licensed facilities

Data gap: Adequacy of facilities as perceived by health administrators, staff, and patients

Emergency services: Medical emergency ambulance service, (MEAS)	Cardiac and CVA are major reasons for MEAS visits to Rosemont	Cardiac and CVA are major reasons for MEAS visits, followed by accidents and home falls

Data gap: Number of persons using MEAS and their age, sex, race, and ethnic characteristics

Intra-community health services

Health practitioners	Rosemont has no: Obstetric, gynecologic, or family practitioners Bilingual health practitioners	Lack of ob/gyn and family practitioners No bilingual health practitioners

Clinics

Third Street Clinic	Health providers feel immediate health needs include Ill infant, child, adolescent, and adult assessment, treatment, and follow-up Dental assessment and restoration Counseling, referral, and treatment for substance abuse Group health teaching Support groups for single parents and senior citizens	Inadequate health services for Ill persons (all ages) Dental assessment and restoration Counseling and treatment for substance abuse Health education Self-help/support groups
	Additional needs of the clinic include recruitment and retainment of health providers	
	Many Rosemont residents use the clinic routinely, people feel welcomed and comply with medical care	Rosemont residents state care at Third Street Clinic is acceptable and accessible
	Residents agree that additional services are needed	

(*continued*)

TABLE 7-5.   (Continued)

Categories of Data	Summary Statements/ Measures	Inferences
Data gap: Number of persons requesting services that health providers feel are needed Characteristics of persons requesting medical care services		

Rosemont Health Center	Director of clinic feels immediate needs are
	  Formation of counseling and support groups
	  Orientation program and inservice for staff (all are volunteers)
		Highly acceptable, accessible and affordable care for STD
		Inadequate counseling and support groups
		Lack of orientation and inservice for the staff
		Lack of procedure manuals and posted protocols for emergency care
		Lack of safety procedures including visible emergency cart and proper syringe disposal

Data gap: What do staff perceive as needs?

Social facilities

Extra-community

Hampton Community Counseling Center (HCCC)	HCCC offers counseling to adolescent drug users. Most patients are middle or upper class males; all are white Staff feels that they are meeting community needs Rosemont residents are unaware of the center	HCCC is close to Rosemont and offers needed counseling for substance abuse, yet HCCC is not used by Rosemont residents

YMCA Indo-Chinese Refugee Program	Cultural-orientation programs for asian immigrants; staff perceive immediate needs are for programs on the following
	  Substance abuse
	  Basic life survival skills (*e.g.,* employment, self-health care)
	Many Rosemont residents use the YMCA services; all agree the programs are excellent but state the waiting period for classes is long and frustrating
		Insufficient number of cultural programs resulting in long waiting periods and frustration

(*continued*)

TABLE 7-5.   (Continued)

Categories of Data	Summary Statements/ Measures	Inferences
Intra-community		
Churches		
South Main	Extensive social service programs; social program for homosexual males despite resistance from older members.	Social outreach programs offered by both churches. Only South Main offers program for homosexual males although older members of South Main resent the program.
Westpark	Extensive social service program. No social programs for homosexual males	
Lambda Alcoholic Anonymous (AA)	Active AA program for homosexual males; membership exceeds 120	Active chapter of Lambda AA

- In CT 402 it was found that
    The median household income of $4776 is only 25% of the median income in CT 403 and Hampton
    The majority of families (54%) have incomes below the poverty level
    Half of all households are headed by females
    One-third of all families receive public assistance/welfare
- In CT 403 the following factors exist
    The median household income of $16,019 is much greater than that of CT 402, as well as that of Hampton
    Only 5% of families have incomes below the poverty line
    Only 11% of all households are headed by females
    Only 4.3% of families receive public assistance/welfare
- Striking differences also exist between the labor force characteristics of CT 402 and CT 403.
- In CT 402 it was found that
    Only 40% of the population is of employable age (16 years or older)
    Most people (67%) work in service or operator/labor occupations
- In CT 403 presented a contrasting picture
    Of the population, 85% is of employable age (16 years or older)
    Most people (76%) work in managerial or professional positions

TABLE 7-6.   ANALYSIS OF THE ECONOMIC INDICATORS
             OF ROSEMONT

Categories of Data	Summary Statements/Measures	Inferences
Financial Characteristics of Households		
Median household income (1980)		Median household income in CT 403 is 400% higher than in CT 402
CT 402 $4,776		
CT 403 $16,019		
Hampton $15,321		
% of families with incomes below poverty level (1980)		In CT 402, over half of all families have incomes below the poverty level
CT 402 53.7%		
CT 403 5.4%		
Hampton 7.1%		
% of families on public assistance/welfare		In CT 402, 36.4% of all families are on public assistance/ welfare compared to 4.3% in CT 403 and 3.4% in Hampton
CT 402 36.4%		
CT 403 4.3%		
Hampton 3.4%		
% of female head of households (1980)		In CT 402, half of the households are headed by females
CT 402 49.2%		
CT 403 11.1%		
Hampton 15.4%		
Business/industry characteristics (1980)		
CT 402	Nearly equal percentage of wholesale/retail (48%) as professional (42%)	In CT 402, equal percentage of wholesale and professional businesses
CT 403	Predominance of professional (48%) over wholesale/retail (37%)	In CT 403, predominance of professional businesses
Labor force characteristics (1980): age (% of persons ≥16 years)		Only 40% of persons in CT 402 are of employable age (≥16) compared to 85% in CT 403 and 71% in Hampton
CT 402 39.8%		
CT 403 85.4%		
Hampton 71.5%		

(*continued*)

TABLE 7-6. (Continued)

Categories of Data	Summary Statements/Measures	Inferences
Wage class: % Private, % government, % self-employed		
CT 402 67%, 18%, 2%		Wage class data similar for CT 402 and CT 403 with the majority of all wages derived from private businesses
CT 403 76%, 12%, 6%		
Occupational groups		
Managerial/professional		
CT 402 7.1%		Striking differences between occupational categories
CT 403 42.1%		
Technical/sales		
CT 402 12.1%		In CT 402, 67% of workers are in service or operator occupations, compared to 14.8% in CT 403
CT 403 34.1%		
Service		
CT 402 44.2%		In CT 403, 76% of workers are in managerial or technical occupations, compared to 19% in CT 402
CT 403 10.5%		
Operators/laborers		
CT 402 23.6%		
CT 403 4.3%		

(Note: No data gaps identified; data in this area is complete.)

SAFETY AND TRANSPORTATION

An analysis of the safety and transportation services in Rosemont are set forth in Table 7-7.

Reviewing the data, the following statements can be made about Rosemont's safety (protection) services and associated concerns

- Grease fires are the major cause of house fires.
- Thefts and burglaries are the major reported crimes, followed by robbery

**TABLE 7-7.   ANALYSIS OF SAFETY AND
TRANSPORTATION SERVICES
IN ROSEMONT**

Categories of Data	Summary Statements/ Measures	Inferences
Safety		
Protection services		
Fire	45 fires during past 90 days, of these 40 occurred in homes (usually a grease fire)	Major cause of fires within last 90 days were grease fires

Data gap:
   Obtain additional data (12 months) and determine if grease fires are major cause
   Document age, sex, and racial characteristics, as well as time of day and associated circumstances

Police	Crime statistics for past 4 years show thefts as the leading crime followed by burglary. Frequency of occurrence is high for both census tracts. Robbery is twice as prevalent in CT 402 compared to CT 403 and vehicle theft is three times more common in CT 403. Residents expressed fear and related stories of muggings and violence especially toward the elderly and male homosexual population.	Thefts and burglaries are the major crimes; the elderly and male homosexuals feel especially victimized

Data gap:
   Assess residents' knowledge about self-protection measures against crime
   Assess residents' interest and past participation in crime prevention programs
   Assess available crime prevention programs

Sanitation		
Sewage	Sewage moratorium exists owing to over capacity of present facility	Inadequate sewage treatment facilities resulting in building restrictions

(*continued*)

TABLE 7-7.   (Continued)

Categories of Data	Summary Statements/ Measures	Inferences
Potable water	No fluoride in drinking water. No routine testing of drinking water for arsenic or heavy metals (elements residents believe may be contaminating the water)	Lack of fluoride in drinking water No routine tests of drinking water for arsenic or heavy metals

Data gap:
  Assess history of fluoride issue. Has fluoride been proposed, voted on? What is present position of health department, city council, civic associations?
  Regarding arsenic and heavy metals: Is Lake Hampton tested for arsenic or heavy metals? What is position and plan of health department, city council, civic associations?

Solid waste	Increased illegal dumping of machinery and appliances; unoperable autos are parked on the streets for months before removal by the city of Hampton.	Potential for accidents, (*e.g.,* trauma, suffocation) as persons explore abandoned objects and automobiles

Data gap: Document laws and fees for illegal dumping? Are signs posted to notify persons of law and associated fines? What actions have been taken by residents, civic associations, businesses?

Air	Rise in air pollution attributed to increase in industrial growth and population density. Residents complain of eye irritation and increased number of respiratory conditions Air Board feels citizens are inadequately informed regarding actions needed during an air stagnation advisory, and individual responsibility to decrease pollution	Increased air pollution. Citizens may be inadequately informed regarding personal actions needed during an air stagnation advisory; to decrease air pollution

Data Gap:
  Assess if public awareness programs have ocurred. If so, when, and response? What do residents understand about air pollution, air advisories, and their role in decreasing air pollution?
  Do residents desire more information about air pollution?

(continued)

TABLE 7-7.   (Continued)

Categories of Data	Summary Statements/ Measures	Inferences
Transportation		
Private (to work)		
CT 402	43% of people drive alone; 24% carpool, and 23% use public transportation	Almost half (43%) drive alone to work, with equal percentages (24%) carpooling or using public transportation
CT 403	64% of people drive alone; 16% carpool, and 11% use public transportation	Most people (64%) drive alone to work, some carpool (16%) and only a few use public transportation (11%)
Transportation disability		
CT 402	6% of persons 16–64 have a disability and 21% of those over age 65	When compared to CT 403, a large percentage of residents in CT 402 have a transportation disability, especially those over age 65
CT 403	0.3% of persons 16–64 have a disability and 11% of those over age 65	

and vehicle theft; elderly persons and male homosexuals feel especially victimized. Both groups related numerous stories of harassment and violence.

- There is no fluoride in Rosemont's drinking water, nor is there routine testing for arsenic or heavy metals, substances that residents fear are contaminating the water.
- Owing to abandoned vehicles and dumping of machinery and appliances, residents, especially children, are at increased risk of accidental injury.
- Air pollution has increased; the Air Control Board feels citizens are inadequately informed about air pollution advisories, as well as personal actions that can be taken to decrease pollution.

Regarding Rosemont's transportation services, the following deductions are made.

- A large percentage of residents in CT 403 drive to work alone (64%) compared to those in CT 402 (43%); however, 48% of the residents in CT 402 use carpools or public transportation to get to work, compared to 26% in CT 403.
- When compared to CT 403, a substantially larger percentage of the population in CT 402 have a transportation disability, especially among those over age 65.

POLITICS AND GOVERNMENT

A rich diversity of political organizations exists in Rosemont. However, at this point in the nursing process—analysis—it is sufficient to describe the organizations and identify key persons. Consider your information about the political system and form of government to be reference material that will be useful at the next stage of the nursing process—program planning for a community.

COMMUNICATION

Ample formal and informal communication sources exist in Rosemont. No analysis is required of the data. Consider this communication data to be reference material that will be useful at the next stage of the nursing process—program planning for a community.

> NOTE: If sufficient information is collected regarding a community's communication system (refer to Table 6-32 in Chapter 6 for components to assess) then there is no need to analyze the data.

EDUCATION

An analysis of Rosemont's *general educational status* (characteristics of school enrollment, years of schooling completed, and language spoken) and *specific educational sources* (*e.g.,* public and private schools both intra- and extra-community) is presented in Table 7-8.

Major differences exist between the general educational status of CT 402 and CT 403.

The status in CT 402 is as follows

- A small percentage of high school graduates (28%) with the majority of persons enrolled in school attending elementary grades. Some 75% of the population has poor English proficiency.

In contrast, the CT 403 data show that

- A large percentage of residents are high school graduates (89%); and the majority of the persons who attend school are in college. Only 19% of the residents have poor English proficiency.

With regard to specific educational sources, Temple Elementary is the primary educational resource in Rosemont. Temple has an enrollment of 924 youngsters. The principal, teachers, nurse, and parents were interviewed during the assessment process. To summarize, the situation at Temple, it has been concluded that

- Problems of truancy exist, especially among hispanic boys
- There are large numbers of academic failures (22% of students last year)
- Large numbers of students have English-skills insufficiencies, further documented by general educational data
- Inadequate working relationships exist between parents and teachers, compounded by the language barrier
- Student health problems consist of
    Dental caries (62% of youngsters)
    Head lice, especially grades kindergarten to second
    Incomplete immunizations
    Poor hygiene
    Inadequate parent follow-through of needed medical care
    Inadequate health education program
- There is parental concern and involvement and a desire to communicate needs to staff

One daycare facility exists in Rosemont—the Busybee. This facility is extremely inadequate. As a result, parents are forced to leave children in conditions that may be crowded and undersupervised.

(*Text continues on page 266*)

**TABLE 7-8. ANALYSIS OF EDUCATIONAL SOURCES
IN ROSEMONT**

Categories of Data	Summary Statements/ Measures	Inferences
Educational status		
Years of schooling completed: % high school graduates		
CT 402 28%		In CT 402, only 28% of persons over age 25 are high school graduates, compared to 89% in CT 403 and 68% in Hampton
CT 403 89%		
Hampton 68%		
School enrollment: % elementary, % high school, % college		
CT 402 59%, 23%, 4%		The majority of persons attending school in CT 402 are elementary grade students, compared to CT 403 where the majority of those attending school are in college
CT 403 15%, 7%, 73%		
Hampton 48%, 23%, 19%		
Language spoken: % of population with poor English proficiency		
Age 5–17 *Age 18+*		In CT 402 some 75% of the population has poor English proficiency compared to small percentages in CT 403
CT 402 76% 74%		
CT 403 11% 19%		
Hampton 21% 26%		
Educational sources		
Intra-community		
Temple Elementary	Grades K to 8th Enrollment 924 Ethnicity 42% black 33% asian 18% hispanic 5% white	Mixed ethnicity, predominance of black children

(continued)

TABLE 7-8. (Continued)

Categories of Data	Summary Statements/ Measures	Inferences
	Principal feels major problems are Truancy Academic failure Principal wants to stop bilingual classes	According to staff, major problems are Truancy Academic failure (22%) Inadequate parent–teacher relationships English insufficiencies Stressed home environments with inadequate adult supervision

Data gap:
　Explore principal's statement about bilingual education. Why the opposition? What is position and policy on bilingual education in HISD?
　What is principal's perception of parental concerns?

| | *Teachers feel* major impediments to student learning are:
Inadequate parent–teacher communication
Poor English proficiency
Stressed home environment
Inadequate adult supervision | Same as above |

Data gap:
　Explore teachers' perceptions of bilingual education.
　What are teachers' perceptions of parental concerns?

| Temple Elementary | *Nurse feels* major health problems of youngsters are
Poor hygiene
Dental caries
Prevalence of head lice
Incomplete immunizations
Lack of parent follow-through for needed medical care | Major student health problems are inadequate
Hygiene
Control of dental caries
Control of head lice
Parent follow-through with needed medical care
Health education |

(continued)

TABLE 7-8.   (Continued)

Categories of Data	Summary Statements/ Measures	Inferences
Data gap: Document age, sex, ethnicity and racial characteristics of children with specific health problems.		
	Nurse feels more health teaching and screening would be possible with parent volunteers. Present policy restricts nurse to clinic, permitting no classroom teaching.	Same as above
Data gap: Document school policy regarding Recruitment and training of parent volunteers The nurse's presence and role in the clinic Explore nurse's attitude toward health education. Discuss options for health programs for students, staff, and parents.		
Temple Elementary	*Parents feel* Temple is a community strength *but* the present staff are insensitive to ethnic and racial needs; attempts to discuss these concerns with Temple's staff have been frustrating.	Parental concern and involvement evident; however, attempts to discuss concerns with staff have been frustrating.
Data gap: Identify officers and key people (committee chairs) of Temple's PTO. Are these officers/key people aware of ethnic and racial needs? Identify students' perceptions of their school. What activities do they enjoy? Are there after-school activities? Who participates? What activities are needed?		
Busybee Daycare	One daycare center in CT 402; no facility in CT 403	Inadequate daycare facilities Parents leave children in crowded homes
Extra-community		
Central Hampton High	Truancy and grade failure reversed with program "Failproof" Increased number of teenage pregnancies	Increased number of teenage pregnancies Increased use of alcohol among high school students

(*continued*)

TABLE 7-8. (Continued)

Categories of Data	Summary Statements/ Measures	Inferences
	Decision by school board not to permit sex education classes	Sex education classes not permitted in high school
	Increased use of alcohol	

Data gap:
 Number of pregnancies last 3–5 years (for comparison) and age, grade level, racial, and ethnic characteristics of girls
 History and reason for Hampton Independent School District (HISD) Board decision to stop sex education
 Document scope of alcohol use and characteristics of users

The major extra-community educational facility is Central Hampton High. The major problems of Central Hampton High, according to the school nurse, include

- Increased number of teenage pregnancies
- Lack of sex education classes
- Increased use of alcohol

Central Hampton has succeeded in reducing truancy and grade failure through a program called "Failproof."

RECREATION

Recreational space and facilities are minimal. A sum of 5.6 acres of public recreational space is available for a population of 13,631 (combined populations of CT 402 and CT 403). The organized sports and recreational programs that are available through churches and associations require membership and usually charge a fee. There are no public recreational programs and the few pieces of public recreational equipment that exist are in need of repair.

COMMUNITY NURSING DIAGNOSIS

In the preceding pages, each subsystem of the Rosemont sample has been analyzed and inferences have been drawn. The final task of analysis is the synthesis of the inference statements into community nursing diagnoses.

A *diagnosis* is a statement that synthesizes assessment data. A diagnosis is a label that both *describes a situation* (or state) and *implies an etiology* (reason).

A *nursing diagnosis* limits the diagnostic process to those diagnoses that represent *human responses to actual or potential health problems that nurses are licensed to treat.* This stipulation is based on the American Nurses' Association (ANA) Social Policy Statement (see the Suggested Readings list). Although no standard format exists, most nursing diagnoses have three parts

- A *description* of the problem, response, or state
- Identification of factors *etiologically* related to the problem
- *Signs and symptoms* that are characteristic of the problem

A *community nursing diagnosis* focuses the diagnosis on a *community* —usually defined as *a group, population, or cluster of people with* at least one *common characterisitc,* (*e.g.,* geographic location, occupation, ethnicity, or housing condition). To derive a community nursing diagnoses, community-assessment data are analyzed and inferences are presented. Inference statements shape nursing diagnoses. Some inference statements form the descriptive part of the nursing diagnosis—these inferences testify to a potential or actual community health problem or concern; for example

- Inadequate antepartal services for Rosemont residents
- High prevalence of dental caries among youngsters at Temple Elementary School in Rosemont

Other inference statements are etiologic and document the possible reasons for the health problem or concern. Etiologic statements are linked to the descriptive statements with a "*related to*" clause; for example

- Inadequate antepartal services for Rosemont residents *related to* Inadequate resources at the Health Department's Sunvalley Clinic to meet antepartal care needs

Inaccessibility and unacceptability of present antepartal services at the Sunvalley Clinic

Lack of obstetric and family practitioners in Rosemont

- High prevalence of dental caries among youngsters at Temple Elementary School in Rosemont *related to*

    Lack of dental assessment and treatment at the Third Street Clinic

    Lack of fluoride in Rosemont's drinking water

    Low median household income in CT 402 and associated limited economic resources for purchasing dental care

    No dental hygiene education offered at Temple Elementary

Finally, the *signs and symptoms* of the community nursing diagnosis are the inference statements that *document the duration or magnitude of the problem.* Examples of documentation include record accounts, census reports, and vital statistics. This final piece of the community nursing diagnosis is linked to the first two parts with an "*as manifested by*" clause; for example

- Inadequate antepartal services for Rosemont residents *related to*

    Inadequate resources at the Health Department's Sunvalley Clinic to meet antepartal care needs

    Inaccessibility and unacceptability of present antepartal services at the Sunvalley Clinic

    Lack of obstetric and family practitioners in Rosemont

    As manifested by: many Rosemont women who deliver at Jefferson Memorial with *no* antepartal care; many Rosemont women who self-deliver at home; and a high infant, neonatal, and fetal death rate

- High prevalence of dental caries among youngsters at Temple Elementary School in Rosemont *related to:*

    Lack of dental assessment and treatment at the Third Street Clinic

    Lack of fluoride in Rosemont's drinking water

    Low median household income in CT 402 and associated limited economic resources for purchasing dental care

    No dental hygiene education offered at Temple Elementary

    As manifested by: 62% of youngsters at Temple Elementary who have dental caries on inspection

Although a single problem is stated, the etiology(ies) and signs and symptoms may be multiple. Also notice that although the health problem inference is drawn from the analysis of one subsystem (such as the health and social services subsystem or the educational subsystem) the etiologies may be, and usually are, drawn from several subsystems. For example, regarding the health problem of dental caries among youngsters at Temple Elementary, etiologic inferences were derived from four subsystems—educational, health and social services, safety and transportation, and economic. This example is the most important lesson of community health nursing. All community factors (subsystems) join to determine the health status of a community. No one subsystem is more important or crucial than any other in determining a community's health.

The process of deriving community nursing diagnoses always remains the same—*first,* assessment data is categorized and studied for inferences that are descriptive of potential or actual health problems amenable to nursing interventions; *next,* associated inferences are identified that explain the derivation or continuation of the problem; and *lastly,* documentation is presented. Additional community nursing diagnoses for Rosemont are presented in Table 7-9. There is no particular order to the list, neither is the list conclusive. Determining the order of priority among community nursing diagnoses is part of problem planning and is dependent on existing community goals and resources—this important skill is discussed in the next chapter.

Deriving community nursing diagnoses requires critical decision making and astute study; it is a challenging and vital task. The completeness and validity of the community nursing diagnoses that have been derived will be tested during the next stage of the nursing process, and will form the foundation of that stage—the planning of a health program.

> NOTE: This is an excellent time to share your assessment data with colleagues and solicit their analysis. Because we each have opinions and values that color our perceptions, group critiquing and analysis of assessment data are one way to foster objectivity.

SUMMARY

Critical analyses of the Rosemont community have been completed using the Community Assessment Wheel (see Figure 6-1) as a guide. Subsequently, community nursing diagnoses were formulated, based on the inferences of the analyses. Although community nursing diagnoses are new to practice, community health nurses have, since the profession's inception, derived inferences from assessment data and have acted on that data. However, the terminology and format that has surrounded these informally produced inferences (diagnoses) have been inconsistent. There is presently considerable discussion,

(*Text continues on page 272*)

TABLE 7-9.   COMMUNITY NURSING DIAGNOSES

Community Response/ Concern/Problem (Actual or Potential)	Etiology "Related to"	Documentation Signs and Symptoms "As Evidenced by"
Stress and anxiety of being criminally victimized	Increased episodes of thefts and burglaries Inadequate knowledge of residents regarding self-protection measures	Police crime statistics of past four years Personal testimony of residents, especially homosexual males and the elderly
Potential for accidents (*e.g.,* trauma and suffocation) as children and adults explore abandoned goods	Illegal dumping of machinery and appliances Abandonment of automobiles Nonenforcement of city ordinances	Parental concern for safety Observation of persons exploring abandoned goods
Potential for health problems associated with air pollution, (*e.g.,* initiation and exacerbation of respiratory conditions)	Increased air pollution Lack of knowledge regarding personal action required During an air stagnation advisory To decrease air pollution	Air Board reports of current air pollution levels Residents' complaints of eye irritation and increased number of respiratory conditions
Truancy and academic failure at Temple Elementary	Large number of students with poor English proficiency Stressed home environment in CT 402, where 50% of homes are headed by females and 54% of families are below poverty level Inadequate communication links between parents and school personnel	Records at Temple Elementary
Inadequate medical care services for children at Temple Elementary	Inadequate ill-person assessment, treatment, and follow-up at Third Street Clinic Lack of family practitioners in Rosemont Inadequate income in CT 402 to purchase medical care Inadequate communication between parents and school staff Lack of health education in Temple Elementary and Third Street Clinic	Records of school nurse at Temple Elementary

(*continued*)

TABLE 7-9. (Continued)

Community Response/ Concern/Problem (Actual or Potential)	Etiology "Related to"	Documentation Signs and Symptoms "As Evidenced by"
Potential for decreased health potential of youngsters at Temple Elementary	Lack of regular health-promotion programs School policy that limits nursing activities to the clinic Lack of needed volunteers for screening tasks	Role and functions of nurse at Temple Elementary
Stress within Rosemont between the homosexual and nonhomosexual populations	Differing lifestyles of homosexual males Lack of acceptance of homosexual male lifestyle	Lack of social programs for homosexual males in Westpark Church Resistance of older church members in South Main to existing program for homosexual males Large percentage of single males in CT 403
Potential for inadequate coping of single parents, the elderly, and persons with STD	Lack of support groups and programs for single parents, the elderly, persons with STD Inadequate resources at Third Street Clinic to offer programs although the need is recognized Inadequate resources at Hampton Health Center to offer programs although the need is recognized	Health providers' perceptions of the Third Street Clinic Health providers' perceptions of the Rosemont Health Center High percentage of deaths owing to homicides and suicides in CT 402
Potential for inadequate medical care at Rosemont Health Center	Lack of orientation and inservice programs for staff Lack of procedure manuals and posted protocols for emergency care Lack of safety procedures	Visual assessment Perceptions of administration
Potential for inadequate cultural assimilation of asian immigrants	Lack of programs to meet present needs Lack of staff at Indo-Chinese Refugee program Increased need for programs Large asian population in CT 402 (19%) Large percentage of population in CT 402 (75%) with poor English proficiency	Perceived needs of asians in Rosemont

(*continued*)

TABLE 7-9.   (Continued)

Community Response/ Concern/Problem (Actual or Potential)	Etiology "Related to"	Documentation Signs and Symptoms "As Evidenced by"
Incomplete immunization status of children at Temple Elementary	Inadequate communication between parents and school's staff Inaccessibility and unacceptability of Health Department's Sunvalley Clinic Inadequate income in CT 402 to purchase immunizations	School health records at Temple Elementary
High infant, neonatal, and fetal mortality rate	Inadequate antepartal care at Sunvalley Clinic Lack of obstetric and family practitioners in Rosemont Lack of bilingual practitioners in Rosemont Inadequate income in CT 402 to purchase essential medical care	Vital statistics
Potential for boredom and associated consequences (*e.g.,* violence, vandalism)	Lack of public, no-fee recreational programs. Minimal public recreational areas and equipment	A total of 5.6 acres of public recreational space in Rosemont Visual inspection of available land and equipment
High prevalence of capitis pediculosis among children at Temple Elementary	Crowded living conditions Knowledge deficit regarding transmission and treatment	Cases reported by school nurse at Temple Elementary
Inadequate primary health care services	Large dependent population (*i.e.,* children and elderly, in CT 402 Large percentage of population in CT 402 below the poverty line Large percentage of population on public assistance/welfare	Census data

and some controversy, regarding the structure and terminology that would be optimal for community-focused nursing diagnoses. In your practice, you will be exposed to various formats for making community nursing diagnoses; evaluate and test the usefulness of each. It is only through collaboration and vigorous testing that a standard format will evolve. In the Suggested Readings list, there are sources that trace the development of community nursing diagnoses, and present suggested frameworks for deriving diagnoses.

SUGGESTED READINGS

Allor MT: The "community profile." J Nurs Ed 22:12–16, 1983

American Nurses' Association: Nursing: A Social Policy Statement. Kansas City, Missouri, American Nurses' Association, 1980 Author.

Dever GE: Community Health Analysis: A Holistic Approach. Germantown, Maryland, Aspen Systems, 1980

Gordon M: Nursing diagnosis and the diagnostic process. Am J Nurs 76:1298–1300, 1976

Griffith JW, Christensen PJ: Nursing Process. St. Louis, CV Mosby, 1982

Highriter ME: A computerized nursing management information system for identification and community follow-up of high-risk infants. In Werley HH, Grier MR (eds): Nursing Information Systems, pp 162–178. New York, Springer-Verlag, 1981

Luce BR, Stamps PL: An approach to accessibility analysis. Am J Public Health 66:581–582, 1976

Muecke MA: Community health diagnosis in nursing. Public Health Nurs 1:23–25, 1984

Price MR: Nursing diagnosis: Making a concept come alive. Am J Nurs 4:668–671, 1980

White KL: Health information systems in relation to basic health care. In Hetzel BS (ed): Basic Health Care in Developing Countries: An Epidemiological Perspective. New York, Oxford University Press, 1978

8

Planning a Health Program

OBJECTIVES

This chapter covers the planning of nursing actions to promote the health of a community. After studying this chapter you will be able to

- Validate your community nursing diagnoses with your community
- Use principles of change theory to direct the planning process
- In partnership with the community, plan a community-focused health program that includes

  Measurable goals and behavioral objectives

  A sequence of actions and a time schedule for achieving goals

  Resources needed to accomplish the plan

  Potential obstacles to planned actions and revised actions

  Revisions to the plan as goals and objectives are achieved or changed

  A recording of the plan in a concise, standardized, and retrievable form

INTRODUCTION

Once a community's health has been assessed, the data analyzed, and community nursing diagnoses derived, it is time to consider nursing interventions that will promote the community's health—to formulate a *community-focused plan*. Community-focused plans are based on the nursing diagnoses and contain specific goals and interventions for achieving desired outcomes. Planning, like assessment and analysis, is a systematic process completed in partnership with the community.

> TIME OUT: Before proceeding, let's stop and consider the word *partnership* and its implications for community health nursing. Recall that a community is a social group determined by geographic boundaries and common values and interests. Community members function and interact within a particular social structure that both creates and exhibits behaviors and values. The norm behaviors and value systems of individuals, families, and the community that you have assessed may be very different from your own individual and family behaviors and values, as well as the shared values of the community in which you reside. This creates a potential conflict. What may appear to you as a primary health problem of the community (for example, the incomplete immunization status at Temple Elementary in Rosemont) may not hold the same importance for the residents of Rosemont. They may be far more concerned about the possibility of being criminally victimized. Hence, there is a real need to *validate* community nursing diagnoses with the community. There is one question to ask: Are the community nursing diagnoses of importance to community residents? Methods of validating community nursing diagnoses will be presented in this chapter.

Validating your community nursing diagnoses with the community residents is the first step toward establishing a partnership. Equally important is the right of community leaders, organizations, and residents to confidentiality of privileged information, and their right to choose *not to participate* in health planning. Communities have the right to identify their own health needs and to negotiate with the community health nurse with regard to interventions and specific programs. In turn, the community health nurse has the responsibility to provide or assist with the development of information needed for this process. The American Nurses' Association's (ANA) *Code for Nurses with Interpretive Standards* provides a guide for the many human rights issues that the community health nurse encounters.

In addition to forming a partnership with the community, the community health nurse must consider the influences of social, economic, ecological, and political issues. Many (if not all) community health issues are directly and profoundly affected by larger policy issues. The high prevalence of dental caries among youngsters at Temple Elementary is related as much to the lack of fluoride in Rosemont's drinking water as it is to the lack of dental hygiene education at the school. In turn, each etiologic antecedent is influenced by city, county, state, and national legislative actions and policies. None of the nursing diagnoses for Rosemont can be considered to be separate from the remaining diagnoses; all diagnoses document the health status of Rosemont and must be considered as a whole during the community-focused planning.

Additional considerations of the nurse who is involved in community-focused health planning are the health needs of populations at risk. Special at-risk groups reside in all communities—pregnant women, infants, children, and the elderly are groups at increased risk to decreased health status. The health needs of at-risk groups must be considered as part of all community health plans.

Lastly, community-focused planning involves an awareness and application of planned change—a process of well-thought-out actions to make something happen. Planned change is discussed in detail later in this chapter.

VALIDATING COMMUNITY NURSING DIAGNOSES

In reviewing the community nursing diagnoses for Rosemont (see Table 7-9), it can be seen that several diagnoses focus on the health status of children, and others on the health of special groups such as the asian and homosexual male populations. Many diagnoses seem to affect all residents such as the stress and anxiety of being criminally victimized. It may be helpful to stop and review your community nursing diagnoses and categorize them according to the population most affected. A categorization of Rosemont's diagnoses appears in the displayed material, *Community Nursing Diagnoses for Rosemont by Population Group.*

Because several diagnoses focus on children; and because the age and dependency status of children place them at increased risk of decreased health status, a decision was made to begin the planning process by validating the diagnoses that focused on children.

PLANNED CHANGE

We all experience change. As you read these words your knowledge level is changing. Yet *planned change* differs from *change* in that actions occur in a

COMMUNITY NURSING DIAGNOSES FOR ROSEMONT BY POPULATION GROUP

Children

- Potential for accidents, (*e.g.,* trauma or suffocation as children explore abandoned machinery)

Specific to children at Temple Elementary

- Truancy and academic failure
- Inadequate medical care services
- Potential for decreased health status
- Incomplete immunization status
- High prevalence of *capitis pediculosis*
- High prevalence of dental caries
- Lack of health promotion information including nutrition, exercise, and safety

Infants

- High infant, neonatal, and fetal mortality rate

Male Homosexuals

- Stress within Rosemont between the homosexual and heterosexual populations (especially the heterosexual elderly)
- Potential for inadequate coping of persons with sexually transmitted diseases (STD)
- Potential for inadequate medical care at Rosemont Health Center

All Rosemont Residents

- Stress and anxiety of being criminally victimized
- Potential for health problems associated with air pollution
- Inadequate primary health care services

---

definite sequence, with each action serving as preparation for the next. Planned change is a well-thought-out effort designed to make something happen; all efforts are directed and targeted to produce change. (Many theorists have written about planned change; several works are listed at the end of this chapter.) Reinkemeyer's stages of planned change are presented in the displayed material. The stages are like a receipt in that to produce change each must be followed strictly and be completed. One theorist, Kurt Lewin, de-

REINKEMEYER'S STAGES OF PLANNED CHANGE

Stage 1   Development of a felt need and desire for the change
Stage 2   Development of a change relationship between the agent and the client system
Stage 3   Clarification or diagnosis of the client system's problem, need, or objective
Stage 4   Examination of alternative routes and tentative goals and intentions of actions
Stage 5   Transformation of intentions into actual change
Stage 6   Stabilization
Stage 7   Termination of the relationship between the change agent and the client system

scribed three stages of planned change: *unfreezing, moving,* and *refreezing,* as shown in the displayed material on Lewin. It is during the unfreezing stage that the client system (*i.e.,* organization, community, at-risk population) becomes aware of a problem and the need for change. Then the problem is diagnosed and solutions to the problem are identified. From these alternative solutions one is chosen that seems most appropriate for the situation. In the

LEWIN'S STAGES OF PLANNED CHANGE AND THEIR APPLICATION TO THE PLANNING PROCESS

Lewin's stages of planned change	*Application to the Planning Process*
>> ◆Unfreezing	◆Unfreezing
	▪ Identification of a need for change
>> >> ◆Moving process	◆Moving process
	▪ Presence of a change agent
	▪ Identification of problems
	▪ Consideration of alternatives
	▪ Adaptation of plan to circumstances
>> >> >> ◆Refreezing	◆Refreezing
	▪ Implementation of the plan
	▪ Stabilization of the situation

moving stage, the change actually occurs. The problem is clarified, and the program for solving the problem is planned in detail and begun. Finally, the refreezing stage consists of the accomplished changes becoming integrated into the values of the client system. In this stage the idea is established and continues to be influential. Lewin also addressed forces that help or hinder change to occur, labeling the helping forces, the *driving forces,* and the hindering forces the *restraining forces.*

Theories of planned change are important because they can be used to guide and direct the planning process.

APPLYING CHANGE THEORY TO COMMUNITY HEALTH PLANNING

To validate our nursing diagnoses and initiate the planning process, Reinke-meyer's stages of planned change have been chosen as a guide.

Stage 1: Development of a Felt Need and Desire for the Change

To initiate a felt need and desire for change within the Rosemont community, those organizations that reported actual or potential health concerns of youngsters were contacted and a meeting was suggested in order to report the findings of the Rosemont community assessment. Meetings were arranged with the staffs of Temple Elementary, the Third Street Clinic, and the YMCA Indo-Chinese Refugee Program. During the meetings input from each staff member was sought regarding their observations and perceptions of child health needs, as well as their desire to become involved in a planned program of health promotion.

Temple Elementary requested the assessment data be shared with representatives of the Parent Teacher Organization (PTO), as well as the school's newly formed parent–teacher liaison group. Both the Third Street Clinic and the YMCA Indo-Chinese Refugee Program requested a presentation to their community advisory boards.

Stage 2: Development of a Change Relationship Between the Agent and the Client System

Both Stages 1 and 2 were completed during the assessment presentations. All staff were keenly aware of child health needs, and each organization desired to

become involved in the planning process. To expedite planning, it was decided to form the *Rosemont Health Promotion Council.* Each of the three
organizations, Temple Elementary, the Third Street Clinic, and the YMCA
Indo-Chinese Refugee Program, decided to send one staff member and one
interested parent to the planning meetings. At this point the community health
nurse functioned as a change agent to guide and facilitate but *not* to direct the
planning process. The council elected a chairperson and agreed on meeting
dates. The purpose of the council was to coordinate interagency planning for a
community-focused health promotion program.

Stage 3: Clarification or Diagnosis of the Client System's Problem, Need, or Objective

Now the time has arrived to validate the community nursing diagnoses. At the
conclusion of each presentation the community health nurse proposed a survey questionnaire to assess the target population's perception of their health
concerns. Revisions were solicited from staff and community groups and the
final agreed-upon questionnaire is presented here. Notice that the questionnaire is directed to parents, yet the nursing diagnoses are focused on children.
Why not ask the children? This suggestion was made by several council participants. Some members felt two questionnaires were necessary—one for the
parents and one for the youngsters. What do you think? Because of the age of
the youngsters (some had not learned how to read) and the associated time
and costs of two questionnaires, it was decided to use one questionnaire and
to direct it to the parents.

Although the Rosemont questionnaire is focused on child health, the
identical format could be used to validate assessed health concerns of the
elderly, well adults, teenagers, or pregnant women. The process of checking
your assessed community data against the perceptions of the target population
can be completed by a survey questionnaire (such as the one in the displayed
material) that can be mailed or given as an interview. Or you may choose to
validate assessed data by interviewing community leaders and civic groups
that are *representative* of the target population. The word representative is
very important. For example, the Temple Elementary PTO would not be representative of parents in Rosemont because, as was noted during the assessment, most parents are not active in the organization.

Before we continue, a few words are needed about composing questionnaires. Everyone is confronted daily with people who are asking questions.
Questionnaires arrive in the mail and people call on the phone. Frequently,
the interviewees never learn the purpose of the questionnaire nor how the

QUESTIONNAIRE TO VALIDATE
COMMUNITY NURSING DIAGNOSIS

Dear Parent;

We are nursing students who are interested in learning more about what you think are the most important health needs of your family. Answering a few short questions will help us plan some information sessions for you about how to keep your family healthy. Please either place a ✓ in the appropriate box or fill in the line. Your participation is voluntary. All information is confidential and you will not be identified in any way. If you have questions, please feel free to call us. Thank you.

Virginia Brown
Ricardo Guerrero
Ann Wang
Alice Washington

1. How many children do you have? _____
2. What are their ages? _____
3. If you have a baby, do you breast feed? Yes [   ] No [   ]
4. If you have a baby, do you bottle feed? Yes [   ] No [   ]
5. What other foods do you feed your baby? _____
   _____
6. What foods do you usually feed your children?
   _____
   _____
   _____
   _____
7. Would you like to know more about what to feed your baby and children to keep them healthy? Yes [   ] No [   ]
8. Would you like to know where you can take your children for health care, both when they are well and sick? Yes [   ] No [   ]
9. Check (✓) the following common problems you would like to know more about.
   [   ] Vomiting
   [   ] Diarrhea
   [   ] Colds and allergies
   [   ] Skin rashes
   [   ] Cuts and falls
   [   ] Head lice
   [   ] Worms
   [   ] Fever
   [   ] Temper tantrums and angry behaviors
   [   ] Refusal to do homework or go to school
   [   ] Poor school grades

(continued)

QUESTIONNAIRE TO VALIDATE
COMMUNITY NURSING DIAGNOSIS (Continued)

10. Other concerns that you would like information about (this can include information for yourself, a friend, or a child):

_____

_____

11. Have you ever felt that you, a sibling, or another adult hurt your child when the child was punished? Yes [   ]   No [   ]

12. Would you like to learn about ways to keep from hurting children when adults are angry? Yes [   ] No [   ]

13. Circle the best days and times for you to attend information sessions.
Monday   am   pm
Tuesday   am   pm
Wednesday   am   pm
Thursday   am   pm
Friday   am   pm
Saturday   am   pm
Sunday   am   pm

14. Circle the best place for you to attend information sessions:
Temple Elementary
Third Street Clinic
YMCA
Other (specify where) _____

---

information will be used. When you draft a questionnaire, begin with introductory information that states who you are and the purpose of the questionnaire. Emphasize that participation is voluntary and that the information given will be confidential. Sign your name and, if the questionnaire is to be mailed, include a phone number where you can be contacted. Write questions that can be answered quickly (the whole questionnaire should not take longer than ten minutes to complete). Ideally, place all questions on one side of a standard 8½-inch by 11-inch piece of paper that, if it is to be mailed, can be refolded so that a return address shows. Before sharing the questionnaire with agencies or community residents, administer it informally to friends and family; any comments made (*e.g.,* "What do you mean by . . . ?" or "I don't understand. . . .") signals the need for further rewriting and clarification.

Because Rosemont has a large population of Spanish- and Vietnamese-speaking residents, staff at Temple Elementary and the YMCA Indo-Chinese

Refugee Program volunteered to translate the questionnaire into these languages. The questionnaire was then ready for distribution.

> DECISION POINT: How should the questionnaire be administered? Should the questionnaire be mailed to all households of children at Temple Elementary? *Or,* should the questionnaire be given to all adults who bring their children to the Third Street Clinic? *Or,* should the questionnaire be used as an interview and given to a *selected* number of parents at Temple Elementary, or to clients at the Third Street Clinic, or to adults attending the YMCA Indo-Chinese Refugee Program? (Recall from Chapter 2 that persons who have been randomly selected can be considered representative of the total population.) What would you recommend? Before making a decision, list each option and consider the benefits and problems of each. Here is some information for your decision-making: Mailed questionnaires have about a 50% return rate that can be increased somewhat with a reminder postcard or telephone call, whereas questionnaires administered as an interview have a 100% return rate. However, interviews require interview*ers* and about five minutes per person per page of questionnaire, whereas mailed questionnaires require less labor, but has the financial cost of postage. *Decisions . . . decisions. . . .*

Following several discussions of the Rosemont Health Promotion Council, it was decided to distribute the questionnaire from Temple Elementary by sending one form home with each child. The questionnaires were color-coded by language, and each child was given a questionnaire in the language that was spoken commonly at home.

Within two weeks, 410 of the 736 questionnaires had been returned. The results were tabulated and summarized by the community health nurse and presented to the Rosemont Health Promotion Council. Examples of the summarized data are presented in Tables 8-1 through 8-4. Why do you think the information was presented by ethnicity? What differences do you notice between family composition and ethnicity, health information desired and ethnicity, and further concerns and ethnicity? Of what importance are these ethnic differences for community health planning?

> NOTE: The Rosemont questionnaires were categorized by ethnicity (surmised from the language commonly spoken in the home. However, depending on the community, responses may be categorized by urban versus rural residence, age of respondents, or other meaningful vari-

TABLE 8-1.   FAMILY COMPOSITION BY ETHNICITY

Number of Children	Hispanic		Vietnamese		Other*	
	n	*%*	*n*	*%*	*n*	*%*
Baby only	82	57	44	61	31	16
Two children	12	8	3	4	112	58
Three children	24	17	10	14	34	18
Four or more children	26	18	15	21	17	8
Total	144	100	72	100	194	100

* Primarily white and black

ables). Once summarized, no preferred day and time emerged for the classes. However, a definite preference was shown for location with all Vietnamese-speaking families preferring the YMCA location and Spanish-speaking clients preferring the Third Street Clinic.

TABLE 8-2.   HEALTH INFORMATION DESIRED BY ETHNICITY

	Hispanic		Vietnamese		Other*	
	n	*%*	*n*	*%*	*n*	*%*
Vomiting	124	86	65	90	22	11
Diarrhea	134	93	71	98	34	18
Skin rashes	114	79	11	15	52	29
Cuts/falls	45	31	60	83	5	3
Colds/allergies	46	32	5	7	62	32
Head lice	24	17	10	14	74	38
Worms	85	59	70	97	10	5
Fever	132	92	69	96	93	48
Tantrums/angry behavior	10	7	4	5	175	90
School refusal	5	3	6	8	165	85
Poor grades	4	3	2	3	132	68
Total respondents	144		72		194	

* Primarily white and black

TABLE 8-3.   PERCENTAGE OF RESPONDENTS NOTING
OTHER CONCERNS BY ETHNICITY

	Hispanic (%)	Vietnamese (%)	Other (%)*
Legal issues (*i.e.,* child support, custody rights)	32	15	64
Finances/budgeting	23	26	51
Child-care programs	82	12	75
Adult health (*i.e.,* weight reduction, birth control)	75	11	68
Employment	82	95	75
Crime prevention, especially prevention of rape and child molestation	88	84	89

* Primarily white and black

Stage 4: Examination of Alternative Routes and Tentative Goals and Intention of Actions

Having validated the community nursing diagnoses, the Rosemont Health Promotion Council was anxious to establish a plan. Much discussion followed the presentation of the questionnaire results. Representatives from Temple Elementary focused on questions 9 and 10 and were anxious to present a series of effective parenting seminars on discipline. Temple also felt the high percentage of white and black families who requested information about school phobias and poor grades merited sessions on that topic. Temple's staff discussed how programs to meet the questionnaire needs were consistent with the school's goal of improved communication between teachers and parents, as well as their "Fail-Safe" program. In addition, recent state programs developed to prevent child abuse were proposed for presentation.

The staff of the Third Street Clinic focused on the high percentage of families with infants and the associated desire for information on nutrition and the care of common health conditions. The Third Street Clinic had recently initiated a Health Baby Program, consisting of evening and Saturday well child and prenatal clinics, as well as a total service day on Friday when clients could drop in without appointments for immunizations and screening tests for blood pressure, vision, and hearing. Informal counseling was also offered on Friday.

TABLE 8-4. PERCENTAGE OF RESPONDENTS
ANSWERING YES TO QUESTIONS 11 AND
12 BY ETHNICITY

	Answered Yes		
	Hispanic *(%)*	*Vietnamese* *(%)*	*Other* *(%)**
Question 11: Have you ever felt that you, a sibling, or another adult hurt your child when the child was punished?	89	92	94
Question 12: Would you like to learn about ways to keep from hurting children when adults are angry?	94	95	98

* Primarily white and black

The goal for the next six months was to invite various service providers, such as optometry and dental-hygiene students, as well as Medicare and State Unemployment Commission representatives, to jointly use the clinic space for information sessions and services. After considering the results of the questionnaire, the staff began to discuss the possibility of offering on Fridays, health promotion classes such as weight reduction, exercise fitness, and information sessions for common conditions. The idea of inviting the Police Department to make presentations on crime prevention and legal rights was proposed and agreed upon by everyone.

Representatives from the YMCA Indo-Chinese Refugee Program felt that, because of cultural taboos against discussing topics such as birth control in public, the information would be best accepted if offered at the YMCA by a respected member of the Vietnamese community. The YMCA was beginning a daycare service for mothers of preschoolers and felt some of the information on child care could become part of the new program, as well as basic child health screening services of development, vision, and hearing. The YMCA representatives were equally concerned that Vietnamese refugees be culturally assimilated into the Rosemont community and wanted to plan interagency programs such as crime prevention and legal rights that would bring the Vietnamese into more contact with other Rosemont residents. The suggestion was made that a program on crime prevention would not only bring residents of different cultures together but also residents of different lifestyles. Keenly aware of the tension and stress between the homosexual and heterosexual populations, a community-awareness program on crime prevention was suggested that would involve all three agencies and all residents of Rosemont. The idea was agreed upon by all council members.

> TIME OUT! Notice that each agency is considering how information learned from the questionnaire can be assimilated into *existing* or *planned programs.* All agencies have budgets and a set number of staff members to deliver services. Agencies must be as cost efficient as possible and will want to consider how to include new services (such as information desired by parents) into an existing program. Community health nurses can facilitate this process by becoming familiar with the organizational structure and purpose of each agency. When you establish a planned-change relationship with an agency, ask about their organizational structure (most agencies have an organizational chart with positions arranged according to authority). Decision-making usually follows the organizational chart, with consent from all levels being required before major changes can be made or a new program can be begun. Learn the names of the staff and their position on the organizational chart. (An organizational chart for the Third Street Clinic appears in Figure 8-1.) Ask for a statement of the agency's purpose and goals. Ask if you can attend a board meeting and pertinent committee meetings. Your purpose is to learn as much about the services and decision-making process of the agency as possible in order to facilitate the planned-change nursing interventions.

COMMUNITY HEALTH GOAL

Now is the time to transform the ideas and proposals of each agency into a community-focused goal and concrete intentions of action. After validating the nursing diagnoses with the community, the community-focused goal was: *To provide health promotion programs on issues desired by the community residents, using methods acceptable to cultural norms and offered in an accessible location at a cost the community can afford.*

This is a very comprehensive statement and can be considered to be an umbrella goal for the Rosemont community under which each agency will have goals. Goals specific to Temple Elementary included

- Reduce truancy 20% by the end of one school year

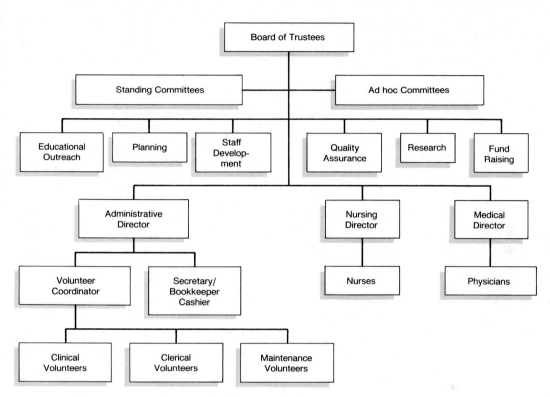

Figure 8-1. Organizational chart—Third Street Clinic.

- Reduce grade failures 20% by the end of one school year
- Increase immunization levels to 95% within one year
- Improve communication between parents and teachers
- Increase parental knowledge on how to protect children from molestation

Goals for the Third Street Clinic that were congruent with the community goal included

- Increased knowledge of community residents regarding crime prevention and legal rights
- Increased knowledge of parents regarding common health problems of children
- Increased knowledge and practice of effective parenting skills
- Increased percentage of adults who practice healthy lifestyle practices, including

Exercise fitness
Weight control
Stress management

Goals for the YMCA Indo-Chinese Refugee Program included

- 100% of children in daycare program screened for vision and hearing problems
- Increased knowledge and correct use of contraceptives
- Increased knowledge of parents regarding common health problems of children
- Increased rate of employed adults by 50%
- Increased rate of employed teenagers by 20%
- Increased knowledge of community residents regarding crime prevention and legal rights

PROGRAM ACTIVITIES

After formulation of goals, the next step is specifying the program activities. *Program activities* map out the actions necessary to deliver the program and thereby reach the goal(s). For example, one goal of the Third Street Clinic was: *increased knowledge of parents regarding health problems of children.* Program activities for the goal might include

- Third Street Clinic staff and the community health nurse will select topics that are congruent with the questionnaire results to be included in classes for parents on common health problems of children.
- Third Street Clinic staff and the community health nurse will select resources (*i.e.,* audio-visuals, pamphlets) for presentation on the selected topics.
- Third Street Clinic staff and the community health nurse will decide on a day, time, and presentation schedule that are congruent with the questionnaire results.

Each program activity deals with planning the program and is written as sequential steps, each step being required to reach the goal. In addition, each program activity needs a date of accomplishment (for example: "By June 15, the Third Street Clinic staff and the community health nurse will . . .").

LEARNING OBJECTIVES

Once program activities have been established, learning objectives are written. *Learning objectives* are derived from a goal and describe the precise behavior or changes that will be required to achieve the goal. Where program activities map out the actions necessary to deliver the program, learning objectives specify what changes in knowledge, behaviors, or attitudes are expected as a result of program activities.

Learning objectives focus on the learner and state what changes the learner can expect as a result of participating in the program. For example, one topic selected for presentation during the classes on common health problems of children was fever assessment and home management. The learning objectives were

- Following the class and practice session on fever assessment and management of the fever at home, each participant will be able to
    Demonstrate how to take a rectal and axillary temperature
    Discuss common causes and dangers of fever during childhood
    State what constitutes a fever
    Explain at least three methods to reduce a fever
    Describe danger signs that require a medical assessment

Both program and learning objectives can be written in sequential steps that are required to reach the goal; or each objective may have different aspects that, when combined, achieve the goal. Goals and objectives need to *measurable.* To make statements measurable, use precise words. Examples of precise terms and less precise terms appear below:

Less Precise Terms (many interpretations)

To know	To appreciate
To understand	To be aware
To realize	To lower

More Precise Terms (fewer interpretations)

To identify	To compare and contrast
To discuss	To state
To list	To decrease by 20%

In addition, strive for each goal and objective to include

- A time frame for attaining the change; for example, "By June 15th . . ."

- The direction and magnitude of the change; for example, "Increase immunization levels to 95%"
- The method of measuring the change; for example, "Following the session, each participant will demonstrate. . . ."

Goals and subparts of the goals (objectives) help to clarify a program and establish the expected changes that will result from the program. Although much has been written on the mechanics of writing goals and objectives (several texts are listed at the conclusion of this chapter), little information exists on the collaborative relationship that must exist between community health nurse and community agency(ies) before meaningful goals and objectives can result.

COLLABORATION

What is meant by a collaborative relationship? Recall from the initial community assessment data that the staff of Temple Elementary had voiced concerns about truancy and grade failure; these same concerns are their first two goals. However, when the nursing diagnoses were validated with the community, parents were more concerned about ways in which they could protect their children from molestation. Could the concerns of the parents and those of the Temple Elementary staff be addressed in the same program? If they could, what would be the program objective? the content objectives? This process is an example of *collaborative planning* and is the essence of community health nursing. You may be wondering how to establish collaborative planning and inform agencies about the usefulness of goals and objectives. Although you may be convinced of the value of planned change, how do you convince others to agree, especially since planned change is not commonly practiced in agencies? *Role modeling* is probably the best strategy. After reviewing the community nursing diagnoses and validating data with an agency, propose goals and objectives that are congruent with the agency's purpose and organizational structure. Solicit input from the group, and continue to revise the goals and objectives until a group consensus is reached.

RESOURCES, CONSTRAINTS, AND REVISED PLANS

Once goals and objectives are written, the next step is to identify available resources and any constraints to the plan. Lastly, revised plans are proposed to the planning group. *Resources* are all the available means for accomplishing a task, including staff and budget, as well as physical space and equipment. For program planning, it is important to identify the *resources needed,* as well as the *resources available. Constraints* are obstacles that restrict or limit actions, and can include a lack of staff, budget, physical space, and equipment. *Revised Plans* are actions that are proposed based on the knowledge of resources and constraints.

Following much discussion and self-examination, each agency of the Rosemont Health Promotion Council formed program goals and objectives. Then, alongside each goal and objective, necessary resources were listed. For example, at the Third Street Clinic, the following resources were identified as crucial to the goal.

Goal

To increase the knowledge of parents regarding common health problems of children

Resources Needed

- Staff member to develop and assemble existing information on common health problems of children
- Staff member to present the information materials in English, Spanish, and Vietnamese
- Physical space and necessary equipment (*e.g.,* thermometers, basins) to teach assessment and home care skills

Resources Available

- Staff members who speak English and Spanish
- Staff nurse with knowledge about the care of children
- Physical space and some necessary equipment
- Staff interest and desire to offer information requested by parents

Constraints

It may be helpful to consider constraints as the mismatch between resources needed and resources available. Constraints at the Third Street Clinic include

- No staff member who speaks Vietnamese
- Discomfort of staff because of inexperience in developing and adapting learning materials
- Time limitations
- Staff felt insecure about their ability to perform group teaching (all previous teaching was one-to-one)
- Lack of resource material (*e.g.,* audio-visuals and brochures on care of common childhood problems)

> NOTE: Universal constraints are *staff* and *money*—agencies never have enough. An additional constraint is *resistance to change.* All people are reluctant to change existing routines and patterns of behavior. Initially, change is uncomfortable and until new roles are learned, there is anxiety. Making people aware of the natural discomfort associated with change can build rapport and establish a collaborative relationship.

When each agency had listed their program goals, activities, and objectives along with resources and constraints, several alternative actions became apparent. For example, a constraint of the Third Street Clinic was lack of staff who spoke Vietnamese. A similar constraint of the YMCA Indo-Chinese Refugee Program was lack of a staff member with necessary knowledge to offer classes on contraception or the care of children with common health problems. Therefore, the following revised plan was proposed:

Revised Plan

A bilingual (English–Vietnamese) staff member from the YMCA would attend the classes offered in English at the Third Street Clinic and then offer the classes in Vietnamese at the YMCA.

Both the Third Street Clinic and the YMCA noted a lack of resource materials as a constraint to program implementation. However further assessment of community health resources by the community health nurse revealed that the Sunvalley Clinic, as part of the Hampton Health Department, had access to various audio-visuals and printed materials on the subjects; however, all materials were in English.

Revised Plan

One Spanish–English-speaking staff member from the Third Street Clinic and one Vietnamese–English-speaking staff member from the YMCA would translate the materials into Spanish and Vietnamese free of charge with the provision that they be given copies of all the translated materials.

An additional constraint to each agency was that their staffs felt unprepared to do group instruction.

Revised Plan

The community health nurse would provide instruction in basic principles of group teaching, including methods of presenting information. In addition the community health nurse would participate in the development and adaptation of materials and the teaching of classes.

For each constraint a revised plan was proposed, discussed and adopted. This is a period of intense collaboration between the community health nurse and community agencies and only at the completion of this stage is the community ready for Stage 5 of planned change—transformation of intentions into actual change behavior. This *transformation of intentions* is the actual program implementation (which is covered in the next chapter). However, before the plan is implemented, it must be recorded.

RECORDING

Community plans must be recorded in a standardized, systematic, and concise form that clearly communicates to others the purpose and actions of the plan, as well as the rationale for revisions and deletions of actions. Discuss with each agency their present recording system and decide on a format and system for recording the plan. The format need not be elaborate and a simple one such as that used at the Third Street Clinic would be adequate *if* agreed upon by the agency (see the displayed material).

SUMMARY

Before concluding, let's review the learning objectives for this chapter and their application to community health nursing. The planning process begins with validation of the community nursing diagnoses—a process that establishes the community's perception and value of community health needs. Next, using theories of planned change, the community health nurse and the

FORMAT FOR RECORDING A COMMUNITY HEALTH PLAN

Agency: *Third Street Clinic*

Community Nursing Diagnoses Specific to Children

- Inadequate medical care services for children
- Potential for decreased health status of children
- Incomplete immunization status of elementary-school-age children
- High prevalence of *capitus pediculosis* among elementary-school-age children

Validation Data

- Questionnaire sent to 736 families and returned by 410

Program Goal

- Increase knowledge of parents in regard to common health problems of children

Program Activities

- Third Street Clinic staff and the community health nurse will select topics to be included in classes that are congruent with questionnaire results.
- Third Street Clinic staff and the community health nurse will select resources (*i.e.,* audio-visuals, pamphlets) for presentation of the selected topics.
- Third Street Clinic staff and the community health nurse will decide on a day, time, and presentation schedule that is congruent with the questionnaire results.

Learning Objectives

Following the class and practice session on fever assessment and home management, each participant will be able to

- Demonstrate how to take a rectal and axillary temperature
- Discuss common causes and dangers of fever during childhood
- State what constitutes a fever
- Explain at least three methods to reduce a fever
- Describe danger signs that require a medical assessment

Resources

- Needed   Staff member to develop and assemble information on common health problems of children
          Staff member to present the information materials in English, Spanish, and Vietnamese

(*continued*)

FORMAT FOR RECORDING A COMMUNITY
HEALTH PLAN (Continued)

Physical space and necessary equipment (*e.g.,* thermometer, basins) to teach assessment and home-care skills

- Available
Staff members who speak English and Spanish
Staff nurse with knowledge about the care of children
Physical space and some necessary equipment
Staff interest and desire to offer information requested by parents.

- Constraints
No staff member who speaks Vietnamese
Discomfort related to lack of experience in developing and adapting learning materials
Time constraints
Insecurities in staff's abilities to implement group teaching experience (all previous teaching was one-to-one)
Lack of resource material (*i.e.,* audio-visuals and brochures on care of common childhood problems)

Revised Plans

- A bilingual (English–Vietnamese) staff member from the Third Street Clinic and one Vietnamese–English-speaking staff member from the "Y" will translate needed materials into Spanish and Vietnamese free of charge, with the provision to have copies of all the translated materials.
- The community health nurse would provide instruction in basic principles of group teaching, including methods of presenting information. In addition, the community health nurse would participate in the development and adaption of materials, as well as the teaching of the classes. (Chapter 13 details the role of teaching in community health and contains valuable information for health education program development.)

---

community form a collaborative partnership to establish program goals and objectives. Lastly, based on resources and constraints, plans are proposed, recorded, and adopted. Although only one example is offered here, the process of community health planning was the same for all eight programs that were developed by the Rosemont Health Promotion Council.

SUGGESTED READINGS

Community Health Planning

American Nurses' Association: Code for Nurses with Interpretive Standards. Kansas City, Missouri, American Nurses Assoc, 1985

Archer SE: Implementing change in community: A Collaborative Process. St. Louis, CV Mosby, 1984

Blum H: Planning for Health: Generics for the Eighties. New York, Human Science Press, 1981

Dignan M, Carr P: Introduction to Program Planning. Philadelphia, Lea & Febiger, 1981

Green LW, Kreuter MW, Deeds SG, Partridge KG: Health Education Planning: A Diagnostic Approach. Palo Alto, California, Mayfield, 1980

Kraegel JM: *Planning Strategies for Nurse Managers.* Rockville, Maryland, Aspen Systems, 1983

Rothman J: Three models of community organization practice. In Cox F (ed): *Strategies of Community Organization.* Hasca, Illinois, FE Peacock, 1979

Spiegel AD, Hyman HH: Basic Health Planning Methods. Germantown, Maryland, Aspen Systems Corporation, 1978

Staropoli CJ, Waltz CF: *Developing and Evaluating Educational Programs for Health Care Providers.* Philadelphia, FA Davis Co, 1978

Objective Writing

Gronlund NE: Stating Objectives for Classroom Instruction, 2nd ed. New York, Macmillan Publishing, 1978

Mager R: Preparing Objectives for Programmed Instruction. San Francisco, Fearon Publishers, 1978

Reilly D: Behavioral Objectives—Evaluation in Nursing. New York, Appleton-Century-Crofts, 1980

Planned Change Theory

Havelock R: *The Change Agent's Guide to Innovation in Education.* New Jersey, Educational Technology Publishers, 1973

Lewin K: Group decision and social change. In Maccoby E (ed): Readings in Social Psychology, 3rd ed. New York, Holt, Rinehart and Winston, 1958

Lippitt G: Visualizing Change: Model Building and the Change Process. LaJolla, California, University Associates, 1973

Lippitt R, Watson J, Westley B: The Dynamics of Planned Change. New York, Harcourt, Brace and World, 1951

Olson EM: Strategies and techniques for the nurse change agent. Nurs Clin North Am 14:307–321, 1979

Welch LB: Planned change in nursing: The theory. Nurs Clin North Am 14:307–321, 1979

9

Implementing
a Health Program

OBJECTIVES

Implementation is the action phase of the nursing process; the carrying-out of the community-focused plan. Implementation is necessary to achieve goals and objectives, but more importantly, the implementation of nursing interventions acts to promote, maintain, or restore health; to prevent illness; and to effect rehabilitation.

This chapter discusses the process of implementing a community-focused health program. Intervention strategies are presented, as well as resources that are helpful in program implementation.

After studying this chapter you will be able to

- Suggest strategies to the community for implementation of health programs

In partnership with the community, you will be able to

- Implement planned programs
- Review and revise interventions based on community responses
- Use interventions to formulate and influence health and social policies that impact the health of the community

INTRODUCTION

Once goals and objectives have been agreed upon and recorded during the planning stage, all that remains for implementation is the actual carrying-out of those objectives. This probably seems straight-forward and simple. Indeed, at this point you will have spent considerable time assessing, analyzing, and planning a program. You will be ready and eager to begin. But it is this very eagerness and the associated impatience of the intervention stage that is a danger. You must take time to consider how you can create a feeling of community ownership, a unified program, and a clear health focus.

COMMUNITY OWNERSHIP

Essential to achieving the desired outcomes of the interventions is the active participation of the community. The meaning of partnership and collaboration was discussed in the preceding chapter, but the present concern is *ownership*. The community needs to feel a sense of ownership of the program or event, which can only come with their participation in the decisions regarding planning and a responsibility for implementation. Herein lies a potential conflict. The profession of nursing is one of nurturing, sustaining, and caring for others. It is part of our profession to do for others what they would do for themselves if they were able. Indeed, most nurses interact professionally with people during an altered health state that requires nurses to do for others; but this is not true in community health nursing. Stepping into the community requires an attitude of *doing with* the people, not doing things to them or for them. When things are done to us or for us, our emotional commitment remains limited.

How might you ensure community ownership for a proposed program and planned interventions? How can you facilitate involvement? In Rosemont, the Rosemont Health Promotion Council functioned to coordinate inter-agency planning for a community-focused health promotion program. When the planning had been completed, the council directed its attention to the coordination of activities for the program's implementation. The important point in this example is that a coordination group was already in place. Usually the planning committee can coordinate implementation.

DECISION POINT: When the Rosemont Health Promotion Council and designated staff in charge of program implementation reviewed the program objectives and needed resources, it was evident that before the program could proceed resources had to be selected. (Resources mean audio-visuals, pamphlets and other material for presentation of the program.) Council and staff members began to ask where such materials could be obtained. What was available in Rosemont? What could you have suggested at this point?

Examining the initial assessment of Rosemont, it was noted that the United Way listed 42 private and publicly supported social service agencies located in Hampton or Jefferson County. The United Way listing included identifying information for each agency, and services and fees. Reviewing the list with the council and participating staff, the community health nurse suggested that selected agency representatives be invited to discuss agency programs and resources that they could make available such as films and speakers. It was found that several could provide relevant material. The March of Dimes was sponsoring a campaign in Hampton to increase public awareness of the importance of a healthy pregnancy for the birth of a healthy child. The Mental Health Association had developed teaching modules on effective parenting, and the police department and the Woman's Center were offering programs on crime prevention. All of these programs had received recently a brief description, including the names of their contact persons, in the *Hampton Herald*. At this point, it was decided to complete program and learning objectives for each of the health promotion goals established by the Rosemont Council. Therefore as various agency personnel discussed their program with the council, decisions could be made on the appropriateness of the material for the Rosemont Community.

> TIME OUT! Do not panic at this point and feel that you must be knowledgeable about all 46 agencies and their programs in the community that you have assessed. Do, at the implementation stage, refer back to your initial assessment and consider logically which service agencies may have resources helpful to the planned program(s). Then contact selected agencies, request information on their purpose and present programs, share with the agency your community-focused program plans and solicit recommendations with regard to materials and resources. A list is presented in the displayed material of voluntary organizations that have professional staff at the national and local levels, and an affiliated or community linkage structure. These voluntary organizations have ongoing programs for a wide variety of health issues and most acknowledge health promotion as a vital part of their mission. The list is not inclusive and is meant to serve only as a guide.

VOLUNTARY ORGANIZATIONS

Name of Organization

American Association of Retired Persons
American Cancer Society
American Heart Association
American Lung Association
American Red Cross
Association of Junior Leagues, Inc.
Boy Scouts of America
Boys' Clubs of America
Cooperative Extension Service
Girl Scouts of America
Girls' Club of America, Inc.

March of Dimes
National Board of the YMCA of the U.S.A.
National Coalition of Hispanic Mental Health
   and Human Services Organizations (COSSHMO)
National Council of Alcoholism
National Health Council
National Kidney Foundation
National Safety Council
National Recreation and Parks Association
National Urban League
United Way of America

In addition, the Office of Disease Prevention and Health Promotion (ODPHP), located within the Public Health Service (PHS) (which in turn is located within the U.S. Department of Health and Human Services [DHHS]) publishes a tremendous amount of information that is designed to promote health and prevent disease among Americans. Special attention is given to facilitating the prevention activities of the five public health service agencies: The Alcohol, Drug Abuse, and Mental Health Administration; the Centers for Disease Control (CDC); the Food and Drug Administration (FDA); the Health Resources and Services Administration (HRSA); and the National Institutes of Health (NIH). Several special programs, termed initiatives, are sponsored by the Office of Disease Prevention and Health Promotion. A partial listing of the initiative programs, services, and information available, as well as an address and phone contact, are listed in Table 9-1.

NOTE: Several libraries are designated as government depositories and therefore have many government publications. The government also has bookstores located throughout the United States. Make yourself familiar with the nearest government depository library and bookstore. The Suggested Readings list for this chapter contains several government publications that are focused on disease prevention and health promotion.

Having discussed the importance of community participation and ownership of the program, the remaining issues to consider are a unified presentation of the program and emphasis on health, not the program.

UNIFIED PROGRAM

Because of limited resources, staff constraints, and, frequently, situations beyond rectification, many good programs are implemented in a piecemeal fashion that minimizes their impact. A *unified program* requires collaboration and coordination between the agency personnel who will implement the program and the program's recipients (the target population). Allowing ample time for publicizing the program, (and how you perform the mechanics of publicity—the *how, where,* and *to whom*) can make a crucial difference in attendance and subsequent impact. After a time and place have been selected (based on initial input from the survey questionnaires), how might you publicize a program? Public service announcements, notification in the newspapers, bulletin inserts for civic and religious associations, flyers sent home with school-age children, and posters and notices in community service buildings and local shopping centers are ways to publicize. The Rosemont Health Promotion Council decided to publicize the first program on child health by sending home a flyer with each child at Temple Elementary. The flyer thanked the parents for their participation during the survey and invited them to programs at the Fourth Street Clinic and the YMCA Indo-Chinese Refugee Center. Public service announcements were made on the radio and feature articles about the Rosemont Health Promotion Council and upcoming programs appeared in the Vietnamese and Spanish tabloids, as well as the *Hampton Herald* and Rosemont Civic Association's newsletter. Posters were placed in local grocery stores, churches, and gathering places. Because the parents on the Rosemont Health Promotion Council had expressed a concern that parents with young children may not be able to attend programs, arrangements were made for infant and toddler childcare, and a separate health program for preschool and school-age children was planned during the adult programs. The program publicity was focused on health promotion for the *whole family* and not just programs for selected family members.

The idea of a holistic health program based on unified goals and objectives is central to the 1979 document, *Healthy People—the Surgeon General's Report on Health Promotion and Disease Prevention* (1979) and its sequel, *Promoting Health/Preventing Disease: Objectives for the Nation* (1980). This comprehensive plan is not a federal plan, to be administered from Washington, but rather a plan to be implemented by the citizens of every community. Attainment of the goals and objectives of this plan by 1990 depends on the participation of state and local health agencies and organizations (both public and private) such as the one you will be working with in your practice, as well as the Rosemont Health Promotion Council. Because the national goals and

TABLE 9-1.   OFFICE OF DISEASE PREVENTION AND
             HEALTH PROMOTION: SPECIAL INITIATIVES

Initiative	Description
Community/Media Health Promotion Initiative	The National Health Promotion Program has used media-based efforts to mobilize community resources for health promotion. Activities for the general public include the HealthStyle campaign, as well as the Healthy Mothers Healthy Babies program. Now attention is being directed to older Americans with the initiative on Health Promotion for the Elderly. This initiative is designed to use the media and community organizations to enhance the health practices of older people with respect to diet, exercise, smoking, alcohol use, and appropriate use of medications and preventive services.*
National Health Information Clearinghouse (NHIC)	The NHIC responds directly to requests for health information from both the general public and health professions. The Clearinghouse is a central source of information and referral for health questions. The clearinghouse answers questions in two ways: by retrieving information from the NHIC's onsite library and database or by forwarding requests to other organizations for direct response. The NHIC staff only provide health information; they cannot give medical advise, diagnose, or recommend treatment. Materials available from the Clearinghouse include health-risk appraisals and a list of physical fitness organizations and centers concerned with health topics. Telephone contact: 1-800-336-4797 toll-free (in Virginia 1-703-522-2590) or write P.O. Box 1133, Washington, DC 20013-1133.
School Health Initiative	Focus is to enhance the health of school children by undertaking comprehensive health-oriented efforts such as the assessment of the fitness level of school children, development of a special review on the use of computers for health education, and an evaluation of curricula developed for school health education.Summary reports on school health are available, as well as information material for a school health program. A listing of reports and published material are available from the Office of Disease Prevention and Health Promotion.*

(continued)

TABLE 9-1.   (Continued)

Initiative	Description
Worksite Health Promotion Initiative	Focus is to enhance the health of employees and their families by offering materials to assist in the development of worksite programs, case studies of the health promotion activities of businesses, a national survey of worksite health promotion activities, and projects to explore the future of work and health. Summary reports on worksite health are available, as well as information material for a worksite health program. A listing of reports and published material are available from the ODPHP.*

* Additional information about these activities and other ODPHP publications may be obtained from the Office of Disease Prevention and Health Promotion, Mary E. Switzer Building, Room 2132, 330 C Street SW, Washington, D.C. 20201, Telephone (202) 245-7611.

objectives offer guidance for local health program implementation, the following text discusses the specifics of national health goals and objectives.

Healthy People Documents

In *Healthy People—the Surgeon General's Report on Health Promotion and Disease Prevention, 1979,* the following goals were identified for the year 1990

- For *infants,* the goal is a 35% lower death rate than the 14.1 deaths per 1000 live births that occurred in 1977 (This would mean fewer than 9 deaths per 1000 live births by 1990.)
- There are also two subgoals for infants
  - To reduce incidence of low-birth-weight infants
  - To reduce birth defects
- For *children, ages 1–14,* the goal is a 20% lower death rate (This would be fewer than 34 deaths per 100,000 population by 1990, compared with 43 in 1977.)
- Subgoals for children are:
  - To enhance childhood growth and development
  - To reduce childhood accidents and injury

- For *adolescents and young adults, ages 15–24,* the goal is a 20% lower death rate (This would mean decreasing the death rate from 117 per 100,000 population in 1977 to fewer than 93 in 1990.)
- Subgoals for adolescents and young adults are
    To reduce death and disability from motor vehicle accidents
    To reduce the misuse of alcohol and drugs
- For *adults, ages 25–64,* the goal is a 25% lower death rate (Decreasing from 540 in 1977 to fewer than 400 per 100,000 population in 1990)
- Subgoals are
    To reduce heart attacks and strokes
    To reduce incidence of cancer
- For *older adults, ages 65 and over* the goal is a 20% reduction in days of restricted activity (Restricted activity days will be reduced to fewer than 30 per year.)
- Subgoals for older adults are
    To increase the proportion of older people who can function independently
    To reduce premature death and disability from influenza and pneumonia

The same report identified improvements in 15 priority areas that were necessary in order to reach the goals. The target areas fit into three categories: *personal preventive services, health protection,* and *health promotion.* Preventive services are usually offered by health care providers and include programs such as family planning, maternal and infant health, immunizations, and control of sexually transmitted diseases (STD). Health protection is the efforts made by government, industry, and other organizations to reduce health hazards in the environment. Programs include toxic-agent control, occupational safety, accident and injury control, and surveillance and control of infectious diseases. Lastly, health promotion denotes programs to educate the public about the risks that are involved in health abuses and to increase public commitment to sensible lifestyles that can add years to life expectancy. Target areas include smoking, alcohol and drug misuse, stress and violent behavior, as well as the benefits derived from good nutrition and physical fitness.

Once health goals were established and published in the *Healthy People* document, the next step was to develop a series of objectives—those step-by-step activities needed to reach goals. Public and private groups worked together; and, in 1980, *Promoting Health/Preventing Disease: Objectives for the Nation* was published.

The objectives—a total of 227 in all—are keyed to the 15 priority areas in the three groups mentioned above (*i.e.,* personal preventive services, health protection, and health promotion). Some objectives apply to more than one target area. Several target areas have numerous objectives; for example, there are nine objectives to control high blood pressure. One such objective is

> *By 1990, no geopolitical area in the United States is without an effective program to identify people with high blood pressure and to follow-up on their treatment.*

This one objective will affect the health of people in each of the five population groups! The target areas that particularly need local involvement and programs are those in health promotion. Health promotion is the most difficult area in which to achieve change and to measure progress, because health promotion requires that millions of citizens change their daily habits and modify their lifestyles. The relationship between smoking and health is obvious and proven, yet millions of Americans continue to puff away their lives. Misuse of alcohol and drugs, control of stress, and violent behavior are additional examples of major target areas that must be addressed to promote health. Cities, counties, regions, and states have used this list of objectives for the nation in many interesting ways. Health agencies are using them to assess existing programs, to project where additional programs are needed, and to restructure existing programs.

A complementary document to the national goals and objectives is *Model Standards: A Guide for Community Preventive Health Services* (1985). This publication offers a format for setting specific community objectives. For example, the following format appears

> *By 19___ (year to be filled in) the incidence of motor vehicle fatalities for children under 15 years of age will be reduced to _____ (level to be filled in).*

This type of format allows each community flexibility in setting both its time frame and level of accomplishment. The *Model Standards* document also includes the 1990 health objectives. (References to all three documents plus additional federal documents dealing with the national health objectives have been included in the Suggested Readings list at the end of this chapter.) You should use the national goals and objectives as a guide in your work. Do the goals and objectives for your community-focused program further the national goals and objectives? When the Rosemont Health Promotion Council reviewed their goals and objectives, each was found to be congruent with the national plan, as well as Rosemont's state's objectives for improved health.

HEALTH FOCUS

There is one remaining question to ask before initiating the program: Does the program focus on health? This may seem to be a strange question. You might wonder, don't all programs focus on maintaining, restoring, or promoting health? Frequently the answer is *no*.

In Rosemont, the council and designated staff had become very involved in planning specific activities and information modules associated with the program. Several programs had been enlarged to include screening programs and health fairs; additional activities were suggested at each council meeting. The initial goal of promoting the health of Rosemont residents had changed seemingly to providing Rosemont residents with lots of activities and information about health. What had happened? Remember, we discussed the impatience and eagerness that is often associated with new programs. This situation is normal. What tends to happen is that committees overemphasize activities and knowledge and forget the initial reason for the program—to improve health. But it should be remembered that it is the sustained day-to-day use of knowledge and lifestyle practices that improve health. Frequently, a program is begun with enthusiastic momentum; media publicity attracts people to screening and information sessions—then the program is over. Objectives are evaluated as successful and another program is planned and implemented. But, was there any real improvement in health? Did the participants *change lifestyle practices?* Will the changes be maintained and continued for a week? A month? A year? Most importantly, are the changed lifestyle or health practices supported by the surrounding *environment and culture?*

Environmental and Cultural Support

Many parents in Rosemont responded affirmatively to the survey questions about discipline. These parents had felt that they or another person had hurt a child when the child was punished; the parents wanted to learn ways to keep from hurting children when adults were angry. The Rosemont Health Promotion Council responded with a series of programs on effective parenting. The effective parenting sessions included information on various nonphysical strategies for disciplining youngsters, as well as role-playing and open-discussion periods. However, as part of the community assessment, the community health nurse had recorded that the Hampton Independent School District used physical punishment as a primary discipline method. Youngsters at Temple Elementary were hit on the buttocks with a wide board that frequently left large bruises. The conflict between the effective parenting programs and punishment methods at Temple Elementary is obvious. What can be done? What do you suggest?

In Rosemont, part of the planned effective-parenting classes included discussion sessions on the difference between discipline and punishment and the importance of inquiring as to discipline and punishment procedures at places parents were leaving their children for supervision, including childcare facilities, the school, and babysitters. Parents were asked their feelings about the school district's policy on physical punishment. Although some parents were unaware of the school district's policy, most were aware of the punishment but felt the procedure could not be changed. After a discussion of parental rights and responsibilities, a group of parents made an appointment with the principal of Temple Elementary to discuss the situation. (Following additional meetings with school board members, an open public hearing on public school discipline, and letters to state school board officials, the Hampton Independent School District changed the discipline policy to exclude physical punishment. The process took two years.)

Countless such incongruencies exist between healthy lifestyles and existing environmental and cultural practices and policies. Here is one additional example: Recall that one nursing diagnosis for youngsters at Temple Elementary was a high prevalence of dental caries. During the effective-parenting discussions, several parents commented that their children were given hard candy, usually suckers, for good behavior. When the nurse at Temple Elementary was contacted, it was verified that children exhibiting good behavior were given hard candy. This practice was done daily.

> STOP: Identify the environmental and cultural practices and policies that are in conflict with the proposed community-focused health program that resulted from your community assessment. What can be done to increase community awareness of these conflicts and how can change begin? To focus on health and the maintenance of healthy lifestyles, all of the community must be involved.

The best way to maintain a focus on health and not on the activities of the program is to use your nursing practice model as a guide. The nursing practice model built and described in Chapter Five (see Figure 5-9) defines intervention as primary, secondary, and tertiary levels of prevention. Do the programs proposed for Rosemont address these three levels of prevention?

Levels of Prevention

Recall that *primary prevention* improves the health and well-being of the community and makes the community less liable to stressors. Health promotion programs are primary prevention, as are programs that focus on protection from specific diseases. Usually health promotion is nonspecific and directed toward raising the general health of the total community (*e.g.,* teaching youngsters about nutritious foods, or adult exercise-fitness and stress-reduction sessions). Primary prevention can also be very specific such as protection measures against specific diseases (*e.g.,* immunizations). Additional primary prevention measures include the wearing of seatbelts and the purification of public water supplies.

Secondary prevention begins after a disease or condition is present (although there may be no symptoms). Emphasis is on screening, and early diagnosis and treatment of possible stressors that may adversely affect the community's health. The tine test for tuberculosis, the Denver Developmental Screening test for developmental delays, and blood-pressure assessments are secondary prevention interventions.

Tertiary prevention focuses on restoration and rehabilitation. Tertiary prevention programs act to return the community to an optimum level of functioning. Adequate shelters for battered women, and counseling and therapy programs for sexually abused youngsters are examples of tertiary prevention.

The distinction between prevention levels is not always clear. Is a program on the assessment of fever in children (and the prevention of febrile convulsions and dehydration through use of tepid baths and extra fluids) secondary or tertiary prevention? How would you classify an effective-parenting program? Support groups for single parents? A crime prevention program? Sessions on stress reduction and physical fitness? Can some programs be primary, secondary, and tertiary depending on the needs of the persons who attend? Certainly effective-parenting classes for the parent with a child who has a behavior problem will have a different purpose from classes designed for expectant parents of a first child. Likewise, the corporate executive who has been diagnosed with cardiovascular disease and placed on a low cholesterol diet has very different nutritional learning needs from those of the senior citizen on a fixed income. Few programs are purely on one level of prevention.

The important point is to evaluate your programs (the implementation phase of the nursing process) and ask if the nursing interventions are consistent with the nursing practice model. If the focus is prevention, then are the programs directed towards prevention?

SUMMARY

Having considered the importance of *community ownership* of the program, the need to offer a *unified program,* and maintaining *a focus on health,* there remains one process—*evaluation.* Before a program is implemented, the evaluation of the program must be established. Chapter 10 explains why this final stage of the nursing process is essential *before* implementation.

SUGGESTED READINGS

Aging and Health Promotion: Marketing Research for Public Education. (1984)
   Presents recommendations for health promotion messages and activities for older people. (For sale by the National Technical Information Service, PB84-1211150)
Health Information Terms. (1984)
   Lists subject terms, or keywords, in the database of the National Health Information Clearinghouse (NHIC). Used by the NHIC as a thesaurus to index and retrieve descriptions of organizations that provide health information.
Healthy People: The Surgeon General's Report on Health Promotion and Disease Prevention. (1979) Government Printing Office Stock No. 017-001-00416-1
   Sets forth priorities for the nation's health by identifying specific goals in 5 stages of human development and 15 priority areas.
Healthy People: The Surgeon General's Report on Health Promotion and Disease Prevention—Background Papers. (1979) Government Printing Office Stock No. 017-011-00417-1
   A series of articles that examine the past successes, future challenges, and unanswered questions relating to key topics in prevention. Also discussed are psychological factors influencing health and the economic dimensions of prevention.
Model Standards: A Guide for Community Preventive Health Services. Washington DC, American Public Health Assoc, 1985 ($8 a copy)
   Offers a format for writing specific community health objectives in several hundred aspects of 34 program areas of public health.
Prevention Profile. (1984)
   Presents data to help measure the nation's progress toward the health promotion and disease prevention goals for 1990. (Single copy free from the National Health Information Clearinghouse.)
Proceedings of Prospects for a Healthier America: Achieving the Nation's Health Promotion Objectives. (1985)
   Provides background papers and recommendations from meetings of groups from health care settings, business, voluntary associations, and schools. Helps to identify approaches to developing materials, initiating programs and stimulating collaboration to implement the health promotional objectives set forth in *Promoting*

Health/Preventing Disease: Objectives for the Nation. (Copies free from the National Health Information Clearinghouse.)

Promoting Health/Preventing Disease: Objectives for the Nation. (1980) Government Printing Office Stock No. 017-001-00435-9

Identifies specific and measurable objectives for the 15 areas set forth in *Healthy People.*

Staying Healthy: A Bibliography of Health Promotion Materials. (1984) Government Printing Office Stock No. 017-001-0049-9

Describes publications available from the Public Health Service in the field of health promotion and disease prevention. Arranged by subject, it includes consumer pamphlets, guides for health professionals, films, and Spanish-language materials. (Single copy free from the National Health Information Clearinghouse.)

Strategies for Promoting Health for Specific Populations. (1981)

Examines the health promotion needs, and priorities of minorities. Includes recommendations on reaching Asian/Pacific Americans, Black Americans, Hispanic Americans, elderly Americans, and American Indians. (Single copy free from the National Health Information Clearinghouse.)

10

Evaluating
a Health Program

OBJECTIVES

Evaluation is measurement. During evaluation information is collected and analyzed to determine its significance and worth. Changes are appraised and progress is documented. This chapter discusses evaluation and the nursing practices that are necessary to plan and implement evaluation. After studying this chapter you will be able to act in partnership with the community to

- Establish evaluation criteria that are timely and comprehensive
- Use baseline and current data to measure progress toward goals and objectives
- Validate observations, insights, and new data with colleagues and the target population
- Revise priorities, goals, and interventions based on evaluation data
- Document and record evaluation results and revisions of the plan
- Conduct evaluation research with appropriate consultation

INTRODUCTION

The nurse evaluates the responses of the community to a health program in order to measure progress that is being made toward the program's goals and

313

objectives. Evaluation data are also crucial for revision of the data base and the community nursing diagnoses that were developed from analysis of the community assessment data.

Do you feel as if we are talking in circles? Evaluation is the final step of the nursing process, but it is linked to assessment, which is the first step of the nursing process. Nursing practice is cyclic, as well as dynamic, and for community-focused interventions to be timely and relevant, the community data base, nursing diagnoses, and health program plans must be evaluated routinely. The effectiveness of community nursing interventions depends on continuous reassessment of the community's health and on appropriate revisions of planned interventions.

Evaluation is important to nursing practice; but, of equal importance is its crucial role in the functioning of health agencies. Staffing and funding are frequently based on evaluation findings, and existing programs are subject to termination unless evaluation evidence can be produced that answers the question: What has been the program's impact on the health status of the community? Recent years have witnessed a growing focus on program evaluation; training programs on evaluation have become commonplace, evaluation has become big business. Unfortunately, evaluation is sometimes practiced separately from program planning. It may even be tacked onto the end of a program just to satisfy funding sources or agency administration. The problems of such an approach are evident. Effective community health nursing requires an integrative approach to evaluation; it is a unique aspect of the field.

THE EVALUATION PROCESS

When evaluation is discussed, the terms *formative evaluation* and *summative evaluation* are used. Formative evaluation focuses on measuring the daily functions and activities of a program. Emphasis is on immediate data gathering and analysis to improve the program and its management. For example, when the first effective-parent training program was offered in Rosemont from 8–9 pm, only five parents attended. These parents stated that the time was too late for them to return home and complete bedtime activities for their school-age children. As a result of this formative evaluation, the time was changed to 7–8 pm, and attendance increased to 20 parents. Summative evaluation, in contrast, refers to activities that are associated with long-term effects of a program (for example, did the program change the participants' health practices, attitudes, or knowledge?) In the case of effective-parenting classes, summative evaluation criteria might include: parental self-reports of changes in their attitudes toward physical punishment and discipline practices before and following the program, any alteration in discipline policies at Temple Elementary, and change in the number of reported incidences of child abuse. Both types of evaluation are important and strategies exist to obtain each.

Before considering specific evaluation strategies, it is important to evaluate the "evaluability" of the program. To do this, review the program plan and ask

- Are program activities stated in precise words whose concepts can be measured?
- Has a time frame for attaining the change been included?
- Are the direction and magnitude of the change included?
- Has a method of measuring the change been included?
- Are the data that will be needed to measure the objectives available? At a reasonable cost?
- Are the program activities that are designed to meet the objectives plausible?

If you find in your practice that any of these questions cannot be measured in one of your plans, review Chapter 8 and amend the plan to make it as concise and complete as possible.

> NOTE: A positive response to each of the above questions would be an *ideal* state that few programs attain. Therefore, do not despair if your program is less than perfect, but rather strive to increase your sensitivity to the issues that need to be considered in program planning in order to achieve optimum program evaluation.

COMPONENTS OF EVALUATION

Why collect evaluation data? To whom will the evaluation data be given and for what purpose will it be used? What programs or activities will result from or be discontinued as a result of evaluation data? Before a strategy or method of evaluation can be selected, the reasons for and uses of the evaluation data must be established. An evaluation strategy appropriate for answering one type of evaluative question would not be useful for another. For example, if the Rosemont Health Promotion Council wanted to know the *relevancy* to community needs of a program on crime prevention, then questions would be asked of the participants concerning the usefulness and adequacy of the information that was given. Possible questions would cover a range of topics:

Did the information make a difference as to how residents protect themselves from crime? what protection behaviors do the residents practice now that were not practiced before the program? did the program answer the residents' questions? did the program meet *perceived needs?* However, if the council wanted to know the *impact* of the crime prevention program, (such as if the program decreased the incidence of crime experienced by the participants) then self-reports and community crime statistics would be monitored. Usually questions of evaluation focus on the areas of *relevancy, progress, efficiency, effectiveness,* and *impact.*

Relevancy

Is there a need for the program? *Relevancy* determines the reasons for having a program or set of activities. Questions of relevancy may be more important for existing programs than for new programs. Frequently a program is planned, such as a blood pressure screening, to meet an expressed community need. Then it is continued for years without an evaluation of relevancy. The question should be asked routinely—is the program still needed? Clearly, evaluation is not just necessary for new programs, but it is needed for all programs. A common constraint to beginning a new program is inadequate staff or budget. A remedy to that constraint can be a relevancy evaluation of existing programs. Staff and budgets from a program that is no longer needed can be redirected to the new program.

Progress

Are program activities following the intended plan? Are appropriate staff and materials available in the right quantity and at the right time to implement the program activities? Are expected numbers of clients participating in the scheduled program activities? Do the inputs and outputs meet some predetermined plan? Answers to these questions measure the progress of the program.

Cost Efficiency

What are the costs of a program? What are the benefits of the program? Are program benefits sufficient for the costs incurred? Cost efficiency evaluation measures the relationship between the results (benefits) of a program and the costs of presenting the program (*e.g.,* staff salary, materials). Cost efficiency evaluates whether or not the results of a program could have been obtained less expensively through another approach.

Effectiveness

Were program objectives met? Were the clients satisfied with the program? Were program providers satisfied with the activities and client involvement? Effectiveness focuses on formative evaluation, and the immediate short-term results.

Impact

What are the long-term implications of the program? As a result of the program, what changes in behavior can be expected in six weeks, six months, or six years? Effectiveness measures the immediate results, whereas impact evaluation measures whether or not the program activities changed the initial reason for the program. The fundamental question is: has health improved?

EVALUATION STRATEGIES

Several methods exist to evaluate programs. No one method is best nor does any one strategy address all the issues of relevancy, progress, cost efficiency, effectiveness, and impact. For example, the case-study method is designed to focus on program relevance, but has limited use in evaluating cost efficiency. Similarly, cost-benefit analysis evaluates cost efficiency, but does not adequately address any of the other issues. Even evaluative research, which frequently is revered as the pinnacle of evaluation techniques, is of little use for answering questions of progress or cost efficiency. Program evaluation requires a knowledge of the various evaluation methods and careful decision making as to which method can meet evaluation goals.

Case Study

A *case study* looks inside a program to determine adequacy to meet stated needs. The case-study method provides insight into an entire program and unlike many forms of evaluation can be started at any time during the program. The type of data that is collected during a case study includes observation of program activity, reports prepared by the program, unstructured conversations with program personnel, statistical summaries of program activities, structured or unstructured interview data, and information collected through questionnaires. *Subjective data* and *objective data* can both be collected. Subjective data include information collected primarily through observations of participants or program staff. Objective data are collected from organization or program documents or structured questionnaires and interviews. The distinction between subjective and objective is not readily perceptible. All questionnaires, regardless of how carefully written, have a subjective component, and likewise, "objective" records or documents are all written by people and therefore introduce a "subjective factor." It is optimum to have a mix of both objective and subjective data.

Observation

Observation is one method of collecting data for a case study. Observation can be *participatory* or *nonparticipatory.* The participant observer assumes a working role in the agency or organization and collects data about the program while working within the group. The nonparticipant observer remains an "outsider," does not assume a working role within the agency, and reviews and examines the program for designated periods.

The types of observations that are made are determined by the questions that have been asked about the program. For example, if the question is one of relevancy, the observer would concentrate on the *who, what, why,* and *when* of the program. *Who* is using the services? Record the demographics of age, ethnicity, geographic location, educational level, and employment status. *What* services are the participants receiving? (For example, what services are offered in the well child clinic? Immunizations? Physicals? Health teaching? Screening? How often are the services offered and what are the ages of the children who use the services?) *Why* is the population using the offered services? (Availability? Affordability? No other options?) Lastly, *when* are the services accessed? (Do people come at appointed times? Only when ill? Or do people tend to cluster at opening and closing times?)

Some data can be collected from agency records, other information can be collected by informal conversations with the participants—both the professional health care providers and the clients. When interviewing, always have a checklist of topics you want to consider, arranged in a logical sequence, along with the who, what, why, and when questions. Informal conversations, sometimes referred to as "unstructured interviews," afford the opportunity to *explore* with the participants their perceptions of the program. The results of unstructured interviews provide specific areas from which a "structured" interview can be developed. Recall from Chapter 8 that an interview is administered by an interviewer as opposed to a questionnaire, which is self-administered. (If a questionnaire is written, review the process in Chapter 8.) Observations and interviews share the problem of selective perception.

Selective perception

Selective perception is the natural tendency of everyone to consciously classify into categories the behaviors or statements of others. These categories have been established by our cultural values, learning, and life experiences. To a certain extent, this process is desirable because it limits the number of observations that need conscious consideration and permits the rapid and effective handling of information. For example, if it was observed that a client waited one hour for a scheduled appointment, most people, based on the common orientation to time, would classify that observation as a negative aspect of the clinic's functioning.

Herein lies the major problem of selective perception. Statements and behaviors are classified according to the selective perception of the observer, which may be completely different from the selective perception of the client or the health providers. The most dangerous effect of selective perception in program evaluation is when the observer has a preconception that a program will be successful or unsuccessful. This can produce a self-fulfilling prophecy because the biased observer may unconsciously record only data that support the preconceived belief. Both selective perception and self-fulfilling prophecy are sources of subjective data that were discussed earlier. Perhaps the most important point is that you should be aware of the problem of selective perception and share your observation and interview data with a mixed group of clients and health providers. Ask the group for categorization and summation implications.

Interactiveness

Interactiveness is an additional event to be aware of during all observations. When an observer, whether participant or nonparticipant, observes and records program activities, the person's presence affects and shapes the activities observed. Productivity may increase because the staff are aware of being observed, as well as concerned about client satisfaction or dissatisfaction. All evaluation strategies can have an interactive component, but perhaps the interactive consideration is strongest in case studies because of the presence of an observer.

Two additional techniques of the case study method are *nominal group* and *Delphi technique*. (References to both techniques and examples of their application are presented at the conclusion of this chapter in the *Suggested Readings* list.) Both techniques are based on the belief that the individuals in a program are the most knowledgeable sources on its relevancy.

Nominal group

The *nominal group* technique uses a structured group meeting, during which all individuals are given a judgmental task such as to list the functions of the program, problems of the program, or needed changes in the program. Each member is asked to write a response on paper and to not discuss it with other people. At the end of 5 to 10 minutes, all members present their ideas and each idea is recorded (without discussion) so everyone can see all the suggestions. Once all ideas have been presented, a discussion is begun, during which ideas are clarified and evaluated. After the discussion a vote is held to determine the order in which the group wants to address different areas. The nominal group technique allows all individuals to present their ideas before the entire group. Involving the entire group both decreases selective perception and promotes individual cooperation with the group's decisions because people feel themselves to have been involved in the decision-making process.

Delphi technique

The *Delphi technique* tends to be used in large-survey studies but also is useful as a case-study method. Delphi involves a series of questionnaires and feedback reports to a designated panel of respondents. An initial questionnaire is distributed by mail to a preselected group (this could be all nursing staff, a group of clients, or program administrators). Independently, respondents express their thoughts through the questionnaire and return it. Based on the responses of the group, a feedback report and a revised version of the questionnaire is sent to the respondents. Using the feedback information, the respondents evaluate their first answers and complete the questionnaire again. The process continues for a predetermined number of feedback rounds.

Usefulness to evaluation

The case-study method of program evaluation can help answer questions of *relevance.* Questioning clients and health providers helps explore perceptions of how well the program is meeting its defined goals, as well as ascertaining problem areas and possible solutions. The case-study method would not point to any one solution but rather would offer several possible choices.

Questions of *progress* can also be addressed through the case-study method. The extent to which a program is meeting predetermined standards of service indicates progress. Because the case study provides an examination of the program, much can be learned if program activities are already in place.

Cost efficiency of the program is difficult to evaluate using a case-study method. First, to evaluate if the program could have been offered more economically, a comparable program must exist; and second, the case-study method is designed to look at only one program. The method is not formatted to look at two programs and compare them. However, judgments can be made as to the operating efficiency of the program. These must be based on the experience and knowledge of the evaluator and cannot be based on comparisons with other operating programs.

Effectiveness determines if the program has produced what it intended to produce immediately following the program, as opposed to *impact,* which measures long-term consequences. Although the case-study method may determine aspects of effectiveness such as whether or not the aims of the program have been met in the short-run, it is very difficult to measure long-term consequences unless the case study method is conducted over a long period that allows a retrospect (look backward) at the program.

Surveys

A *survey* is a method of collecting information and can be used to collect evaluation information. Surveys are usually completed by self-administered questionnaires (the process used in Rosemont to determine community perception of health information needs) or by personal interviews. Surveys are formulated to describe (*descriptive surveys*) or to analyze (*analytic surveys*) relationships. (Actually most surveys can be used to both describe and analyze.)

Surveys can be used to describe the need for a program, the actual operations of the program, or a program's effects. Along with the descriptive information, questions of analysis can be answered through a survey. For example, a survey could be used to *describe* the composition of the groups that attend crime-prevention or weight-reduction classes, as well as to *analyze* the relationship between descriptive data of sex and weight-reduction success.

Surveys are usually performed for summative evaluation. Did the program accomplish what it was proposed to do? Was the program perceived as successful by clients? By personnel? If the program was considered successful, what parts were most helpful? Least helpful? What should be changed? Left unchanged? The questions asked by the survey are determined by the initial list of questions asked about program evaluation.

Like the case-study method, the answers on surveys come from the perceptions, values, and belief systems of the respondents. The response given to questions of program usefulness by the nurse who planned and implemented the program may be very different from the answers of the participants. Awareness of perception bias can direct evaluation efforts to consider the perceptions of all persons (providers, clients, and management) involved in program implementation.

Surveys that are used to measure program evaluation must be concerned with the *reliability* and *validity* of the information collected. Reliability deals with the repeatability, or reproducibility of the data (that is, if the same questions were asked of the same people one week later, would the same responses be recorded?). Validity is the correctness of the information. If questions are written to evaluate knowledge and the answers of the respondents reflect behaviors then the questions are not valid. The questions are not valid because they do not measure what they claim to measure. (Refer to Chapter 2 for further explanation of issues of reliability and validity, and methods that can be used to evaluate the reliability and validity of your questionnaire or interview schedule.)

Usefulness to evaluation

Surveys can be very valuable to answer questions of *relevance* or the need for proposed or existing programs, especially if the *perception* of clients, providers, and management are solicited. In like fashion, *progress* can be measured. People critiquing surveys as an evaluation strategy may be concerned with the "subjectivity" of the survey—indeed, individual perception affects every response to every question. However, most decisions that are made are based on "subjective" judgments, not "objective" reality. The important concern is to understand whose "subjective impression is being used as a basis for judgement;" it is imperative for community health nurses to ensure that clients' perceptions are represented alongside those of health providers and management.

Cost efficiency, effectiveness, and *impact* are difficult to measure by using a survey. Although a survey can measure the perceived efficiency of the program, or ideas on alternative ways of operating to make the program most cost efficient, these perceptions are formed only in the context of the existing program—there is no other comparison program against which recorded perceptions can be measured. A survey can provide information on the characteristics of program activities that are perceived by the respondents to have caused changes in their health status, *but* these impressions are reported in the absence of any comparison group. A comparison group is especially important with regard to effectiveness and impact because it is impossible to tell if an alternative program (or no program at all) might have been more or less effective in accomplishing the same objectives.

TIME OUT! You may be wondering—if a comparison group is so important and if perceptions cloud the evaluation with "subjective impressions"—then why use surveys at all? Two pluses exist in surveys: a great deal of information for program evaluation can be obtained, especially about the activities of the program from the perception of several groups; and important evaluation data can be inferred *if* the instrument (questionnaire or interview schedule) is reliable and valid. Once again, you are referred to Chapter 2 for a review of the importance of reliability and validity, as well as information on how to establish the reliability and validity of any questionnaire, interview, or test.

Experimental Design

Completed correctly, an experimental study can provide an answer to the crucial questions: Did the program make a difference? Are health behaviors, knowledge, and attitudes changed as a result of the program activities? Is the community healthier because of the programs offered by the Rosemont Health Promotion Council? However, the problem with experimental studies in program evaluation is that they require *selective implementation,* meaning that people who participate are selected through a process such as random assignment to a control group and an experimental group. For many ethical, political, and community health reasons, selective implementation is difficult to complete, and is sometimes impossible. Despite these problems, the experiment remains the best method to evaluate summative effects of a program and the only way to produce quantified information on whether the program made a difference.

STOP! Refer to Chapter 2 and review the steps of the research process.

Indeed, each issue such as a theoretical framework, sampling, reliability, and validity must be addressed if an experimental design is proposed for evaluation.

The following designs are the most feasible and appropriate to health care settings. Apply the research process to each design.

Pretest-posttest one-group design

The pretest-posttest design applied to one group is illustrated in Figure 10-1. Two *observations* are made, the first at Time 1 and the second at Time 2. The observation can be the prevalence of a health state (*i.e.,* the percentage of

	Time 1		Time 2
Experimental group	Observation 1	Experiment	Observation 2

Figure 10-1.   Pretest-posttest one-group design.

adults in Rosemont who exercise regularly, teenage pregnancy rate, cases of child abuse, etc.), knowledge scores, or other important health facts in the community. Between Time 1 and Time 2, an experiment is introduced. The experiment may be a planned program to a target group (*i.e.,* teen-sexuality classes) or a community-wide focus (*i.e.,* a crime-prevention program). The evaluation of the program is measured by considering the difference between the health state at Time 1 and the health state following the program at Time 2.

If the experiment in Figure 10-1 was teen-sexuality classes to 10th grade girls at Hampton High School and Time 1 was a teen pregnancy rate of 5 per 100 and Time 2 (one year later) was a teen pregnancy rate of 3 per 100 among the girls taking the classes, would you agree that the teen sexuality program was responsible for the decrease in teenage pregnancies? What other information do you need to know in order to decide? (Are there other factors that could account for the decrease in the teen pregnancy rate? Perhaps family-planning programs have been focused on the teenager, or local churches and social service agencies have sponsored teenage-sexuality programs. Teen access and use of contraceptive methods may have increased or laws regarding teen access to contraceptive methods may have changed.) Each of these factors cannot be eliminated as unassociated with the decrease in the teen pregnancy rate. To eliminate other possible explanations for program effectiveness, a control group must be added.)

Pretest-posttest two-group design

A pretest-posttest with a control group design is illustrated in Figure 10-2. The design has both an experimental group and a control group. At Time 1 an observation is made of both the experimental and control groups. Between Time 1 and Time 2 an experiment is introduced with the experimental group. At Time 2, second observations are made on both the experimental and control groups. Program evaluation is the difference between Observations 1 and 2 for the experimental group when compared to the comparison group (which has been selected to be as similar as possible to the experimental group). Will

	Time 1		Time 2
Experimental group	Observation 1	Experiment	Observation 2
Control group	Observation 1		Observation 2

Figure 10-2.   Pretest-posttest two-group design.

the pretest-posttest with a control group design eliminate the effect of outside factors that occurred simultaneously with the experiment and that might account for the change between Observation 1 and Observation 2? (The very problem that plagued the pretest-posttest one-group design.) Yes, *if* the experimental and control groups are similar.

To explain, let's return to Rosemont and the idea of a teenage-sexuality class for 10th grade students at Hampton High School. If a group of 10th grade students, similar in social, economic, and geographic characteristics, were randomly selected and then randomly assigned to the experimental or control group, then it could be assumed that any other factors that influenced the experimental group would also affect the control group. However, frequently the decision is made that all students must be given the same program, thereby eliminating a comparison group. At the Rosemont Health Promotion Council, when the information was received that *all* 10th graders must be given a teen-sexuality program that had been proposed by the school nurse as a response to an increasing number of teen pregnancies, the suggestion was made that perhaps another high school could be used as a control group. How would you respond to that suggestion? Perhaps another high school class of 10th graders could be used, *if* the students were similar in social, economic, and geographic characteristics to the students at Hampton High (an unlikely situation). Another possibility mentioned by the Rosemont Health Promotion Council was to offer the program in one school year to one half of the Hampton High 10th graders (using the other half as a control), then in the following year to offer the program to the remaining students. This method would ensure that all students would be given the program, but would also allow for an experimental pretest-posttest design for evaluation. A third method that was suggested to ensure an experimental design was to give the control group sexuality information, and give the experimental group sexuality education *plus* assertiveness training. The assertiveness training would differentiate the groups and allow an experimental design. All the suggestions were discussed with school officials, and it was decided to offer a traditional sex-education class to half the 10th grade students (the control group); the remaining students (the experimental group) would get the traditional sex-education material, but would receive in addition classes on assertiveness training and value clarification. This design will not allow for evaluation of traditional sex-education classes versus no information, but rather it will provide all students with the health information (an ethical compromise) and allow for evaluation of a traditional program on sexuality versus traditional education plus assertiveness and values clarification information (an approach to reduce teenage pregnancies that is supported in the literature).

> PAUSE TO CONSIDER: Notice that the decision to offer information on assertiveness and values clarification as part of teen-sexuality classes was based on documentation from the literature. Rosemont is not the first community to offer health promotion programs. Many communities have assessed the health status and perceived health needs of the residents, and have followed up with planned and implemented programs that have been evaluated and the results reported in the literature. A function of community health nursing is the review and synthesis of the results of similar programs and the presentation of this information to the community for use in decision making. After the program topics have been decided, you should begin a literature review to study the ways in which other communities have addressed and evaluated similar programs.

Usefulness to evaluation

When completed correctly, the experimental design is the best evaluation technique for assessing the effectiveness and impact of a given program. No other evaluation approach can assess the true value efficiency, effectiveness, and impact. An experimental design can yield data on whether or not a program has produced the desired outcomes when compared to the absence of such a program, or, alternatively, that one program strategy has produced better results with regard to the desired outcomes than some other strategy. However, the experimental design is not useful for evaluation of program progress or program cost efficiency.

Monitoring

Monitoring measures the difference between the program plan and what has actually happened. Monitoring focuses on the sequence of activities of the program; specifically, *how* the program is to be implemented (the activities), by *whom* (the personnel and other resources), and *when* (the timing of activities). Monitoring is usually done with a chart and, although there are several different styles of charts, all arrange activities in a sequence and specify the time allotted to completing each task. Figure 10-3 shows an example of a monitoring chart.

Monitoring charts

To construct a monitoring chart for your program plan, information is needed on the *inputs* (resources necessary to carry out the program such as personnel, equipment, and finances), the *process* (the program activities, their sequencing, and timing) and *outputs* (the expected results of the program, including immediate and long-term health effects). It is helpful to make a list of inputs, processes, and outputs.

> NOTE: You have already recorded this information as part of your program plan. Refer back to Chapter 8 and note that *resources, program activities,* and *learning objectives* were listed for the proposed class on common health problems of children. *Resources* are the same as *inputs; program activities* correspond to *processes;* and *learning objectives* designate expected *outputs.* So all that remains is to place the data into a chart for monitoring.

Figure 10-3 lists the inputs, processes, and outputs for the proposed program in Rosemont, along with a time sequence for beginning and completing each event.

It is difficult to decide on the amount of time that will be needed to complete any task. After assessing the organizational structure and management methods of the agency, you can determine the approximate amounts of time that will be needed to complete the activities of the program. Monitoring charts are easy to formulate and provide useful information for measuring program evaluation *if* the chart is realistic. The publications in the *Suggested Readings* list include references to several other types of monitoring charts, including the Gantt, Program Evaluation and Review Technique (PERT), and Critical Path Method (CPM). These provide a slightly different variation of the basic time-sequencing activities-monitoring chart that appears in Figure 10-3.

Usefulness to evaluation

A monitoring chart measures progress and can be used to evaluate whether or not a program is on schedule and within budget. Perhaps no other evaluation

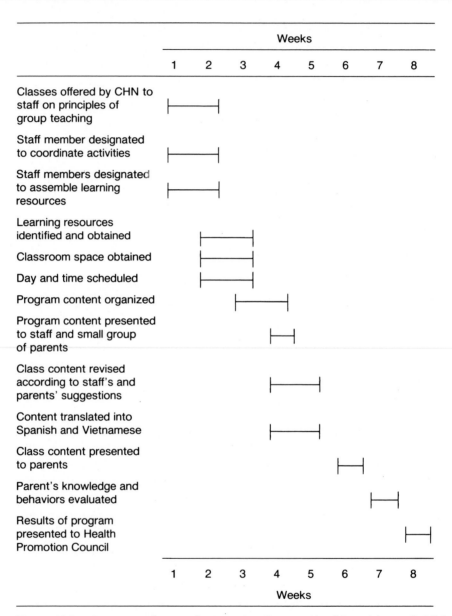

Figure 10-3.   Sequence of events for program: Common health problems of children.

method is as perfectly suited to *progress evaluation* as the monitoring chart. In addition, monitoring can provide information on the *cost efficiency* of the program by measuring the average cost of the resources required per client served. The *effectiveness* of the program can be measured by monitoring the chart if the chart records "outputs achieved." Monitoring charts cannot determine *program relevance* or the long-term *impact* of a program.

Cost Benefit
and Cost-effectiveness Analyses

Much has been written and discussed about the escalating cost of health care services and on ways that cost can be reduced. Chapter 1 is testimony to the various alternative approaches to health care delivery that are being tried in order to contain cost and yet increase access and maintain quality. Every program has a dollar price both in terms of the resources (*i.e.,* personnel and equipment) needed to offer the program, and the dollar benefits to be gained from improved health (*i.e.,* increased worker productivity).

Two of the most common methods of analyzing the economic costs and benefits of a program are *cost benefit analysis* (CBA) and *cost effectiveness analysis* (CEA). Both CBA and CBE are formal analytic techniques for comparing the negative and positive consequences of a program. Both techniques list all costs (direct and indirect) and consequences (negative and positive) of a particular program. The distinction between CBA and CEA is based on the value that is placed on the consequences of a program. In CBA, consequences or benefits of a program are valued in dollar terms; this makes it possible to compare different projects because all measurement is made in dollars. Therefore, the worth of a project can be judged by asking if dollar benefits exceed dollar costs and, if so, by how much.

In contrast, CEA does not place a dollar value on either the consequences or the costs of a project. Another outcome is used for programs whose benefits or costs are difficult to measure. (For example, a primary prevention program to decrease teenage suicide is planned. But how could a dollar value be placed on each suicide prevented?) Therefore, CEA, unlike CBA, does not determine if total benefits exceed total costs.

However, CEA can be used to compare programs with similar goals and objectives. (For example, two different primary prevention approaches to decrease the incidence of teenage suicide share the same benefits, so only costs need be compared—a CEA.) A CEA can also be used if the costs of alternative programs are the same or if only a given amount of money exists and the objective is to select the program with the greatest benefits (not measured in dollar terms). The decision is obvious—select the program that produces the most effectiveness—the most benefits per dollar spent or the least cost for each unit (individual, family, community) benefited.

The choice between CBA and CEA depends on the type of questions and programs considered. Neither technique is superior to the other. Both techniques can be used in planning for future programs or as an evaluation strategy of present or past programs. The actual procedures for completing a CBA or CEA are beyond the scope of this book; however, several references that include the procedural steps are listed in the Suggested Readings list. Obviously both CBA and CEA are strategies for measuring program cost efficiency and do not address the issues of relevancy, progress, effectiveness, or impact.

SUMMARY

Several methods of evaluation have been presented and discussed. No one method will evaluate components of *relevancy, progress, cost efficiency, effectiveness,* and *impact* equally well. It is important to be knowledgeable about different methods of program evaluation and to discuss the benefits and limitations of each with the community as the program is being planned and *before* program implementation occurs. Figure 10-4 presents a summary table of appropriate evaluation methods for program components to be evaluated. Once evaluation components are selected, then the methods (*i.e.,* case study, experimental design, monitoring charts) become part of the program plan.

You may be wondering which evaluation methods were used to evaluate the health promotion programs in Rosemont; a variety were used. To evaluate the relevancy of the health promotion programs (*i.e.,* crime prevention, effective-parenting classes), nominal group meetings were scheduled, and both health providers and consumers attended. In addition, the use rates and demographics of the participants using the health promotion programs were assessed as were the participants' perceptions of the value of the information. Program progress was evaluated with monitoring charts such as the one presented in Figure 10-3. The effectiveness and impact of individual programs

Components	Case study	Survey	Experimental	Monitoring
	Method			
Relevancy	yes	yes	no	no
Progress	yes	yes	no	yes
Cost efficiency	no	no	yes	yes
Cost effectiveness	some	no	yes	some
Impact	no	no	yes	no

Figure 10-4.   Examination of the appropriateness of different evaluation methods for program components.

was evaluated with knowledge, attitude, and behavioral intent surveys (*i.e.,* questionnaires, interviews, tests) given to participants before the program, immediately after the program, and at a predetermined follow-up time (*i.e.,* six weeks, three months following the program). As often as was feasible, an evaluation research design was followed such as a one-group pretest-posttest. Additional measures of effectiveness and impact were community statistics on crime, child abuse, and teenage pregnancies before as compared to after the program, as well as health policy changes that affected the residents of Rosemont (*i.e.,* access of minors to contraceptives, discipline practices in the public schools, financial eligibility requirements for health services). Cost effectiveness analysis was completed on several of the programs.

You are ready *now* for program implementation and the reinitiation of the nursing process, namely assessment of the program's effects. As you implement the planned program, data will be added to the community assessment profile, which will demand addition, deletion, and revision of the community nursing diagnoses and the associated program plans and interventions. Let's take a final look at the Community-as-Client Model (see Figure 5-9) and ask: Will the planned programs assist the community to attain, regain, maintain, and promote health? strengthen the community's ability to resist stressors? make the community more competent and self-reliant?

A FINAL TIME-OUT! It is fitting that the final chapter of this section on the application of the nursing process in community health nursing end with questions. Community health nursing is the constant questioning, prodding, probing, and pondering of the health status of a population. While individual and family health are always important, the uniqueness of the community health nursing field is the application of nursing techniques to the health of a community. Each community is unique, and special. There is no other community quite like the one in which you are applying community health nursing. We have enjoyed sharing the uniqueness of Rosemont with you and the application of the nursing process to community health nursing.

SUGGESTED READINGS

Delbecq AL, Van De Ven AE, Gustafson DH: Group Techniques for Program Planning: A Guide to Nominal Group and Delphi Processes. Glenview, Illinois, Scott, Foresman, 1975

Moscovice IS, Armstrong P, Shortell S, Bennett R: Health services research for decision-makers: The use of the delphi technique to determine health priorities. J Health Polit Policy Law 2(3):388–410, 1977

Shortell S, Richardson W: Health Program Evaluation. St Louis, CV Mosby, 1978

Starkweather DB, Gelwicks L, Newcomer R: Delphi Forecasting of Health Care Organization. Inquiry 12(1):37–46, 1975

Starpoli C, Waltz C: Developing and Evaluating Educational Programs for Health Care Providers. Philadelphia, FA Davis, 1978

Suchman E: Evaluation Research: Principles and Practices in Public Health Service and Social Action Programs. New York, Russell Sage Foundation, 1967

Veney JE, Kaluzny AD: Evaluation and Decision Making for Health Services Programs. Englewood Cliffs, New Jersey, Prentice-Hall, 1984

Weiss C: Evaluation Research Methods of Assessing Program Effectiveness. Englewood Cliffs, New Jersey, Prentice-Hall, 1972

PART III

Roles in
Community Health Nursing

11

History and Dimensions of Public Health Nursing

INTRODUCTION

This chapter contains two articles reprinted from the *American Journal of Public Health.* They originally appeared as a special feature, "Public Health Then and Now," during the 75th anniversary of the American Public Health Association. The authors, who are public health nurse scholars, have brought to life the legacy of public health nursing, using two different, but complementary, perspectives.

No attempt has been made to cover the history of the specialty areas such as school nursing or occupational health nursing, but we hope rather to present a general history of the field of public health nursing. In the two articles is presented a view of public health nursing in the context of social change.

OBJECTIVES

Unit I: Public Health Nursing: In Sickness or in Health?, examines the history of public health nursing between 1900 and 1930, and Unit II: Public Health Nursing Comes of Age, follows its history to the 1980s. After reading this chapter you will be able to

- List social forces that affected the growth and development of public health nursing

- Describe the effects that social forces (for instance, war, industrialization) had on public health nursing
- Describe major milestones and decisions that affected the development of public health nursing
- Compare early public health nursing functions to contemporary descriptions
- Describe the similarities and differences of public health problems and concerns in 1900 and today
- Describe two recent major events that are having significant impact on public health nursing

Unit I: *Public Health Nursing: In Sickness or in Health?*

KAREN BUHLER-WILKERSON, RN, PhD*

INTRODUCTION

By the last decade of the nineteenth century, American cities were experiencing a major transformation. Those first affected were the northern coastal cities where the concentration of immigrants and industry linked poverty to disease and dirt. Population growth alone required major adjustments in the lives of most city dwellers. With immigration accounting for much of this urban growth, ethnic, cultural, religion, and economic differences accentuated the separation between old and new inhabitants.[1,2]

For many, the advent of the germ theory of disease simply heightened these concerns. Realizing, that individual health depended to some extent on the health of the population generally, the hazards of infectious diseases became an increasingly tangible concern. The knowledge that the diseases of workers—who sewed clothes in their filthy tenement homes or who processed food—could spread to decent, clean, and respectable citizens served as

* Reprinted from the American Journal of Public Health 75(10):1155, 1985

powerful incentive for renewed efforts to eliminate the menace of illness among the poor.[3]

Like most city dwellers, the urban poor usually chose to stay at home during illnesses, relying on traditional healing methods or, perhaps, the services of a dispensary physician.[4] Compared to the middle and upper classes whose diseases were supervised by the frequent visits from the family physician either in their homes or, to a lesser extent, in the well-ordered surroundings of a hospital's pay ward or private rooms, treatment of the sick poor during illness seemed careless at best.

A few lady philanthropists, in New York, Boston, Philadelphia, and Buffalo, found these grim realities intolerable. Motivated by their shared "vision" of the good society, they hired trained nurses to bring care, cleanliness, and character to the homes of the sick poor.[1] As was the case with so many philanthropic activities, these nurses were expected to bring a message with their medicine. Disciplined and well-bred women, they were to raise the "household existence" with their "delicate instruction and firm convictions," and to protect the public from the spread of disease with forceful, yet tactful lessons in physical and moral hygiene. The image of the visiting nurse climbing the tenement stairs to save the indigent from illness and bad habits struck the fancy of a wide variety of social reformers.[5]

As knowledge of these visiting nurses' work spread, the number of agencies organized to provide their services rapidly increased. These early visiting nurse associations, as they were called, began as small undertakings in which a few wealthy "lady managers" financed and supervised the work of one or two nurses. In most associations the nurses worked six days a week, eight to ten hours a day, and were able to visit daily eight to twelve patients. The ailments they encountered were commonly infectious, often acute, and always complicated by the families' social and economic circumstances.[1,5]

Usually, after only a brief interval of tension, even the dispensary and private physicians, who cared for the sick poor in their homes, came to appreciate the work of visiting nurses. In the context of a widespread debate on "charity abuse" of health care facilities, the rapid acceptance of the visiting nurse may have been based on the rising cost of hospital care and the effort to reduce the number of charity patients seeking hospitalization.[6] In their search for paying patients, hospitals valued any program that helped them shed their image as a "once charitable enterprise."[7] Obviously, one way to relieve hospital burdens—caused by what some contemporary spokesmen asserted was excessive and indiscriminate charity—was to provide the poor with more care in their homes, while simultaneously teaching them how to stay healthy.[8] From the perspective of the sick poor, the visiting nurse brought much needed care and relief from the often extreme burdens of illness. Thus, as the result of a complex set of social, medical, and economic needs, the visiting nurse, seemingly assured of success, entered the twentieth century with a clear sense of purpose, backed by a supportive constituency anxious to promote what appeared to be an unambiguously valuable undertaking.

THE NEW PUBLIC HEALTH CAMPAIGN

It was the changing emphasis of the "public health campaign" that would, within the first decade of the 20th century, create a bond between these visiting nurses and public health.[9] By 1910, death rates, especially for infectious disease, were declining and public officials showed no hesitation in claiming their share of the success. Many others agreed, that it was through public hygiene that these diseases had been successfully combated: care of the water, food, and milk supply; removal of garbage, ashes, and dirt; the cleaning of streets; disposal of sewage; better housing; and the control of contagious disease. But freedom from disease no longer depended simply on community effort or the construction of more public works. Winning the fight against disease now required moving from public hygiene to personal hygiene. This new campaign would focus on the affairs of the household and conduct of the individual's life. There was nothing to be gained by uplifting the masses, it was argued, unless each individual in the mass was to lift himself or herself.[9–13]

If public health was indeed an increasingly private matter, then the task ahead required translating the knowledge of scientific medicine into terms of personal effort and responsibility. Education, declared C.-E.A. Winslow, a leading proponent of this view, was a keynote of the modern campaign for public health. The "new idea" of this campaign was to bring "hygienic knowledge right to the individual in his home," where the information taught could be adapted to the particular circumstances of each individual and presented in the words of the kitchen or the sitting room.[14]

In actuality, this idea of a "health visitor" originated with Florence Nightingale and was first discussed in this country in 1893 at the International Congress of Charities, Correction and Philanthrophy.[15] In her widely read paper, "Sick Nursing and Health Nursing," she outlined the details of this new scheme, which she had helped initiate in England in 1892. In the Nightingale plan, these health missionaries were to be ladies with special training and practical instruction.[16,17]

The only significant variation in the American version of the Nightingale plan was to make the teacher of positive health the visiting nurse, not a lady health missionary. Already well established in the homes of the poor, the visiting nurse was the logical choice, as one medical authority suggested, to serve as "the relay station, to carry the power from the control stations of science, the hospital, and the university to the individual homes of the community."[18] She was "preeminently fitted" for this function, explained C.-E.A. Winslow, because she was a woman and therefore possessed the patience and tact necessary to bring hygiene into the life of the tenements. Unlike the social worker, she knew the human body and what he described as its reaction to external conditions and to the hygienic conduct of life. Her approach was far superior to that of the physician because she was trained to see the body as a whole, while the physician's vision was distorted by a preoccupation with special pathological conditions.[19]

Most nurses shared this viewpoint, and some even went so far as to suggest that this new field of health nursing differed so greatly from sick nursing that it might one day constitute a distinct profession. Why not, queried one editorial in the *Public Health Nurse,* "come boldly forth, one and all, and claim the right to exercise the promotion of health as a profession?"[20]

Asserting their independence, these nurses declared an end to "the old teaching" of the nurse as the handmaiden of the physician. She was instead an associate or co-worker of the physician who helped him produce results he could never accomplish alone. While some physicians still expected to find the nurse waiting "at his elbow," more progressive physicians could be counted on, stated nursing leader Mary Gardner, to gladly give these nurses "a helping hand" by strengthening their new position with the patient.[21-24]

Health nursing seemed particularly well suited for those nurses seeking the opportunity for autonomous practice. Although these nurses still carried out the doctors' orders, their new working conditions made it possible to discriminate as to doctors, cooperating with those working for "a higher standard of public welfare" while standing in but "remote and casual relation with those who have no such aims or desire."[23] These nurses appeared to be crossing the invisible and ill-defined line between medicine and nursing, as they believed it their business to select those cases requiring diagnosis, sending them where this might best be accomplished.

In the case of the tuberculosis patient, for example, the nurse was, according to Ellen LaMotte, an early leader in the field, "singularly independent." There were no special orders; the doctor knew what should be done and the nurse knew what to do. Further words were, she claimed, unnecessary.

Patients could go for months without seeing the doctor or even change physicians, and it would have no significant impact on their daily regimen. It was the nurse who was in charge of the patient's care, who was there through the long months of illness, and who moved the patient from doctor to doctor. Some exploitative or ignorant physicians reacted to such behavior on the part of nurses with antagonism and opposition, but, according to LaMotte, they were simply "holdovers from a passing regime." In such cases the nurse simply proceeded with her duty even if at seemingly cross purposes with the physician.[23] As those nurses entering this new field suggested, what they intended to do was certainly not, in the words of nursing leader Adelaide Nutting, "nursing in the ordinary sense of that term."[25]

PREVENTION PROGRAMS, SERVICES

Visiting nursing willingly added these new preventive tasks to their traditional responsibilities of caring for the sick at home. By 1910, the majority of the large urban visiting nurse associations had initiated preventive programs for school children, infants, mothers, and patients with tuberculosis. While pleased by this sudden growth of their new enterprises, the ladies who managed these associations found themselves overwhelmed by the need for correspondingly rapid increases in their sources of support. As a result, not only was the focus of these programs a radical departure, but the methods used by the lady managers to finance them were equally unprecedented. Unable to finance any large new programs, the ladies used two methods to entice others to pay for these new works—the joint venture and the demonstration. In the joint venture, the visiting nurse association provided the nurses while some other voluntary organization provided the money. Demonstrations were a bit more risky, since in those instances the visiting nurse association initiated the program on a small-scale, experimental basis, assuming that when its worth was clear to "the public," the necessary funds would be provided.[26]

School nursing best illustrates the demonstration approach to expansion. In many cities, physicians had been hired by the city to inspect school children and to exclude those with contagious diseases. Initially, this approach presented few problems, but as the number of children excluded grew rapidly, many boards of education began to seek other solutions. By 1902, the situation in the New York City schools was out of control with 15 to 20 children per school being sent home daily. At the suggestion of Lillian Wald, a nurse from the Henry Street Settlement House was sent to four schools to demonstrate how, through home visiting, the illnesses of these children could be cured. The experiment was successful, and at the end of a month the Board of Health hired 12 nurses to continue this work. The efficiency of the program was further documented by a dramatic decrease in absenteeism.[1,27,28]

Visiting nurse associations also assumed an important role in the campaign against tuberculosis. Tuberculosis was seen as a "house disease" of the very poor, and its elimination required the personal cooperation of patients and their families. By the turn of the century, it had become clear that, although medical science was now able to provide a great deal of information about tuberculosis and specific guidance as to its prevention, no prompt or simple medical solution was forthcoming. The campaign would need many more clinics and sanatoriums, but more importantly any progress required overcoming of public apathy and ignorance.[1,29]

The visiting nurse seemed ideally suited for this task and, not surprisingly, visiting nurse associations were among the first voluntary societies working to combat tuberculosis.[1,23] Many quickly found, however, that this was their most expensive program, since the patients tended to be poverty stricken and often required much time-consuming teaching. Recognizing the magnitude of this undertaking, visiting nurse societies were careful, as one Boston lady manager put it, to "avoid allowing anyone to place responsibility for the whole tuberculosis movement with their organization."[30,31] The glory of the visiting nurse association, would come, they hoped, from initiating the work, not in bearing its long-term financial burden. Financing this educational campaign was, from these lady managers' perspective, the responsibility of the growing number of voluntary societies for the prevention of tuberculosis and, ultimately, the city government.

Thus, the role of visiting nurse associations in the development of the campaign against tuberculosis was most frequently that of partners in a joint venture. Typical of this approach was the work initiated by John and Isabel Lowman in Cleveland. John Lowman was a member of the Western Reserve Medical School faculty, and Isabel Lowman an active member of the Board of the Cleveland Visiting Nurse Association. Concerned about the lack of services for tuberculosis patients, the Lowmans went to Germany and France in 1903 to study treatment of consumption. Following their trip, John Lowman began to open tuberculosis dispensaries—four by 1905—while Isabel Lowman and her committee on tuberculosis began to raise money to provide Visiting Nurse Association staff to visit the dispensary's patients. With the help of the Lowmans, the Cleveland Anti-tuberculosis League was organized in 1905, and by 1908 was able to assume all expenses for these tuberculosis nurses. In September 1910, the League's report to the mayor on tuberculosis conditions in the city resulted in the creation of a Bureau of Tuberculosis within the Department of Health. By 1913, all tuberculosis nursing was being financed by the city, which saw itself, as one health officer suggested, as having "come to the rescue and provided funds for the support of the work."[32]

For the visiting nurse, these circumstances created a time of unlimited possibilities. Visiting nurses could be found working for department stores, factories, insurance companies, boards of health and education, hospitals, settlement houses, milk and baby clinics, playgrounds, and hotels, as well as for visiting nurse associations. Not surprisingly, the number of agencies seeking their services had increased from only 58 in 1901 to nearly 2,000 by 1914.[33,34]

VOLUNTARY VERSUS OFFICIAL HEALTH AGENCIES

The outcome of this rapid growth in preventive services varied from city to city with voluntary and "official" government agencies assuming essentially unpredictable, often overlapping, responsibilities. As the confusion grew so did the debate as to the relative functions of the voluntary or "nonofficial" versus the official health agencies. The central concern was one of control.[22,35] As Haven Emerson, a former Health Commissioner of New York City, later remembered, "competition and rivalry in methods, resources and accomplishments became as keen as in selling soup or advertising tooth paste."[12]

While locally voluntary and public agencies negotiated their rather idiosyncratic relationships, publicly the struggle for consensus continued in the journals. The views of the public health nursing leadership and their predominately voluntary organizations most commonly appeared in the *Public Health Nurse,* while those of the public health physicians and their official agencies were usually expressed in the *American Journal of Public Health.*

In these articles, voluntary organizations characterized themselves as fulfilling a set of responsibilities that they could accomplish with "peculiar fitness and effectiveness." They saw their purpose as assisting or supplementing official activities through education, research, demonstration, and standardization. Health officers, they claimed, could not attend to the details of their administrative work and simultaneously conduct the needed investigations. Nor could the health department be justified in using tax money to test new methods of work. It was therefore the task of the voluntary agency to conduct these experimental programs. Once the work of a particular program was established, public interest aroused, and the most effective methods established, the official agency could, they argued, easily obtain expansion funds for their continuation as part of a governmental program.[36,37]

Thus voluntary agencies saw themselves as a cornerstone of public health work. As Isabel Lowman described it, they were "an experimental laboratory whose cost in energy and money must ever be a surtax on the good will of the private individual."[36] While admitting that at some point all health activities might conceivably be taken over by public health departments, the voluntary agencies claimed that the time had not yet come. Organizations for community health were far from complete and health officers were far from wise, contended these voluntary agencies, while the public was not educated to the point of recognizing the need to provide sufficient money for health programs.[37]

In contrast, some health officers tended not to see the activities of voluntary health organizations as supportive or cooperative, but as competitive and self-serving. The growing popularity of public health, declared Francis Curtis, Chairman of the Newton, Massachusetts Board of Health, caused clever people to see it as a means for justifying the existence of their nonofficial agencies.[38,39] According to such public health officials, private health organizations had "mistaken their functions and misunderstood their relationship to government." Such organizations needed to be put in their proper place: "standing back of and helping the official agencies, placing themselves at the disposal of the health officer and permitting him to direct their activities according to his plan."[38,39]

As might be expected, debate over the proper domain of public health practice was not confined to these struggles between voluntary and public organizations. Attempts by health departments to extend the focus of their concerns also often resulted in conflict with the medical profession. Inevitably, most health officers found themselves forced to abandon claims to any curative activities that might be construed as threatening the economic well-being of private physicians. Consequently, despite much ongoing discussion, health department and school health services become increasingly preventive.[40–42]

What they chose for themselves, they not surprisingly chose for their employees and, accordingly, many health officers believed the work of the public health nurse was hygienic, not therapeutic. Thus, an inescapable, though seemingly unexpected, consequence was the limitation of the activities of these publicly supported nurses to the prevention of disease, leaving the care of the sick to the visiting nurse associations. Some health officers even went so far as to suggest that nurses who spent any significant amount of their time providing bedside care should not even be classified as public health nurses.[24,43]

The nursing leadership, many of them superintendents of visiting nurse associations, were outraged by such assertions. Visiting nurses, they insisted, had always been teachers of prevention and hygiene and had in fact "blazed the trail" for all of the health departments' new preventive programs. But, unlike their narrowly focused critics, they had possessed the wisdom to see the value of caring for the sick as a means of gaining access to families in greatest need of health education. Were the assertions of health officers that visiting nurses were not public health nurses made, they wondered, "to keep the visiting nurse in her place, outside the sphere of public health work?" If so, these efforts were in vain, for the visiting nurse was as much a public health nurse as any nurse employed by the health departments.[44-47]

By the 1920s, many nursing leaders were campaigning for the creation of an institutional framework that would allow the public health nurse to care for both the healthy and the sick. Realizing that separating the curative and preventive functions of the public health nurse had been a mistake, they argued for an "amalgamated" organization that would unite both the voluntary and publicly funded agencies.[26] Even though these views were substantiated in numerous demonstration projects and major reports throughout the 1920s and 1930s, nurses gained few allies in their efforts to create such agencies. In most communities, relationships between these organizations remained haphazard, with gaps and duplication in services the inevitable outcome.[33,48,49]

With health departments, school health services, and visiting nurse associations providing a perplexing assortment of both curative and preventive nursing services, the meaning of public health nursing became increasingly obscure to both its practitioners and the public.[48,50] The legacy of this dilemma still haunts contemporary public health nursing.[51]

DOMAIN OF
PUBLIC HEALTH NURSING

Thus, during its first 50 years, the domain of the public health nurse came to include almost every health aspect of life from the care of the sick to the prevention of disease. Unmistakably, to the public and voluntary agencies who sought their services, these nurses seemed an economical and appropriate way to help the poor. By the late 1920s, however, public health nursing had reached a turning point. From the perspective of the visiting nurse associations, the circumstances that had created the need for their organizations 20 years before were simply no longer of major concern to most communities. With fewer immigrants, declining death rates from infectious diseases, and the growing centrality of the hospital, the work of the visiting nurse seemed increasingly inconsequential. While they fought for a role in the evolving health care system, most had little success.[26] Despite visiting nurse associa-tions often-stated interest in extending their services to the whole community —sick, well, rich, and poor—their clients remained the poor and their major programs remained the care of the sick at home.[48,52,53]

In contrast to the experience of most visiting nurse associations, public health nursing within official agencies was undergoing a period of steady expansion. By 1924, with 54 per cent of all public health nurses working for official health agencies, it seemed inevitable that these organizations would remain the major source of employment for the field.[54]

But health departments and boards of education were not managed like visiting nurse associations, as a cooperative effort of ladies and nurses guided, of course, for the most part by the nurses. In contrast, the work of the public health nurse in these organizations reflected more the policy of their organiza-tion or desires of the health officer than the "visions" of the nurses. This break with custom and loss of authority was, not surprisingly, of great concern to many leading public health nurses.[26] While the leadership continued its cam-paign for the creation of a publicly funded comprehensive nursing service, the concerns of nurses in most official agencies were confined to the teaching of prevention.[48]

Thus, within both public and voluntary organizations, public health nurses found it increasingly difficult to create the kind of institutional setting that would allow them to offer every kind of nursing service to patients in their homes. Despite their failed ideal, public health nurses went on caring for at least some of the public—in sickness or in health—but rarely the same nurse for both.

REFERENCES

1. Brainard A: The Evolution of Public Health Nursing. Philadelphia: W.B. Saunders, 1922
2. Boyer P: Urban Masses and Moral Order in America. Cambridge: Harvard Univer-sity Press, 1978
3. Duffy J: Social impact of disease in the late 19th century. *In:* Leavitt J. Numbers R (eds): Sickness and Health in America. Madison: University of Wisconsin Press, 1978; 395–402
4. Rosenberg C: Social class and medical care in 19th century America. J Hist Med Allied Sci 1974; 29:32–54
5. Fulmer H: History of visiting nurse work in America. Am J Nurs 1902; 2:411–425
6. Rosner D: Health care for the 'truly needy': nineteenth century origins of the concept. Milbank Mem Fun Q 1982; 60:355–385

7. Rosner D: A Once Charitable Enterprise: Hospitals and Health Care in Brooklyn and New York, 1885–1915. Chicago: University of Chicago Press, 1980
8. The hospital deficit. Trained Nurse Hosp Rev 1904; 32:115
9. Winslow CEA: The untilled fields of public health. Science 1920; 51:23–33
10. Ferrell J: The trend of preventive medicine in the United States. JAMA 1923; 81:1063–1069
11. Frankel L: Science and public health. Am J Public Health 1915; 5:281–289
12. Emerson H: Meeting the demand for community health work. Public Health Nurse 1924; 16:485–489
13. Field W: Civic control of public health nursing. Public Health Nurse Q 1914; 6:70–80
14. Winslow CEA: The Evolution and Significance of the Modern Public Health Campaign. New Haven: Yale University Press, 1935
15. Billings J. Hurd HM (eds): Hospitals, Dispensaries and Nursing: Papers and Discussions in the International Congress of Charities. Correction and Philanthropy. Section III, Chicago, June 12–17th, 1893. Baltimore: Johns Hopkins Press. 1894
16. Nightingale F: Health teaching in towns and villages: rural hygiene. *In:* Seymour L: Selected Writings of Florence Nightingale. New York: MacMillan, 1954
17. Monteiro LA: Florence Nightingale on public health nursing. Am J Public Health 1985; 75:000–000
18. Their Health is Your Health, a fund raising booklet for Henry Street Nurses' Settlement. New York, 1934
19. Winslow CEA: The New Profession of Public Health Nursing and Its Educational Needs. Speech, 1917, Winslow Collection. Yale University Library. New Haven, folder 119:128
20. The profession of promoting health. Public Health Nurse 1919; 11:10–12
21. Wald LD: Windows on Henry Street. Boston: Little Brown, 1934
22. Gardner M: Public Health Nursing. New York: MacMillan, 1916
23. La Motte E: The Tuberculosis Nurse: Her Function and Her Qualifications. New York: Putnum's Sons, 1915
24. Royer BF: Public health nursing vs. bedside work. Public Health Nurse 1923; 15:231–234
25. Nutting A: Nursing and health. Visiting Nurse Q 1910; 2:10–13
26. Buhler-Wilkerson K: False Dawn: The Rise and Decline of Public Health Nursing, 1900–1930. PhD dissertation, University of Pennsylvania, 1984
27. Struthers (Rogers) L: The School Nurse. New York: Putnum, 1917
28. Dock LL: The school nurse experiment in New York. Am J Nursing 1902; 3:108–110
29. Shryrock R: National Tuberculosis Association 1904–1954: A Study of the Voluntary Health Movement in the United States. New York: National Tuberculosis Association, 1957
30. Visiting Nurse Society of Philadelphia: Annual Report, 1907

31. Graves S: Instructive District Nurse Association: 1885–1912. MSN thesis, Boston University, 1970
32. Bower I: Public Health Nursing in Cleveland, 1895–1928. Cleveland: Western Reserve University, 1930
33. Goldmark J: Nursing and Nursing Education in the United States. New York: MacMillan, 1923
34. Waters Y: Visiting Nursing in the United States. New York: Charities Publication, 1909
35. See for example the series of articles: Relative functions of official and non-official agencies: a symposium. Am J Public Health 1920; 10:940–972
36. Lowman I: The relation of private and municipal antituberculosis activities. Public Health Nurse Q 1914; 6:40–51
37. Hatsfield C: Relative functions of health agencies: viewpoint of the non-official agency. Am J Public Health 1920; 10:948–952
38. Curtis FG: Relative functions of health agencies: relation between official and non-official health agencies. Am J Public Health 1920; 10:956–960
39. McCombs CE: Public health and private health agencies. Am J Public Health 1919; 9:951–955
40. Rosenkrantz BG: Public Health and the State: Changing Views in Massachusetts, 1842–1936. Cambridge: Harvard University Press, 1972
41. Rosen G: The Structure of American Medical Practice: 1875–1941. Philadelphia: University of Pennsylvania Press, 1984
42. Duffy J: The American medical profession and public health: from support to ambivalence. Bull Hist Med 1979; 53:1–22
43. Hill HW: Is the visiting nurse a public health nurse? Public Health Nurse 1923; 15:231–234
44. For an interesting discussion of these developments see, Melosh B: The Physician's Hand: Work, Culture, and Conflict in American Nursing. Philadelphia: Temple University Press, 1982
45. Tucker K: Whither? Public Health Nurse 1919; 11:700–702
46. Fox E: Is a visiting nurse a public health nurse? Public Health Nurse 1919; 11:575–578
47. Theory or experience? Public Health Nurse 1919; 11:579–581
48. National Organization for Public Health Nursing: Survey of Public Health Nursing: Administration and Practice: New York: Commonwealth Fund, 1934
49. East Harlem Nursing and Health Service: A Comparative Study of Generalized and Specialized Health Services, 1926: New York: Garland Publishing Company, 1984 (reprint edition)
50. Welch M: What is public health nursing? Am J Nursing 1936; 36:452–456
51. Williams C: Community health nursing—what is it? Nursing Outlook 1977; 25:250–254
52. Reverby S: Something besides waiting: the politics of private duty nursing reform

in the depression. *In:* Lagemann E (ed): Nursing History; New Perspectives, New Possibilities. New York: Teachers College Press, 1983; 133–156

53. Davis M: Nursing service measured by social needs. Am J Nursing 1939; 39:35–40
54. Tattershall L: Census of public health nursing in the United States. Public Health Nurse 1926; 18:266

EDITOR'S NOTE

Although Wilkerson ends on a somewhat negative note, we are reminded that the public health nurse has been in the vanguard of health promotion and disease prevention since the turn of the century. Roberts and Heinrich, who bring our history to the present, describe additional public health concerns and functions such as social activism and primary health care. Other activities within the public health nurse's purview described in Unit II include community assessment, coordination of services, patient–family advocacy, and health education.

Unit II: *Public Health Nursing Comes of Age*

DORIS E. ROBERTS,
RN, PhD,
AND JANET HEINRICH,
RN, DrPH*

INTRODUCTION

A decade ago, the World Health Organization's Committee on Community Health Nursing defined the emerging role of public health nursing in primary health care.[1] The report focused attention on untapped nursing potentials and added impetus to the dynamic movement that had begun 10 years earlier with the first Child Health Nurse Practitioner.

By 1974, public health nursing had come a long way since the early 1930s, when it was struggling to assert itself as a full-fledged member of the public health system while coping with differences both within the profession and

* Reprinted from the American Journal of Public Health 75 (10):1162, 1985

within the organizational structure of practice. Although the importance of specialized preparation for home visiting had been recognized from the beginning, the majority of nurses in service had little or no academic preparation in public health. And, as Wilkerson points out,[2] the shifting of service from the voluntary visiting nurse structure to the official agency not only relegated decision making for nursing services to health officers, it splintered general nursing into preventive and sick care and fomented rivalry between "visiting" and "public health" nurses which further undermined the possibility of comprehensive health care. It was not unusual to find a nurse assigned to the health department placarding homes for communicable diseases, quarantining children from schools, and advising mothers to have their infants vaccinated, while, at the same time, a visiting nurse took care of the ill patient or the mother and baby, with communication between the two components relying haphazardly on the individual nurses involved.

There were exceptions, of course, in localities where the visiting nurse agency had contracted with the health department to provide the combined services and in rural areas where public health nurses were often employed as "town" or "district" nurses and provided care to both the sick and well in the community.[3,4] Pioneering work by the American Red Cross had demonstrated how effective nurses, properly trained and supervised, could be in providing broad-based county-wide health care to rural communities. (By 1930, there were 636 rural nursing services administered entirely by the Red Cross or in partnership with county health units; from 1919 to 1930, the Red Cross operated 2,972 generalized public health nursing services throughout the country but, by policy, transferred the programs to local agencies as they developed and were able to assume these responsibilities.[5]) Nevertheless, separation of "bedside" care from disease prevention and casefinding services prevailed, and increased with the expansion of city and county health departments.

ECONOMIC CRISIS AND RECOVERY

The weight of the Great Depression, felt by American families across the country, seriously affected all types of public health services as well. Communities were neither financially nor conceptually prepared to address the enormity of the problem. Decreased funding brought drastic personnel reductions, salary cutbacks, and curtailment of the most basic services. Many public health nurses, facing the effects of poverty, malnutrition, sickness, and deprivation, became social activists.

Federal relief and employment programs under The New Deal finally brought new hope and incentives to public health. Surveys identified the health and medical needs of the nation and work was provided for the unemployed. Over 10,000 nurses were given employment under the Civil Works Administration, assigned primarily to official health agencies.[6] While this facilitated rapid program expansion by recipient agencies and gave the nurses a taste of public health, the nurses' lack of field experience created major problems of training and supervision for the regular staff.

The Sheppard-Towner Act of 1921, aimed at improving maternal and child health care, had stimulated the organization of state health departments. The subsequent Public Health Title VI of the Social Security Act of 1935 went far beyond: through state grants, it strengthened and extended state health organizations; accelerated the growth of local health services; provided funds for the recruitment, training and supervision of public health personnel; and promoted the expansion of services in research, prevention, treatment, and control of pressing health problems.[7]

The public health nursing leaders who had helped draft this legislation were ready to plan its implementation.

- Katherine Tucker, General Director of the National League for Public Health Nursing (NOPHN) worked with the Roosevelt Administration to include bedside nursing care for the indigent in the Emergency Relief grant program.[8]
- Sophie Nelson, Director of Nursing for the John Hancock Insurance Company, was loaned to the US Public Health Service to survey public health nursing needs and advise the Surgeon General of the US Public Health Service on ways public health nurses might contribute to the work of that organization.
- Pearl McIver, Director of Nursing in the Missouri State Health Department, gave consultation on critical community needs for health care. In 1933, Ms. McIver joined the Public Health Methods and Research Division of the US Public Health Service and, soon after, was transferred to the States Relations Division as the first public health nursing consultant for state health departments.[9] (The 1944 PHS reorganization established an Office, later Division, of Public Health Nursing in the new Bureau of State Services.) Referring to Ms. McIver's appointment in the PHS, McNeil states this was ". . . the beginning of a new era in public health nursing."[10]

Pearl McIver was pragmatic, courageous in criticizing unnecessary deterrents to program development, and unswerving in her faith that nurses could improve the health and well-being of individuals, families, and entire communities. Convinced that the scope and quality of local services depended heavily on wise leadership at the state level, she labored to see a well-prepared nursing director in every state health department. To achieve this, she often assigned nursing consultants to help establish the position or to substitute for an incumbent on study leave. She created an organizational structure that enabled nurses assigned to regional offices and categorical programs of the US Public Health Service to relate professionally to the Service's Central Office of Public Health Nursing, a design which became the prototype for many state agencies.[11] Working closely together, Ms. McIver and Naomi Deutsch, Director of Nursing in the US Children's Bureau, promoted a unified approach to community nursing services and planned with states for the use of grant-in-aid funds for staffing rapidly developing programs and for preparing nurses in public health. The results of these joint efforts ". . . demonstrated what two able, experienced nursing administrators, with a small staff of well selected consultants and the support of professional organizations could accomplish when they are concerned about delivery of services."[10]

By the end of the decade, an upsurge in public health nursing was clearly evident. All of the 48 States, as well as the territories of Alaska and Hawaii, and the District of Columbia had established public health nursing programs. According to the 1938 census, there were 19,379 nurses employed full time by state and local agencies, including 3887 by Boards of Education; this represented a 24 per cent increase over the previous census of 1931.[12,13] The largest increase (40 per cent) occurred in local health departments, setting the pattern for the next decade. At the same time, there were still 1077 counties (over one-third of the total) and 26 cities (population 10,000 and over) with no local public health nursing services.[14]

The two national agencies established to promote public health—the National Organization for Public Health Nursing (NOPHN) and the American Public Health Association (APHA)—had formed strong productive ties, as shown in joint statements adopted on minimum qualifications, definition of nursing functions, and standards of practice.[15] Protocols for service records, recording procedures, and cost studies had been prepared and were widely used. The Association of State and Territorial Directors of Public Health Nursing (ASTDPHN)—later changed in 1965 to the Association of State and Territorial Directors of Nursing (ASTDN)—had been organized. This group, working closely with the federal government, professional organizations and the Association of State and Territorial Health Officials (ASTHO), effectively influenced the development of health personnel and services for the nation, states, and local communities.

The training and preparation of public health nurses was of continuing concern. From its inception in 1912, the NOPHN had taken responsibility for promoting educational standards for this specialty. By 1935, 16 approved post-graduate courses in public health nursing were offered by colleges or universities; five years later, this number had grown to 26.[8,11] During the mid-1930s, guidelines for curricula and student field experiences were revised and schools of nursing were urged to include public health in their basic program, to enhance the quality of nursing practice in *all* settings. In 1932, while these efforts were in progress, a survey of public health agencies[8] revealed that only 7 per cent of the nurses employed in public health were adequately prepared. (A nurse was considered to have adequate preparation for public health work if she had completed at least 30 hours of credit in a program approved for public health by NOPHN.)[16]

This problem was given high priority when educational funds became available through the Social Security Act. Those funds alone in 1936 enabled 1000 nurses to complete educational programs in public health.[9] Even so, this was only a beginning step toward reducing a persistent, knotty problem.

In October 1938, Dr. Thomas Parran, Surgeon General of the US Public Health Service, addressing the Annual Meeting of APHA, reported, "Greater progress has been made in public health during the past two years than in any similar period in our history."[7] He then described the health status of the nation as shown by the recent National Health Survey which had revealed: grossly insufficient preventive services, alarming malnutrition, one-third of the population with little or no medical care, excessive disease and death rates in low-income groups and, while threats of communicable disease were diminishing, the chronic diseases—syphilis, tuberculosis, heart disease, cancer and stroke—had become the chief causes of death. In spite of the recent advances, the ability of public health agencies to cope with these new concerns, given the existing patterns of organization and distribution of services, was questioned.

The rural sanitation movement of the 1920s had promoted the development of local health units, from 109 in 1920 to 505 by 1930. The Depression slowed this growth, however, so that only 41 new units were established during the ensuing five years. Progress had been made through state grants but, by the end of the decade, few states had more than half of their counties covered by local full-time public health services.[7,17]

WORLD WAR II

Influenced largely by responses to the Depression, the course of public health was soon to make an abrupt change. As the nation became involved in World

War II, attention focused sharply on safeguarding the health of military personnel, of families in cantonment areas, and of workers in essential industries. Maternal and infant care, nutrition, sanitation, and control of syphilis and tuberculosis were targeted programs; categorical programming was intensified.

To plan and coordinate activities related to the war effort, the national nursing organizations joined forces to form the Nursing Council on National Defense (NCND). The Subcommittee on Nursing in the Office of Defense (SNOD) was responsible for recruitment and assignment of nurses in military and civilian services for defense. These two groups worked closely together to protect the health of the public at home as well as those sent abroad.

With medical and nursing staffs in hospitals greatly depleted, many patients who would normally have been hospitalized had to be treated at home. Families, already stressed, were expected to care for critically ill members, help with home births, or care for mothers and infants discharged early from the hospital. These family caretakers needed much instruction, support, and assistance with direct nursing care and looked to the public health nurse for this help. Both official and voluntary agencies set aside restricting policies in order to meet these needs. The American Red Cross organized courses in home nursing and training programs for nurse's aides. By the end of 1942, over 500,000 women had completed the American Red Cross home nursing course, and nearly 17,000 nurse's aides had been certified. These numbers continued to escalate so that, by the end of 1946, over 215,000 nurse's aide certificates had been awarded.[5] Volunteers were used in clinics, hospitals, and public health agencies more widely than ever before. As schools of nursing with federal subsidies graduated larger classes, more nurses became available for all types of service.

Public health problems were particularly acute in communities selected for military camps. Local resources were quickly overwhelmed by the influx of servicemen's families and other transient groups. Requests for emergency help poured in to the Office of Civilian Defense (OCD) from military headquarters as well as from state and local health departments. In response, the US Public Health Service recruited and assigned doctors, nurses, and engineers, often in teams, to areas in greatest need. During the war years, nearly 250 public health nurses were assigned to official agencies in 35 states, the District of Columbia, and Puerto Rico.[9]

In 1943, passage of the Emergency Maternity and Infant Care (EMIC) Act enabled the US Children's Bureau to take a vital part in determining both the quality and quantity of services for mothers and babies.[18] These federal funds paid for the cost of medical, hospital, and nursing care for wives and babies of servicemen, but eligibility for reimbursement required local services to meet standards set by the Children's Bureau. Demonstration programs for the control of tuberculosis, venereal disease, and malaria were initiated; protocols for the referral and follow-up of draftees rejected for health reasons were firmly fixed in ongoing programs.[7] Public health nurses played a vital role in all of these programs. Nurses coordinated activities, mobilized community resources, and adjusted services to meet emergencies without losing the essence of ongoing programs. The leadership of such notables as Marion Sheahan, Katherine Faville, Elizabeth Fox, Alma Haupt, Mary Beard, Marion Howell, and Pearl McIver gave direction to public health nursing during the war years and guided its development long afterwards.

The most effective strategy designed to increase the supply of nurses for wartime needs was framed by US Representative Frances P. Bolton of Ohio who, having witnessed the effects of nursing shortages in World War I, had funds earmarked for nursing education in federal appropriations for 1941. This support covered courses for basic, postgraduate, and graduate education and, in its two years of operation, enabled schools to increase enrollments by 13,000 students in basic programs and 4200 in graduate programs; approximately half of the graduate students specialized in public health.[7] This experience stimulated legislation for the US Cadet Nurse Corps program, passed in 1943 and administered by the Division of Nursing Education of the US Public Health Service, under the direction of Lucile Petry Leone. This highly successful program enrolled the quota of 65,000 cadet nurses during its first year and 30,000 the second and final year.[8] When hostilities ceased in the fall of 1945, the program was phased out but, during its short span, nursing education changed dramatically. Traditional curricula had been critically evaluated and shortened, experimental junior college programs were begun, and the number of basic baccalaureate programs had increased markedly, with most including some public health content.

THE IMMEDIATE POST-WAR YEARS

Hopes for a "return to normalcy" after the war did not materialize as veterans returned to their communities, families resettled, and schools and industries tried to cope with myriad complex changes. The health system felt the brunt of these adjustments. Military experiences had heightened public expectations of health care. Local health departments faced sudden increases in emotional problems, accidents, alcoholism, and other disabling conditions not previously considered to be in their domain; many scientific breakthroughs made traditional patterns of practice obsolete. For example, newly available antibiotics were effective in preventing and treating infectious diseases, rheumatic fever, venereal disease, etc. Development of the photofluorogram assisted mass casefinding for tuberculosis. Categorical programming, public participation in health decisions, renewed pressures for health insurance, construction of hospitals and health care facilities, and the extension of full-time local health services to all were dominant issues.

Fears that federal funding of state services would be withdrawn after the war were unfounded; instead, funds were increased and sharply focused to impact on categorical programs: tuberculosis, venereal disease, cancer, and mental health were spearheaded in every region. Registers were established for statistical analyses, casefinding and follow-up purposes; protocols for preventive services and care of patients, families, and high-risk groups were revised and referral systems strengthened. Local health councils were formed, patterned after the National Health Council, to study, coordinate and strengthen the total health care system in their jurisdictions. Funding was again available for training personnel and, in many instances, study programs were set up to prepare specialists in the field. The GI Bill enabled veterans to return to school and to major in almost any field. Many nurses took advantage of this, thereby obtaining a baccalaureate or master's degree, with many specializing in public health. In contrast, categorical funding focused on public health training in the respective disease entities, usually in a three- to six-month study program.

In addition to updating their knowledge of disease, there were many other gains for public health nurses in these new ventures. They were able to work intensively with the community in interdisciplinary teams and to apply epidemiologic concepts to populations at risk in a way that individual and family services did not permit.

In 1942, APHA's Subcommittee on Local Health Units, chaired by Haven Emerson, had found that only two-thirds of the population was covered by full-time local health units, and that the number of personnel was too sparse to provide even the basic services—communicable disease control; hygiene of maternity, infancy and childhood; health education of the general public; vital statistics; laboratory; and environmental sanitation. Double the existing number of public health nurses were needed to reach the recommended minimum requirements of one nurse per 5000 population, and that ratio should be doubled again if home care of the sick were added. That report, published in 1945,[17] had substantial impact upon the growth of local health departments, thus opening up more job opportunities for public health nurses. Beginning in the post-WWII years and extending into the 1950s, state health departments as well as the federal government became more active in promoting the establishment of local health departments. Several states, notably New York and California, strengthened their own matching grants, using substantial amounts of state tax money to induce local political jurisdictions to establish departments headed by full-time health officers and staffed by nursing directors and supervisors with approved qualifications.

By 1950, 56 per cent of the 3070 counties in the continental United States were covered by full-time local health services.[19] Five years later, this figure had increased to 72 per cent.[20] Although the growth of agencies providing public health nursing services was marked throughout this period, the increase in public health nursing staff was proportionately greater (Table 11-1).

Organizational changes of considerable importance to nursing were also occurring. A study sponsored by the National Health Council[8] documented the duplication of effort and uneven performance of many voluntary nursing agencies. One of its recommendations was to reduce the proliferation of community nursing services, and—accepting the concept of the generalized public health nurse serving a designated population as most effective—to encourage mergers among private agencies and better coordination with public agencies. Implementation of these recommendations hastened the development of the "combination service"—a partnership of voluntary and official agencies aimed at delivering comprehensive public health nursing services to the community. This ideal proved difficult to administer, however, because of conflicting organizational policies. Some found the combination untenable and, after a trial period, returned to their original separate structures. On January 1, 1960, 47 combination agencies were reported; by 1968, there were 100, but 11 years later, only 52 were still functioning.[14,21]

TABLE 11-1. NUMBER AND PERCENTAGE INCREASE
OF AGENCIES EMPLOYING NURSES FOR
PUBLIC HEALTH AND FULL-TIME
NURSES EMPLOYED

Year	Agencies		Nurses	
	Number	*% Increase*	*Number*	*% Increase*
1938	5901		19,502	
1957	8010	35.7	28,599	46.6
1968	9995	24.8	42,541	48.7
1979	13,753	37.6	69,085	62.4

Passage of the Hill–Burton Hospital Construction and Survey Act in 1946 provided matching grants for construction of public health as well as hospital facilities. The Act was instrumental in moving health departments, including nursing offices and clinics, out of dilapidated buildings, backrooms, and basements. This did much to boost morale of the nurses and to increase the status of public health nursing in the community.

Far-reaching happenings were also taking place that would influence human health and health care delivery around the world. In 1946, the Constitution of the World Health Organization was drafted and made ready for ratification by the United Nations. US Surgeon General Thomas Parran was highly influential in the organization of WHO and saw to it that Elmora Wickenden, Executive Secretary of the National Nursing Council, was included in the International Health Conference convened in June 1946 to draft the WHO Constitution. From the start, public health nursing was a distinct unit in the WHO Division of Public Health Services, included in all regional offices and in country missions and many team projects as they were developed. WHO has undergone structural and programmatic changes since its founding, but public health nursing has continually played an important role in the organization.

THE PROSPEROUS 1950s

The decade of the 1950s began on a note of excitement, prosperity, and expansion for nursing and public health and for the United States in general.

As is usual with rapid change, incongruities were common—for example, rural communities voted simultaneously on bonds for the closure of open sewers and for water fluoridation to prevent dental caries; infant mortality rates in coal mining communities were as much as 127 per cent higher than the national rate; and within states, one found very progressive health departments serving urban populations adjacent to counties with no official health agency.[22,23]

Activities within the NOPHN reflected concerns for the future of voluntary agencies and for bedside care of the sick, in particular, since most tax-supported agencies were again adhering narrowly to preventive services and health supervision. The Metropolitan and the John Hancock Life Insurance companies and the American Red Cross—all important sources of income for voluntary agencies—discontinued their support early in the 1950s. This was a significant loss. The insurance companies had subsidized agencies for the care of policy holders. The American Red Cross, between 1913 and 1947, had established 3109 public health nursing services in about 1800 counties. At the end of 1947, when the decision was made to discontinue the program, there were still over 100 in operation; by June 1950, these had either been transferred to local agencies or closed out. Thereafter, the American Red Cross was primarily involved in demonstrations and experiments in nursing service.[5]

Mounting interests in nurse-midwifery, equality and advancement of black nurses in public health, cost analysis methods and studies, inclusion of nursing services in health insurance plans, and better coordination of organized nursing as a whole were other major considerations. After more than two years of discussion and mutual planning, this latter activity culminated in 1952 with the formation of a new structure for professional nursing. Three organizations—the NOPHN, the National League for Nursing Education (NLNE), and the Association of Collegiate Schools of Nursing (ACSN)—were dissolved and their functions distributed between the American Nurses' Association (ANA) and the new National League for Nursing (NLN).[8] Henceforth, the professional development of public health nursing would be directed primarily by NLN, supported by and in collaboration with the Public Health Nursing Sections of APHA and ANA.

In 1948, Dr. Esther Lucile Brown's study of nursing education, undertaken for the National Nursing Council, had rocked apprenticeship patterns of nurse training and substantiated the need for professional education, *i.e.,* basic preparation in collegiate programs leading to a baccalaureate degree with advanced graduate preparation for teachers, administrators, supervisors, and researchers.[24] These recommendations solidly supported directions already advanced by NOPHN: the inclusion of public health concepts in the basic baccalaureate curriculum and graduate preparation for public health practice. The Brown report marked an exciting turning point for nursing and it was thought to be for public health nursing as well.

Soon after its formation, the NLN set about implementing the Brown recommendations, declaring that all basic collegiate nursing programs should integrate social and public health concepts throughout the curricula and prepare their students for first level positions in public health. Specialized preparation was to be given at the master's degree level with certificate programs gradually eliminated. All of these objectives were important for the upgrading of public health nursing practice and for bringing the profession in line with peer groups in nursing and in public health. Unfortunately, there was no testing of the plan and the time given for transition was too short for so immense a task.

Short courses, of one- and two-week duration, in public health concepts were devised for faculty all over the country. Public health faculty hastily rearranged schedules and looked for agencies to provide field experiences for the increased numbers of students. This effort was further complicated by the requirement that only baccalaureate graduates with public health preparation could serve as clinical preceptors. Up to this time, experienced public health nursing supervisors and senior staff had coached students, but many did not meet the new requirements. Therefore, young nurses minimally qualified, often with little or no work experience, were employed by the schools as field instructors. In addition, hospital clinics, outpatient departments and similar services largely concerned with individual patient care were used for clinical teaching in public health, thereby reducing and even excluding student contacts with agencies responsible for community health. Unknowingly, this well-conceived, goal-directed program dealt public health nursing a blow from which it has not entirely recovered 30 years later. The contextual fiber of public health, *i.e.*, the group and larger community, was lost to many simply because students and young faculty alike, steeped in the one-on-one tradition of nursing, were not adequately taught basic concepts of public health or provided opportunities to see and use those concepts in practice. For too many, "public health" nursing became synonymous with "out-of-hospital" nursing.

Many public health agencies suffered similar detrimental effects. The spark of having students as an integral function of the agency and the challenges of learning and change that accompany teaching responsibilities were soon lost. Add to that the employment of graduates poorly prepared in public health and it is little wonder that a period of dissatisfaction, criticism, and alternate approaches to public health nursing services was on the horizon.

These events might have had more damaging consequences but for a few counteracting influences. Ruth C. Freeman's textbooks on public health nursing practice and supervision—standard references in most schools—were explicit regarding the basic strategies of public health. As an educator, service director, and consultant, she also helped numerous schools, agencies, and individuals cope with the perplexing problems of the educational change. Another positive influence was the Nurse Training Act of 1956, which provided traineeships to prepare nurses for administrative, supervisory, and teaching positions. These funds enabled many students to enroll in schools of public health, as well as in schools of nursing, where the educational content concentrated on the sciences of public health and the community as an entity. Several State Directors of Nursing, including Marion Sheahan (New York), Anne Burns (Ohio), and Rena Haig (California), among others, counseled schools on agency needs, and helped states and local agencies adopt management strategies to align merit system classifications with NLN's recommendations. Statistically, the gains made during this period were clear. From 1940 to 1960, there was a steady increase in the proportion of nurses employed in public health who were educationally prepared in public health. By 1957, this figure had reached 38 per cent, with over 28 per cent having baccalaureate degrees and 27 per cent having both public health and baccalaureate degree preparation.[25] Nevertheless, the general complaint of service directors was that the newly prepared baccalaureate graduates were unable to function in public health without long intensive inservice training. Moreover, having succeeded in raising job qualifications for professional nurse staff, it was difficult to justify the need for continuing education in processes intrinsic to public health.

During the 1950s, international health services were initiated to accelerate the development of public health and nursing in many countries. A Division of International Health was created in the Office of the Surgeon General, US Public Health Service, with goals similar to those of WHO. Public health nursing was included in the core of the program at headquarters and in team assignments to participating countries. Margaret Arnstein, Mary Forbes, and Virginia Arnold worked diligently with Dr. Henry van Zile Hyde to plan and implement the Division of International Health. Virginia Ohlson, under the Supreme Command of Allied Powers (SCAP) and the Rockefeller Foundation, gave leadership in helping Japan and other asian countries develop progressive nursing programs.

Field experiences gained earlier through the US Department of State, the Pan American Sanitary Bureau, the United Nations Relief and Rehabilitation Administration (UNRRA), and post-war country restoration strategies under the military had prepared nurses for these new undertakings. To supplement these experiences, intensive multidisciplinary training programs were created to help personnel understand the culture, health problems, work patterns, and related social conditions they would face in carrying out their assignments.

Several events occurred during the decade that gave all public health nurses a feeling of presence and unaccustomed recognition. In 1951, Ruth B. Freeman was appointed to the Executive Board of APHA, the first nurse to attain such an elected position.[10] In 1955, the prestigious Lasker Award was presented to Pearl McIver, Lucile Petry Leone, and Margaret Arnstein, as a group, for their contributions to public health administration. In 1959, Marion Sheahan was named President-Elect of APHA, clear evidence of the high esteem in which she was held.

REVOLUTION IN HEALTH CARE, THE 1960s

The phenomenal post-war growth of the US population passed the 200,000,000 mark in the 1960s, and by 1965 the very young (under the age of 5 years) and the elderly (age 65 and over) each represented approximately 10 per cent of the total population. While a stable economy, buoyant employment, and space explorations contributed to the general public confidence, many observers noted rising racial tensions, urban disorganization, increasing environmental pollution, widespread poverty, and serious inequities in medical care. In 1961, President John F. Kennedy sought legislation to reduce unemployment, protect civil rights, and provide medical care for the aged under social security. It was 1964, however, before the Congress dealt authoritatively with these problems, in response to President Lyndon B. Johnson's War on Poverty and plans for a Great Society. The Economic Opportunity Act provided funds for neighborhood health centers, Head Start, and numerous other community action programs. Categorical funding expanded programs for maternal and child health (maternity and infant care, children and youth projects), mental health and mental retardation, and public health training; it also initiated Regional Medical Programs for heart disease, cancer and stroke.

In 1965, Congress amended the Social Security Act to include health insurance benefits, providing hospital and home nursing care for the elderly (Medicare) and expanded care for the indigent (Medicaid). Although falling short of a national health insurance plan, these programs made a variety of health services available to the population least well covered by health insurance.

As in previous years, state and national nursing organizations had urged passage of the bill, but had pleaded for the inclusion of preventive services and home health care. The bill as passed did not allow for health promotion or preventive care, and reimbursement of home care of the sick was limited to those treatments specifically prescribed by the physician. Organizational consequences of these new programs varied: demands for nursing care spiraled and many small voluntary agencies—unduly stressed by payment restrictions, prolonged delays in reimbursement, and related problems—had to close. The large majority, however, forced to change, ultimately reaped untold benefits such as modernized fiscal management procedures; revised and standardized care procedures; more efficient utilization of personnel, supplemented where possible by practical nurses, homemakers and home health aides; and expanded nursing programs to include physical therapy, occupational therapy, specialized nutrition, social services, and more. Many local and some state health departments rapidly changed their policies to include reimbursable home care of the sick—with considerable concern expressed over the neglect of preventive care. In 1960, only 250 official health agencies offered nursing care of the sick on a continuing basis.[26] By 1968, this number had increased to 1328 showing that over 50 per cent of all official agencies providing public health nursing services were including sick care in their program.[27] Undoubtedly the most alarming effect of Medicare legislation was the proliferation of proprietary home health agencies and nursing homes throughout the United States. Entrepreneurial groups with no previous interest or experience in health care saw profit-making opportunities and quickly moved into this facet of the health industry.

Early on, APHA and NLN developed a joint accreditation program for community agencies providing home care. Later, in 1970, the National Association of Home Health Agencies was organized to develop standards for personnel and services and, still later, health planning agencies began monitoring community needs for home health care.

Other legislation further compounded the health organization puzzle. While regional medical programs melded service, teaching, and research for cancer, heart disease, and stroke, they splintered state health department programs; model cities and anti-poverty programs supported community health centers, made health care accessible to underserved populations and brought these groups into the planning. New autonomous health planning agencies attempted to take over functions long the provinces of state and local health departments. The 1960s brought a new world of health care delivery, operationalized concepts of health care as a right, but focused that care on diagnostic and therapeutic services. In fact, in 1967, when state nursing directors voiced their concern over preventive care, they were advised to "stop worrying about the health of the community and aim efforts at the target areas of disease and disability."[28]

Combined health and social welfare programming, robust categorical grants, and reorganizations at the federal level prompted parallel changes in the states. Super agencies began to emerge, with the state health department one arm among myriad others. Functions were changing as well; direct state involvement in local public health practice eroded as federal controls increased and multiple support mechanisms became more available to local health departments and independent community projects for the disadvantaged flourished. The authority of state directors for nursing services also underwent change, as nurses in categorical programs became increasingly autonomous and as the director's position broadened to include responsibilities for nursing in hospitals, Office of Economic Opportunity programs, and recruitment and training projects. By 1970, several nursing directors headed divisions of local health services or other multidisciplinary programs. Some of the concerns during this period, as reflected in ASTDN resolutions, included

- The need for greater representation of nurses on planning councils, policy making, and program development boards

- Proposals to strengthen existing agencies instead of creating new ones
- A call for studies of various staffing patterns to improve coverage and cost-effectiveness
- The need for outreach services for better utilization of health centers
- Development of measures to evaluate the quality of health services
- Revamping of the merit system classifications
- Making full use of federal traineeships for all disciplines providing health care[28]

At the local level, assessment of community needs, planning comprehensive health care, coordination of services, and patient–family advocacy were activities within the purview of public health nursing. But community assessment skills were limited and, for the most part, neither the hospitals nor the young, consumer-administered services welcomed outside assistance. Even more important, extensions of hospital services, Medicare programs, and the new community health agencies—all directed primarily toward identifying and treating illness—brought many clinical nurses into the field of public health. Consequently, the 1968 census showed 42,541 nurses employed in community services, a 49 per cent increase over the 1957 total of 28,599; however, the percentage with public health preparation remained at 38 per cent,[25] despite traineeship funds, which became available through the Nurse Training Act of 1964 for specialty preparation including public health. Nurses with baccalaureate preparation had increased by 12 per cent, up from 28.8 per cent in 1957 to 40.7 per cent in 1968 (Table 11-2).

Two additional factors added to the changes of the 1960s.

- One was the nurse practitioner movement, which began in 1965 at the University of Colorado and was to open a new era for nursing in primary health care. The term "nurse practitioner" (NP) refers to a registered nurse who is prepared at the certificate or master's degree level in the diagnosis and treatment of common illnesses, including such skills as history taking, physical examination, ordering laboratory tests, and having responsibility for medical management and supervision of patients with specified conditions. Although conceived as a public health nurse with extended clinical skills, the nurse practitioner soon became the clinical nurse ready to function in any care setting. Many public health nurses obtained practitioner training and, on returning to their communities, focused on increasing sparse clinical services, *i.e.,* establishing clinics, screening and follow-up programs with physician backup and referral. This was particularly true for rural areas,

TABLE 11-2.   PER CENT OF FULL-TIME REGISTERED
NURSES IN PUBLIC HEALTH WITH
BACCALAUREATE OR HIGHER DEGREE
AND PER CENT PREPARED IN PUBLIC
HEALTH NURSING, 1948, 1957, 1968,
1979

Year	Number Reporting	% Baccalaureate or Higher Degree	% Completed Public Health Nursing Preparation
1948	22,075	16.0	31.1
1957	28,599	28.8	38.4
1968	42,541	40.7	38.5
1979	49,362	46.9	42.3

(Source: Refs. 14 and 25)

inner-cities, and populations with a concentration of health-related needs
and little medical care.

Initially, there was strong resistance to nurse practitioner programs,
from both nursing and medical professions alike, with nurses fearing a dimi-
nution of their caring, instructive, and supportive functions and with physicians feeling threatened by the invasion into their traditional functions of
history taking, physical examination, and treatment of patients.[29,30] Nor did
approval come easily; medical and nurse practice acts were examined, jobs
restricted, and competing programs such as those for physician assistants
(PA) confused the picture further. But there were sustaining influences for
the NP concepts among nurses, doctors, legislators, policy makers, service
administrators, and consumers, and acceptance grew as graduates demonstrated that their new skills substantially strengthened and logically extended conventional nursing practice.

- Evaluation of the effectiveness of public health programs was the other
commanding feature of the decade. Historically, public health nursing had
relied on case studies and quantitative reports of services provided for evaluation purposes. By 1965, federal regulations required states to submit plans
for reducing major health problems following a prescribed format, the
POME (statement of problems, objectives, methods and evaluation), to give
reasonable assurance that funds would be used appropriately. Like others,

nursing directors now faced questions of service never before asked, requiring support data which had never been systematically collected.

As early as 1938, Margaret Arnstein had urged the use of selected health states to determine service effects. By 1963, although methods had been developed to document patient benefits related to nursing care, they were time consuming, costly, and their inferences open to question.[31-33] Still more tribulation was in the offing; as small studies were undertaken to examine patient progress, many notions of service effectiveness remained unconfirmed.[31]

The paralyzing effect of these combined forces was partially offset by regional and state work conferences on evaluation processes, and by a few innovative demonstrations of community nursing.[34-37] More research and experimentation were critically needed. Although more funds for nursing research and research training had become available through the Nurse Training Act of 1964, the findings were not yet available.

RESEARCH, REDIRECTION, REAFFIRMATION IN THE 1970s

The issues of the 1960s continued into the next decade, but signs of changing perspectives were already evident. Scientific breakthroughs had made contraception safe, economical, and widely acceptable, giving countries a means of addressing problems of population explosion and giving women needed family planning prerogatives. Genetic influences were now better understood, enlarging the etiology of disease production and enabling more precise genetic counseling. Human behavior was being recognized as a causative factor in many diseases and life experiences a determinant in the development of disease and disability as well as in recovery.[38] "Humanism" was in the ascendancy and "the caring process" considered therapy in its own right. A fresh look at categorical programs identified undue competition and duplication of services; block grants and planning across categories were to be emphasized. Prevention of disease regained prominence, eventually becoming one of five major themes of the federal program.[39]

Because the focus of care in the 1960s had been on the individual and family, the old question of "what is public health nursing?" was asked more frequently and more stridently than ever before. In response, a multidisciplinary committee of APHA's Council on Health Manpower revised the recommended qualifications for nurses in public health and, attempting to differentiate functions of clinical nursing and public health nursing, introduced the public health nurse specialist, prepared at the master's degree level, to function as an expert in public health.[40]

These tenets and strategies reinforced public health nursing; attitudes of nursing administrators and service plans soon began to reflect new directions. At their September 1969 annual meeting, the ASTDN had given high priority to the need for "studies and demonstrations in new and improved models of community nursing practice based on scientific analyses of health problems." Two years later, at their 1971 meeting, there was a refreshing note of confidence as project directors described service evaluation and research projects being carried out in the states. These included: comparison studies of pediatric nurse practitioner care, demonstrations of primary health care in isolated rural areas, and systematic evaluations of new staffing patterns, of school nursing services, and of prenatal patient care. Program evaluation no longer aroused apprehensions; peer review, record audits, outcome measures, accountability, and quality assurance had become familiar processes.[28]

During the next few years, alternative service patterns became common and a plethora of studies, related primarily to expanded nursing roles, appeared in the public press as well as in medical, public health, and nursing journals. Not all study results were favorable, but many exceeded expectations. The scope of nursing practice, published in 1971 by the US Department of Health, Education, and Welfare,[41] and the 1972 report of the Canadian experience with NPs[42] gave credence to the overall movement and made nursing's role in primary health care explicit. The enlarged concept was spreading to all areas of nursing—maternal and child health, family and adult care, geriatric and care of the chronically ill—and in all care settings. The number of programs preparing nurses for these new functions increased nearly six-fold, from 36 in 1970 to 198 in 1977.[43] Although these programs had graduated over 10,000 NPs, even this number was inadequate to meet all the employer requests.

These developments were seen as a means to extend medical and nursing care and to utilize the competencies of both professions more completely and economically. They also legitimized functions that public health nurses had been doing for years, and added new skills as well.

The WHO Expert Committee on Community Health Nursing, in 1974, envisioned health care for all populations as a realistic goal.[1] The World Health Assembly responded to the Expert Committee's proposals the following year in a resolution which cited "nursing and midwifery as primary providers and teachers of basic health care" and encouraged all member countries to involve nurses and midwives in developing programs. Then, in 1978, the International Conference on Primary Health Care developed a clear definition of the term with guidelines to accelerate progress, and "Health for All by the year 2000" became the motto.[44] In spite of the Conference's comprehensive, community-based definition, most health professionals, including those in the US, interpreted primary health care to mean first contact preventive and curative care of the individual.

The patient–community concept is elusive, complex, and difficult to operationalize, particularly by health practitioners grounded almost exclusively in individual care. In 1979, almost half (49.6 per cent) of nurses employed by state and local health departments had no public health preparation. The 1979 Census showed a total of 56,993 registered nurses employed full- or part-time by 5802 state and local health agencies; 25.6 per cent functioned primarily in clinical areas. In addition, 21,636 nurses were employed by 7656 boards of education.[14] A reorientation would be needed if primary health care were to impact on high-risk populations and affect health status at the community level. The 1971 statement of qualifications of nurses for public health[40] depended on schools to encompass community concepts in their curricula and agencies to demonstrate those concepts in practice. Role extensions in diagnostic and therapeutic techniques, however, had tended to reinforce patient–family concepts at the expense of the community in both educational and practice settings. The first attempt to correct misconceptions and put the two main avenues to public health into juxtaposition within a conceptual frame was a national conference on "Redesigning Nursing Education for Public Health" in 1973.[45] The organization of the Association of Graduate Faculty of Community Health/Public Health Nursing followed in 1978; in 1979, a position paper by ASTDN described relevant competencies for public health. A statement defining the role of public health nursing[46] and another describing a conceptual model of community practice[47] were developed in 1980 by the Public Health Nursing Section of APHA and by ANA's Division on Community Nursing Practice, respectively; "Guidelines for Community-based Nursing Services"[48] have been developed by a joint committee of ANA and APHA, appointed in 1983. Numerous papers were presented and articles published during the 1970s and early 1980s elucidating the problem and suggesting solutions aimed at enlarging the principles and practices of community health in the basic curriculum, as well as strengthening the epidemiologic-sociologic focus in graduate study, service environments, and research.[49-52] Controversy reigned over whether or not to approve only graduate programs in schools of nursing, thus underestimating benefits of diverse multidiscipline experiences offered by schools of public health.

International concerns and activities paralleled those in the US. Programs and task forces were sponsored by both WHO and the International Council of Nursing (ICN) to stimulate primary health care in a community context in regions and countries around the globe.[53,54] And guidelines were developed and tested to assist faculty to intensify their teaching content in community health.[55]

Public health nursing and nursing generally were on the move, contributing significantly to the hospice movement, birthing centers, drug abuse programs, day care centers for the elderly, and rehabilitation nursing in long-term care. (In 1975, 10 states took part in a federally funded statewide educational project directed by ASTDN on rehabilitation nursing in long-term care.) In some instances, they developed home health agencies to provide 24-hour support services for families caring for chronically ill and disabled members. Both longitudinal and cross-sectional research was in progress to find ways for improving the distribution of health care as well as advancing the quality of care.[43,56,57] As the 1970s ended, concern over escalating health care costs mounted.

PATTERNS OF CHANGE

As controls were applied to health expenditures, implementation of the aggressive prevention strategies intended in the late 1970s suffered in competition with surging costs of hospitalization, new intensive care therapies, and complicated medical procedures. In addition, goals for improving the quality of care changed to the provision of minimal, safe practice. Slow economic growth and persistent inflation brought curtailment of Medicare/Medicaid coverage, nutrition supplements for school children, food stamps for the marginally poor, and other support programs which had benefited the health and welfare of many. At the same time, the use of outpatient services, health maintenance organizations (HMOs), and private medical care was encouraged. Home health services and nurse practitioner care, having been found cost-effective, were also given priority.[39] Self-help, self-support, and self-improvement were pushed while increased governmental assistance was an outmoded concept.

One of the movements that seemed to catch on in the early 1980s was health education of the public designed to achieve more healthful behavior and life-styles. Advances in health knowledge—instantly reported by television, radio and the press—caught the attention of the public at large and of the business world which saw unlimited mutually beneficial opportunities in the thriving health industry; commercial centers sprang up to: promote exercise and weight control; reduce smoking, alcohol and drug use; increase family-focused activities; and improve social supports and relationships. Consumer groups pressed for laws to confine cigarette smoking to designated areas and to enforce tougher laws against driving under the influence of alcohol. The extent to which public health nurses stimulated or took part in such activities is unknown and, for this reason, a task force was appointed in 1984 by the PHN Section of APHA to "explore the issue and delineate specific health promotion activities of public health nurses in the community."[58] The Section was also concerned with a variety of other issues, such as: the management and productivity of community services, populations at risk for prevalent social and health problems, legislation for community nursing centers, violence in families, theory development in public health nursing, and research.

Early in 1985, two events took place which could direct public health nursing practice through this century and into the next. On January 14, the Secretary of Health and Human Services announced the establishment of a new Center for Nursing Research "to enlarge the body of scientific knowledge that underlies nursing practice, nursing service administration and nursing education."[59] In making this announcement, HHS Secretary Margaret Heckler added that this action was taken to implement the 1983 recommendations of the Institute of Medicine, National Academy of Sciences, for nursing and nursing education for the future and for meeting the needs for nursing research.[59]

The second event also occurred in January during the meeting of WHO's Executive Board, following a discussion of the report of the Expert Committee on the Education and Training of Nurse Teachers and Managers.[60] Summarizing the event, Dr. Halfdan Mahler, Director-General of WHO, stated that it is now evident that nurses are ready to become agents of change in primary health care throughout the world, taking an important role in the Health for All movement.[61] Changes will need to be made, he said, in reorienting nursing curricula to the main social and health needs of society, developing crash training programs for teachers and directors of schools of nursing in primary health and Health for All goals, strengthening bonds between schools of nursing and community health services and preparing administrators and managers to direct those services. Real change, Dr. Mahler indicated, requires reappraisal of health manpower policies for the inclusion of nurses as leaders and managers of primary health care teams and their participation at all levels of planning for national and community health. WHO is actively supporting these directional changes.

Public health nursing in the United States has gone through periods of expansion, recession, and consolidation.

- It has advanced numerically and professionally.
- It has attained recognition as a vital part of the total health care system.
- Its prominence is bound to increase with the continuing shift of health care from hospitals to homes and community settings.
- It is equipped to meet the multi-faceted, diverse needs of US populations with a mix of clinical and public health specialists.
- It has the ability to strengthen concepts of prevention and methods of practice through research.

The public is more health conscious than ever before and ready to support innovative approaches to health care. Health professionals are being challenged to find ways of providing quality, effective, preventive health care for all. The test of public health nursing is to marshal community resources to achieve this goal.

REFERENCES

1. World Health Organization: Community Health Nursing. Report of a WHO Expert Committee. Technical Report Series 558. Geneva: WHO, 1974
2. Buhler-Wilkerson K: Public health nursing: in sickness or in health. Am J Public Health 1985; 75:000–000
3. Dreher M: District nursing: the cost benefits of a population-based practice. Am J Public Health 1984; 74:1107–1111
4. Buhler-Wilkerson K, Reverby S: Can a time-honored model survive the dilemma of public health nursing? (editorial) Am J Public Health 1984; 74:1081–1083
5. Kernodle PB: The Red Cross Nurse in Action, 1882-1948. New York: Harper & Brothers, 1948; 300–305, 362–364, 408–418, 467–473
6. Woodward ES: Federal aspects of unemployment among professional women. Public Health Nurs 1934; 26:300–303
7. Furman B: A Profile of the US Public Health Service 1798–1948. US Dept of Health, Education, and Welfare, National Institutes of Health, DHEW Pub. No. (NIH) 73-369. Washington, DC: Govt Printing Office, 1973; 394–396, 405–409, 423–424, 452
8. Fitzpatrick ML: The National Organization for Public Health Nursing 1912-1952: Development of a Practice Field. New York: National League for Nursing, 1975; 110–115, 129, 138–140, 166–201
9. McIver P: Development of Public Health Nursing in the US Public Health Service. Prepared for the Bureau of State Services, PHS, January 1953; 1–3, 6, 8–10. (unpublished)
10. McNeil EE: A History of the Public Health Nursing Section, 1922–1972. Washington, DC: American Public Health Association, 1972; 7, 8, 11

11. Gardner MS: Public Health Nursing. New York: MacMillan Company, 1936; 191–205, 111–113
12. Reid M: 1938 Census of Public Health Nurses. Mimeographed report B-2561. Washington, DC: US Public Health Service, 1939
13. US Public Health Service, Division of Public Health Nursing: Total Number of Public Health Nurses Employed in the US on January 1 of the Year 1938 to 1942. Mimeographed report, Washington, DC, PHS, 1943
14. US Public Health Service, Division of Nursing: Survey of Community Health Nursing. DHEW Pub. No. (HRA) 82. Washington, DC: Govt Printing Office, 1979
15. American Public Health Association/National Organization for Public Health Nursing: Minimum Qualifications for those Appointed to Positions in Public Health Nursing. Am J Public Health 1931; 21:526–528
16. US Public Health Service, Division of Public Health Nursing: Total Number of Nurses Employed in Public Health Work in the United States, in the Territories of Alaska and Hawaii, and in Puerto Rico and the Virgin Islands, on January 1, 1937 to 1952. Mimeographed report, August 1952. Washington, DC: Public Health Service, August 1952
17. Emerson H: Local Health Units for the Nation. New York: Commonwealth Fund, 1945; 12–15
18. Lesser AJ: The origin and development of maternal and child health programs in the United States. Am J Public Health 1985; 75:590–598
19. US Public Health Service, Bureau of State Services: Directory of Full-time Local Health Units. Washington, DC: USPHS, 1950
20. US Public Health Service, Bureau of State Services: Directory of Full-time Local Health Units. Washington, DC: USPHS, 1955
21. US Public Health Service: Nurses in Public Health. PHS Pub. No. 785. Washington, DC: Govt Printing Office, 1960
22. Ennes H (ed): A Critique of Community Public Health Services: Discussions of the birth, care, growth of community official health services. Am J Public Health 1957; 47 (suppl), 1–48. (Abridged report of the National Advisory Committee on Local Health Departments, Working Conference, held in Cincinnati, Ohio, March 19, 1957 in conjunction with the National Health Forum of the National Health Council.)
23. Kerr LE: Birth: problems associated with the creation of effective community official health services. *In:* A Critique of Community Public Health Services. Am J Public Health 1957; 47 (suppl):9
24. Brown EL: Nursing for the Future. New York: Russell Sage Foundation, 1948
25. US Public Health Service, Division of Nursing: Nurses in Public Health. Bethesda, MD: DHEW, 1969; 14, 57, 41
26. Bryant Z: The public health nurses' expanding responsibilities. Public Health Rep 1961; 76:857–860
27. US Dept of Health, Education, and Welfare, Division of Nursing: Surveys of Public Health Nursing 1968–1972. DHEW Pub. No. (HRA) 76-8. Bethesda, MD: USPHS, Nov 1975

28. Garrett M *et al:* The Forty-Year History of the Association of State and Territorial Directors of Nursing 1935–1975. Indianapolis: Indiana State Board of Health, 1976; 38, 49–61, 36–48

29. Bates B: Nurse-Physician Dyad: Collegial or Competitive? Three Challenges to the Nursing Profession. Selected papers from the 1972 ANA Convention. Kansas City: American Nurses' Association, 1972

30. Yankauer A, Sullivan J: The new health professionals: three examples. Ann Rev Public Health 1982; 3:249–276

31. Roberts DE: How effective is public health nursing: Am J Public Health 1962; 52:1077–1083

32. Freeman RB: Measuring the effectiveness of public health nursing service. Nurs Outlook 1961; 9:605–607

33. Donabedian A: Quality of care: problems of measurement: II. Some issues in evaluating the quality of nursing care. Am J Public Health 1969; 59:1833–1836

34. Milio N: 9226 Kercheval. Ann Arbor: University of Michigan Press, 1970.

35. Lewis CE, Schmidt G, Waxman D: Activities, events, and outcomes in ambulatory care. N Engl J Med 1969; 280:645–649

36. Silver HK, Ford LC, Stearly SC: Program to increase health care for children: Pediatric Nurse Practitioner Program. Pediatrics 1967; 39:756–760

37. Kauffman MC, Cunningham A: Epidemiologic analysis of outcomes in maternal and infant health in evaluating effectiveness of three patient care teams. Am J Public Health 1970; 60:1712–1725

38. Cassel J: The case for prevention. In Redesigning Nursing Education for Public Health. DHEW Pub. No. (HRA) 75-75. Bethesda, MD: Bureau of Health Manpower, USPHS, 1974

39. US Dept of Health, Education, and Welfare, Public Health Service, Office of the Secretary, Forward Plan for Health FY 1978–82. DHEW Pub. No. (OS) 76-50046. Washington, DC: Govt Printing Office, 1976

40. American Public Health Association, Council on Health Manpower: Educational Qualifications of Public Health Nurses. Am J Public Health 1971; 61:2505–2509

41. US Dept of Health, Education, and Welfare, Public Health Service: Extending the Scope of Nursing Practice: A Report of the Secretary's Committee to Study Extended Roles for Nurses. Washington, DC: Govt Printing Office, 1971

42. Health and Welfare Canada: Report of the Committee on Nurse Practitioners (presented by Thomas J. Bondreau, chairman). Toronto: Health and Welfare Canada, 1972

43. US Dept of Health, Education, and Welfare, Public Health Service, Division of Nursing: Longitudinal Study of Nurse Practitioners, Phase III. DHEW Pub. No. (HRA) 80-2. Washington, DC: Govt Printing Office, 1980; 5–36

44. World Health Organization: Primary Health Care, Alma Ata, 1978. Health for All Series, No. 1. Geneva: WHO, 1978

45. US Dept of Health, Education, and Welfare, Public Health Service, Division of Nursing: Redesigning Nursing Education for Public Health. DHEW Pub. No. (HRA) 75-75. Washington, DC: Govt Printing Office, 1973

46. American Public Health Association: Position Paper No. 8132(PP): The Definition and Role of Public Health Nursing in the Delivery of Health Care. *In:* APHA Public Policy Statements, 1948–present, cumulative. Washington, DC: APHA, current volume

47. American Nurses' Association, Division of Community Health Nursing Practice: A Conceptual Model of Community Health Nursing. Kansas City: ANA, 1980

48. American Nurses' Association, Division of Community Health Nursing Practice: Guidelines for Community-based Nursing Services. Kansas City: ANA, in press

49. Williams CA: Community health nursing—what is it? Nurs Outlook 1977; 25:250–254

50. Wood J, Ohlson V: Graduate preparation for community health nursing practice. *In:* Miller N, Flynn B (eds): Current Perspectives in Nursing, Social Issues and Trends. St. Louis: C. V. Mosby, 1977

51. Anderson ET, *et al:* The Development and Implementation of a Curriculum Model for Community Nurse Practitioners. DHEW Pub. No. (HRA) 77-24. Bethesda, MD: USPHS, Division of Nursing, 1977

52. Goeppinger J: Primary health care; an answer to the dilemmas of community nursing. Public Health Nurs 1984; 1(3):129–140

53. International Council of Nurses: Report of the Workshop on the Role of Nursing in Primary Health Care, held in Nairobi, Sept 30–Oct 1, 1979. Geneva: ICN, 1979

54. World Health Organization, Division of Health Manpower Development: Nursing in Support of the Goal "Health for All by the Year 2000." Report of a meeting, Nov 16–20, 1981. Geneva: WHO, 1982

55. World Health Organization: A Guide to Curriculum Review for Basic Nursing Education, Orientation to Primary Health Care and Community Health. Geneva: WHO, 1985

56. Eyers SJ, Barnard KE, Gray C: Child Health Assessment Part III, 2–4 Years. Seattle: University of Washington, School of Nursing, 1979

57. Highriter ME: Public health nursing evaluation, education and professional issues, 1977–1981. *In:* Ann Rev Nurs Res 1984

58. American Public Health Association: Special Task Force on PHN's Visibility in Health Promotion. Public Health Nursing Section Newsletter 1985; p 6

59. US Dept of Health and Human Services, Public Health Services: Nursing Research. HHS News Release, Jan 14, 1985

60. World Health Organization: Education and Training of Nurse Teachers and Managers with Special Regard to Primary Health Care. Report of a WHO Expert Committee, Technical Report Series 708. Geneva: WHO, 1984

61. World Health Organization, WHO Features, No. 97: Nurses Lead the Way. Geneva: World Health Organization (Media Service), June 1985

EDITOR'S NOTE

Recall from Unit I that education was described as a "keynote" of modern public health and that caring for the sick at home was a *means of gaining access to families in greatest need of health education.* Compared with making a home visit strictly to perform a task (*e.g.,* to change a dressing) can you see how different your approach would be in order to identify *family* needs?

Can you see also how by knowing several families the public health nurse can begin to identify clues as to the *community's* health? How can a community assessment be begun to set in motion the mobilization of community resources to meet these needs?

In Unit II, the American Red Cross' early model and the World Health Organization's (WHO) support for primary health care provide us with on-going challenges of how public health nursing can truly focus on the community, the "contextual fiber" of public health nursing. Chapters 12 through 15 will illustrate the community approach through descriptions of the major roles of practice, teaching, managing and conducting research.

12

The Role of the Community Health Nurse

OBJECTIVES

Community health nursing is a synthesis of nursing practice and public health sciences that is applied to maintain, restore, and promote the health of populations. Indeed, the skill of considering the community as a client is the uniqueness of community health nursing and the focus of this chapter. After studying this chapter you will be able to

- Implement the role of community health nurse by using the skills of primary care, community advocacy, consultation, and research.

INTRODUCTION

The community health nurse integrates the skills and knowledge of nursing and the public health sciences to promote and preserve the health of populations. The community is the *primary* client. Even though care is frequently given to individuals, families, and groups, the community health nurse always considers the impact and consequences of these cases upon the health of the community.

When a child with diarrhea is brought to a pediatric clinic, the immediate concern is for treatment and relief of the child's symptoms, coupled with education of caregivers about homecare comfort measures, symptoms indicating complications, and the creation of a follow-up appointment schedule. The community health nurse delivers direct patient care to the child and family, but then stops to consider the community.

> CONSIDER: Have other children with diarrhea appeared in clinic this week? If the answer is yes, did the children share some characteristics such as being of a similar age? Did they attend the same school or daycare center? Did the youngsters live within close proximity of each other? How does the number of children with diarrhea seen in clinic today or this week compare to last week or last month? What could be the likely pathogen that is causing the diarrhea and how is that pathogen transmitted?

Depending on the answers to community-focused questions, the child with diarrhea may be found to be an isolated case, or may represent a pattern of youngsters with diarrhea caused by a shared etiology. This may include inadequate sanitary conditions or practices, crowding, or inadequate nutrition. To treat the community cause(s) of the diarrhea, the community nurse considers the community assessment data, community organization structure, and likely avenues for intervention. Frequently, to eliminate the cause of the diarrhea will require political and legal activity to change existing policies and procedures that affect health. As you learned in Chapter 3, political activism to initiate change is an important role in community health nursing.

The community health nurse assesses *patterns.* The patterns may be individuals or families with shared health concerns, as in the example of the child with diarrhea, or the patterns may be demonstrated in a lack of agreement between community assessment data and use of health care services. For example, during the process of a community assessment a large population of young Indochinese families was documented as living in the community served by the multiservice health center. However, though the pediatric clinic was heavily used by the Indochinese, there were no Indochinese women attending the prenatal clinics.

To determine why the discrepancy existed between community demographics and health service use, the following community-focused questions were asked:

- What is the birth rate among the Indochinese? (This information can be obtained from vital statistics.)

- Are the pregnant Indochinese women receiving prenatal care? If yes, where, when, and from whom is the care received?
- What are the cultural beliefs and health care practices during pregnancy?
- What type of care provider and setting is preferred during pregnancy and birth?

By asking these questions of the Indochinese mothers who brought their children to pediatric clinic, the community health nurse learned that cultural beliefs and practices forbid the examination of a woman by a man during pregnancy. The only prenatal care providers at the multiservice health center were male obstetricians. The Indochinese women with financial resources and transportation obtained prenatal care in an adjacent community from a female nurse midwife or obstetrician; the women with inadequate resources received no prenatal care and were delivered at home with family assistance.

The community health nurse extends her care of individuals and families to include the impact on the health of the total community. Table 12-1 compares the focus and functions of the community health nurse and the family nurse clinician. As noted, the primary focus of the community health nurse is the community, with the individual and family being secondary. The expansion of nursing skills and processes to the community as client can be practiced from any work setting, including acute care and emergency departments, although most often the community health nurse is based in an ambulatory setting.

Knowledge from the public health sciences of epidemiology, demography, and biometry are used in the application of the nursing process to the maintainance and improvement the health of the total population. Several skills are crucial to the role of community health nurse, including *primary care, community advocacy, research,* and *consultation.*

PRIMARY HEALTH CARE

Primary health care is one method of delivering care. Primary health care begins when the individual or family makes contact with the health care system and a decision is made on what actions are necessary to resolve the health problem. Primary health care is much more than first contact; it includes all the services necessary to prevent disease, maintain, and promote health, including rehabilitation. Primary health care is continuous and comprehensive and includes identification, management, and referral. Primary

**TABLE 12-1.   COMPARISON OF THE COMMUNITY
NURSE PRACTITIONER AND FAMILY
NURSE CLINICAL ROLES WITHIN THE
NURSING PROCESS FRAMEWORK**

	Community Nurse Practitioner	Family Nurse Clinician
Primary focus	Community	Individual/family
Secondary focus	Individual/family	Community
Inferences	Assessment of community-oriented health record	Assessment of problem-oriented patient record
Intervention (planning and implementing)	Identify community priorities and objectives	Identify patient priorities and objectives
	Mobilize resources, individuals, groups in self-help endeavors	Manage diet, drugs, exercise and overall therapeutic program
	Organize groups to effect increase in knowledge of health-affecting practices	Teach patient and family
Evaluation	Identify appropriate and effective measures to meet community objectives	Identify appropriate and effective measures to meet patient objectives
	Identify indicators of improved health status	Identify indicators of improved health status

(Anderson ET, Gottschalk J, Grimes D, Ives J, Skrovan C: The development and implementation of a curriculum model for community nurse practitioners. Publication No. HRA-77-24. Hyattsville, Maryland, U.S. Department of Health and Human Services, 1977)

health care for the community is consistent with the World Health Organization (WHO) (1978) definition of

Essential health care made universally accessible to individuals and families in the community by means acceptable to them, through their full participation and at a cost that community and country can afford. (World Health Organization)

STOP . . . Consider the words you just read: What is meant by *essential?* Are contact lenses and cosmetic surgery essential? . . . That is an easy answer. Far more difficult—are organ transplants and in utero surgery essential?

What determines *accessibility?* The clinic location? Hours of operation? Services provided?

What denotes *acceptability?* The sex, race, and ethnicity of the care provider? The method of service delivery? Finally, *who* determines *what* is *essential, accessible,* and *acceptable* for *whom?*

The WHO definition offers guidance to our field for dealing with these difficult questions in their phrase—*through their full participation.* It is the community-as-client focus and the emphasis on involvement of the community as a whole that guides the delivery of primary health care in community health nursing. In all her duties, whether administering an immunization to a child, offering nutrition information to pregnant women, or facilitating the establishment of a self-help group for bereaved parents, the community health nurse involves her community in each step of the nursing process, and documents the effects of nursing practice on its health.

COMMUNITY ADVOCACY

Advocacy is accountability. An advocate presents the case of another. Community advocacy requires knowledge, awareness, and sensitivity to the unique needs of the community—needs that may not be health services.

Example of Advocacy

A nurse was offering primary health care to youngsters as part of a contractual agreement with the county health department. Immunizations, developmental screening, physical assessment, and ill-child diagnosis and treatment constituted the major nursing care. Over time, the nurse noticed that many children were brought to clinic because of burns, especially on their arms and legs. Although parents were taught how to change the needed dressings and to observe for signs of infection, the children frequently returned to clinic with infected lesions. Deciding that information was needed on the living conditions of the children, the nurse arranged to make a home visit.

The trip to the home was an arduous two-mile drive on partially paved streets that were too narrow to permit the passage of cars traveling in opposite directions. The home that she was to visit resembled all the houses in the area; it was a small, one-story wooden-frame building set only a few yards from the narrow street. The nurse noticed that two houses in the neighborhood had recently been gutted by fire and that a third home, apparently destroyed several years ago by fire, had become a dumpsite for abandoned appliances and automobiles. When asked about the destroyed homes, the family stated that in the area numerous houses had burnt as firetrucks tried in vain to enter the narrow streets. However, widening of the streets would require destruction of all the homes. This family, like most in the neighborhood, had been on a waiting list for public housing for four years.

The burns on the legs of the family's toddler showed signs of infection; the dressing that had been applied three days ago at the clinic offered little protection to the charred skin. The mother explained that the only store that was within walking distance did not stock gauze or dressing materials. There were no chain supermarkets or drugstores in the neighborhood. One full-service grocery store had opened two years ago but was forced to close after six months because of vandalism. The sole source of heat for the small four-room house was an oil-burning heater; it was this that the toddler had accidentally fallen against. Each of the four children had suffered similar burns; one child's injuries had required skin grafting. When asked about concerns, the mother shared her fears of allowing the children outside to play. Not only was the street dangerous, but recently several children in the area had been molested.

To initiate change, the nurse discussed her concerns with other health providers in the neighborhood, local religious leaders, school principals, and concerned citizens. A group of professionals and citizens met and formed a coalition. A community assessment was completed, followed by a plan of action that focused on political activism that involved city housing, recreation, law enforcement, and transportation departments, as well as agreements with merchants and the business community.

To be a community advocate, the nurse stepped into the community and increased her knowledge, awareness, and sensitivity to community-as-client needs. Then she acted as a change agent by sharing information about the community in order to increase the awareness and sensitivity of others. Finally, the nurse used the political process to effect change.

RESEARCHER

Research is *investigation.* The investigation may concern any of a range of subjects in the nursing-care health-delivery systems such as an immunization or family-planning program, or the cost-effectiveness of home visits to deliver primary care to children and pregnant women. The community health nurse is always looking for patterns and all patterns require further assessment (as in the example of the children with diarrhea). However, hunches and feelings must be validated with data. Assessment data (as in the example of the family without adequate and safe housing) can be used as the justification for intervention programs and policy changes.

Research data should be collected during each community–nurse encounter. During each step of the nursing process, data are collected; data that can be used to study health, answer questions, and improve health care delivery. The research process is described in Chapter 2 and is demonstrated with an example of how the process was used to study the community health problem of infant mortality. The research process can also be used in designing community-based programs. The community-focused program presented below was designed to improve the health of a community by preventing a major health problem.

Example of Investigative Research

Interpersonal violence is epidemic and a major public health problem in America. Battering of women is one form of interpersonal violence. Estimates are that from 20% to 50% of all American women will be battered by their male partner. The literature further documents that battering often begins or intensifies during pregnancy. Indeed, when an interview–questionnaire was completed on 290 healthy pregnant women in public and private prenatal clinics, it was documented that 23% of the women had been battered during or previous to their present pregnancy; and an additional 9% of the women may have been battered (as was suggested by their behavior during the interview); and 4% reported being threatened with battering. Thus, a total of 36% of the women had been battered or were at-risk for battering. The problem of battering during pregnancy had been documented (Helton et al, 1987).

The next question was: How can battering be prevented? Because it is only during pregnancy that most healthy women have frequent, routinely scheduled contacts with nurses, pregnancy seemed to be a logical access point for the health care provider to assess for the potential of or existence of battering and to offer primary care. However, first the knowledge and skills of the health care provider must be increased, if necessary, to include assessment and primary care interventions for the woman at risk of, or experiencing battering. To prepare the health care providers, a slide–tape program was developed that included information on the cyclic nature of violence; conflict versus battering; the effects of battering on women, men, children, and society; how to assess, counsel, and intervene for battering; and the legal, social, and health care services that are available to the woman at risk of, or experiencing battering. Health care providers were offered seminar sessions and a protocol of care to increase their skills. Both pre- and post-knowledge and attitudes tests were administered to evaluate the educational program. In addition, health providers received follow-up instruction and assistance in the implementation of an abuse-assessment program.

After presenting the educational program to health care providers, the general public received public-service announcements, brochures, and media presentations about battering. The public was taught how to self-assess for the risk of intrapersonal violence and to initiate self-referral to community agencies. To evaluate the public's knowledge and ability to self-assess and refer, use of community resources designed to prevent or stop battering (*i.e.,* domestic violence legal services, shelters for battered women, and family counseling and crisis centers) were assessed for use both before and after the community-wide awareness and education program.

Through research a community health nurse, using interview–questionnaire assessment, uncovered a segment of the population within the community that was at risk of or suffering from a threat to well being. The community health nurse, performing in the role of researcher, was then able to formulate, coordinate, and carry out programs to prevent or diminish this threat.

CONSULTANT

Consultation is *problem solving.* The problems may be related to staffing, facilities, equipment, program progression, or finances. The consultant assesses the problem, determines the availability and feasibility of resources, proposes a number of solutions, and often assists in implementation. The primary goal of consultation is to improve the health of the community, although recommendations may be made for initiating research, developing educational programs, or changing policy. Evaluation is an integral part of consultation; without it, there is no measure of success in solving the problem.

As a consultant the community health nurse may function as a liaison with other community agencies or work on planning and implementation boards with regional and state agencies. Frequently, the consultant works within and produces change through the political process. Consultants bring their expertise to a problem, and act to facilitate processes and to mobilize the skills and knowledge of the agency personnel or community. It is important for the citizens who are involved to feel a sense of *ownership* of the proposed solutions. For ownership to occur, group involvement is essential. Each person's comments are important. Both the Delphi and nominal group techniques are excellent strategies to facilitate group problem solving.

Thus, the community health nurse in serving as a consultant is doing work that encompasses the realm of nursing expertise. Demands of this role require not only a solid foundation of knowledge, but also the practical knowledge that is gained through experience in community health nursing. The reality of the role of practitioner in community health nursing can best be described by current practitioners.

Application

To summarize the skills required in the community health nursing, several community health nurses have described their role and practice setting. As you read the following accounts, try to identify how the skills of *primary care, community advocacy, research,* and *consultation* are applied to a community-as-client focus.

A Refugee Camp

Poles of bamboo provided the support for the thatched roofs that covered row after row of low wooden huts, called *cots.* The cots, too, were covered, laden with the red clay dust that is so typical of the dry season. Two, three, or more family members shared a cot while bathing, feeding, and caring for sick family members. One determined if a ward was pediatric or adult by the age of the sick persons. Otherwise, the wards were identical, families sharing a cot and waiting.

Infection, malnutrition, and dehydration racked the people of this refugee camp in Thailand. Fleeing a country that had been ravaged by atrocities, the infirm Cambodians and their families constituted the community-as-client entity. Western health care practices met traditional Eastern methods of healing. Cambodian practices and beliefs seemed strange and peculiar; there was not even a common language with which to discuss the differences. Fluid replacement, antibiotics, and basic sanitation constituted primary health care. The care-giving behaviors of family members were watched carefully to determine acceptable practices. Frequently, culturally preferred practices, as in the practice of cooking, conflicted with total population needs.

The culturally preferred method of cooking was over an open fire. Families gathered together, prepared a fire, then proceeded to cook, socialize, and eat. It was this convening of families that sustained their strength and courage. At first, there were no designated areas for cooking, and there was a lot of dry bamboo that stood cracking in the wind or heaped on the ground. For six months each year there was little or no rain; water was precious. There was no running water, and the drums of water scattered among the camp had to be used first for drinking, followed by use for bathing and clothes washing. Almost always, open fires burned without water nearby for extinguishing them. The threat of a destructive large fire was obvious, and the necessity of setting designated areas aside for open-fire cooking with available water was evident. A change in cooking practices needed to be implemented immediately and enforced. How could the change in behavior be instituted?

The camp was divided into sections of about 100 people, and each section was asked to designate a section leader. These leaders were people who were respected by all families living in the section. The section leaders discussed general grievances with members of the volunteer relief organizations that were running the camp, and policies were adopted to address the situations. When the problem of open-fire cooking was discussed with section leaders, an education-awareness program was begun for camp members. Signs were posted everywhere warning people of the danger of open fires and requesting compliance with careful, safe cooking practices. Section leaders cooperated with the request and explained the situation with all families in the section. Many families complied, many did not. Despite these efforts, a cooking fire did break out of control and destroyed the largest Cambodian refugee camp in Thailand. The campaign of education continued, and change too continued —a change in lifestyle practices that had existed for millennia.

Marianne DeWier, RN, MS
Former Volunteer, International Rescue Committee

A Volunteer Social Service Agency for the Elderly

People in the United States are living longer than ever before. Today, 10% of Americans are over age 65, and by the year 2000, two out of three older Americans will be over age 75. Although 80% of persons over age 65 have one or more chronic health conditions, only 5% of these persons are living in health care facilities at any time. Approximately 8% of the elderly are homebound and being attended by a family member who contributes 80% of the daily care. The remaining 85% of the elderly are living in the community, but frequently experience one or more health conditions and require support and assistance from family and social service agencies. Many social service agencies are voluntary organizations with the purpose of fostering independence, self-care, and active involvement of the elderly with family and community.

In one community, to provide coordinated essential care to the elderly, decrease the complications of chronic disease and thereby enable the elderly to remain at home as active contributing members of society, a community nurse practitioner was recruited and hired by a volunteer social service agency. Essential needs of the elderly included basic needs of adequate housing, healthy food, access to health care, and facilitation of an independent lifestyle. The elderly were referred by health professionals, social service agencies, or through self-referral to the volunteer social service agency. Nursing care began with observation, an interview, and noninvasive physical assessment. Nursing diagnoses were formed jointly with each client and an agreed-upon plan of care was established. Care plans usually included teaching self-care skills; increasing involvement of the family in the elder's care with provisions for associated teaching; emotional support; and if the elder was homebound, respite care. Both the planning and implementation of the care plan required an understanding of community resources and capabilities. The community nurse practitioner functioned as a liaison with other health and social service agencies to coordinate services for individual clients and families, as well as to establish new services or discontinue programs that were no longer needed by the "community of elderly." To communicate the special needs of the elderly, the nurse planned, coordinated, and implemented inservice training sessions for homemakers, social workers, and other health providers on topics that were related to the biologic and psychologic aspects of aging and related health care needs. The nurse established nursing role standards and scope of practice responsibilities.

Janet Harrison, RN, MS
Former Community Nurse Practitioner
Sheltering Arms Agency for the Elderly

A Community in Rural Appalachia

Following a community assessment, several community nursing diagnoses were recorded

- Inadequate prenatal care—most pregnant women received no care or third-trimester-only prenatal care
- Children with developmental delays, and visual and hearing impairments that resulted in difficulties with learning
- Adults with chronic respiratory disease that frequently caused unemployment

The setting was rural Appalachia, and the etiology of most nursing diagnoses was the lack of available and accessible primary health care. A community council was established and a primary care nursing clinic was founded. The clinic was financially supported by both the community and a nearby college of nursing. The clients of this rural Appalachian community had lived in the area for generations and professed strong roots in a heritage that proclaimed the worth of extended family and traditional ways, a reluctance to trust outsiders, and a basic sense of fatalism. Because these people were accustomed to being passive recipients of health care and to only seeking assistance when ill, nursing care was directed to facilitating the development of self-care abilities, including effective problem-solving and decision-making skills. Parents were taught how to assess their children for developmental delays, in addition to the complete visual and hearing screening received in the schools. Adults were taught how to perform early assessment of respiratory distress and exercises to increase pulmonary functioning. Lay midwives were consulted and they supported the clinic activities, encouraging women to initiate early prenatal care.

Nursing care was provided to individuals and families through home visits, clinic appointments, and small-group sessions in the school, town hall, and at the work site. The nurse collaborated with each client to form a partnership relationship that included mutual goal setting and contracted behaviors to increase self-care skills. Crucial to the advisory relationship was a genuine respect for the uniqueness of each client and a willingness by the nurse to begin at the client's perceived level of need.

Frances Snodgrass, RN, MS
Assistant Professor, University of West Virginia
Community Health Nurse, Cabin Creek Nursing Center

Before the School Bell Rang

Two students were describing feelings of nausea and dizziness to the nurse when a graduating senior with mononucleosis phoned to ask when he could return to school. The nurse, having completed an assessment—made a diagnosis of flu—and called for parents to pick up the ill teens, next turns to a 15-year-old who states that she may be pregnant. Privacy is scarce in this office and the small supply closet barely accommodates two chairs for the immediate counseling required for the young girl. However, even the counseling session is interrupted by a boy who presents a possibly sprained ankle. He is given an icepack and asked to remain seated for 10 minutes. The bell rings, and the school day has officially begun.

School nursing seeks to modify or remove health-related barriers to learning and to promote an optimal level of wellness. The focus of school nursing is a comprehensive school health program that meets the existing needs and identifies future needs of the child, the school, and the community. School nurses are responsible for individual health plans that include a growth and development history, screening results, physical assessment, and emotional status, as well as the sharing of the nursing care plans with students, family, health care providers, and school personnel. The school nurse also assesses, plans, implements, and evaluates school health services and community services that include primary, secondary, and tertiary prevention.

The school nurse is aware of the health needs of the youngsters; the school nurse must also be aware of the community resources. The match or mismatch between needs of the youngsters and availability of community and school resources to meet health needs is what documents the need for specific services.

> FACT: Teenage pregnancy is an example of a need for a specific service; it is a major problem in every area of the country. The United States is the only developed country where teenage pregnancy has been increasing in recent years, with the rate for 17 to 19-year-olds at 96 per 1000, compared to 14 per 1000 in the Netherlands, and 44 per 1000 in Canada.
>
> Reasons for the high United States teenage pregnancy rate include restrictions on teenagers' access to contraception and a lack of teaching about birth control in school.

Following assessment of existing health education programs for youngsters on sexuality, the school nurse is in a unique position to collaborate with school personnel and community groups to develop and present programs to meet existing needs. As with any health promotion program, knowledge of existing school and community resources is required, followed by a collaborative relationship with school personnel, families, and community leaders.

Linda Bullock, RN, BSN
School Nurse

Healthy Environment = Healthy Workers

Occupational health nursing applies nursing principles to the tasks of conserving the health of workers and maintaining a safe and healthful environment in occupational settings. Presently, more than 20,000 occupational health nurses (OHN) practice this credo daily. It is the workforce of 50 or 5000 that constitutes the community-as-client entity for the OHN.

The scope of occupational health nursing practice includes primary care to ill and injured workers, counseling and health education, health screening and health promotion programs, program planning, and surveillance programs of workers who have been exposed to identified risks. In addition, the OHN must possess extensive knowledge regarding regulations of the Occupational Safety and Health Administration (OSHA), and workers' compensation laws. A major emphasis of OSHA today is the Hazard Communication Standard or "right to know laws." As a result of the interventions of the American Association of Occupational Health Nurses (AAOHN),

OHNs have now been included among the health care professionals with the right to know of trade secrets associated with hazardous chemicals at the worksite. The OHN is a practitioner who must be an advocate for the workers, as well as a consultant to management with regard to identified health promotion and disease prevention needs of workers.

The primary role of the OHN is to provide comprehensive nursing care to workers at the worksite. Comprehensive nursing care includes care of ill or injured workers, as well as screening and counseling for at-risk factors of illness or injury. More than ever, companies are "cost conscious" and the OHN must speak in terms of "dollars and cents" in order to receive the support of management. Because the purpose of the occupational environment is to produce a product or service, not to provide health care, the OHN must be prepared to show that health promotion programs result in healthy workers with decreased absenteeism and increased production and morale.

Finally, the role of the OHN is to keep abreast of current trends and technologies that affect the practice of occupational health nursing, and to become educationally prepared to work within a changing occupational health environment.

Thelma Maynor, RN, BSN
Occupational Health Nurse

SUMMARY

Community health nurses combine knowledge and skills from nursing and the public health sciences in order to apply the nursing process in the maintainance and improvement of the health of a community. We have discussed the essential nature of the skills of primary health care, community advocacy, research, and consultation to community health nursing. You may be wondering what types of settings are avaialable for practice. Most community health nurses practice in an ambulatory setting such as official agencies (*i.e.,* health departments), private clinics, health maintenance organizations (HMO), independent practice, correctional institutions, schools, or occupational/industrial settings. However, the community-as-client focus can be applied to any practice setting, including long-term care settings and acute care settings.

REFERENCES

World Health Organization: Alma-Alta, 1978—Primary Health Care Report of the International Conference on Primary Health Care. Alma-Alta, USSR, Geneva, Switzerland, World Health Organization, 1978

Helton AS, McFarlane J, Anderson ET: Battered and pregnant. Amer J Public Health, 77:1337–1339, 1987

SUGGESTED READINGS

Archer SE, Kelly CD, Bisch SA: Implementing Change in Communities. A Collaborative Process. St. Louis, CV Mosby, 1984

American Nurses' Association: The Primary Health Care Nurse Practitioner. Kansas City, Missouri, American Nurses' Association, 1985

Elliott C: Is primary health care the new priority? Yes, but . . . Contact 28:3–8, 1975

Goeppinger J: Changing health behavior and outcomes through self-care. In Lancaster L, Lancaster W (eds): Concept of Advanced Nursing Practice: The Nurse as a Change Agent. St. Louis, CV Mosby, 1982

Goeppinger J: Primary health care: An answer to the dilemmas of community nursing? Public Health Nurs, 1:129–140, 1984

Helton A, McFarlane J, Anderson E: Battered and Pregnant. Unpublished manuscript, Texas Woman's University, Houston Campus, 1986

International Council of Nurses and the World Health Organization: Report of the workshop on "the role of nursing in primary health care." Nairobi, Kenya, International Council of Nurses and the World Health Organization, Sept–Oct, 1979

Kark S: The Practice of Community-oriented Primary Health Care. New York, Appleton-Century-Crofts, 1981

Krebs D: Nursing in primary health care. International Nursing Review, 30(5):141–145, 1983

Mahler H: Nurses lead the way. World Health, July:28–29, 1985

Pender NJ: Health Promotion in Nursing Process. Norwalk, Connecticut, Appleton-Century-Crofts, 1982

Pesznecker B, Draye MA, McNeil J: Collaborative practice models in community health nursing. Nursing Outlook, 30:298–302, 1982

Primary health care: A first assessment. World Health, Sept:6–9, 1983

Skrovan C, Anderson ET, Gottschalk J: Community nurse practitioner, an emerging role. Amer J Public Health, 64:847–853, 1974

13

The Teaching Role in Community Health Nursing

OBJECTIVES

The purpose of all community health education is to offer health knowledge to the community—with the intent of causing a voluntary improvement in health attitudes and behaviors. The purpose of this chapter is to present the process and skills of the teaching role in community health nursing. After studying this chapter you will be able to

- Select and use a model to plan a community health-education program
- Prepare a community education program that meets assessed health-education needs
- Implement an educational program for a specific target group, using the principles and theories of teaching and learning

INTRODUCTION

Community health nursing is a synthesis of the nursing and public health practices. But the principles and practices of education are additional elements when the nurse functions in a teaching role in the community. (*Synthesis* is a key word; it facilitates the application of knowledge in new ways.) In this chapter, *education,* and the *practice of teaching* will be explored in the role of the community health nurse.

Public health practice uses the tools of demography, epidemiology, biometry, and environmental health. The community health nurse uses these same tools in order to better comprehend the characteristics of a community. In the practice of teaching in the community, the physical, social, biological, and behavioral sciences are also included. You will use the nursing process to facilitate collection of data, analysis of situations in order to problem-solve and make decisions, planning and carrying out of interventions, and evaluation of effectiveness. In addition, principles of education are synthesized by the community health nurse and used to plan, implement, and evaluate health-education programs.

DIMENSIONS OF COMMUNITY HEALTH EDUCATION

Community health programs focus on the health of a population; they are centered on a target population, not on an individual or family unit. However, in order to have an impact on the whole population or community it is necessary to meet individual, family, and group education needs.

Health maintenance and health promotion are dependent upon the entire community having health as a concern and actively following healthy lifestyle behaviors. However, competent health care providers play a large part in the assurance of a healthy community; the community health nurse must perform an active service role that includes health promotion. The educational component of community health practice is geared to two populations

- The community as client
- The health service provider

Individual clients, groups (*e.g.,* pregnant women, the elderly, teens) and other health providers are the audience for educational programs in the community health setting.

In your practice, as the nurse in the community, you will spend much time in teaching. To teach is to impart knowledge, instruct, and guide. In the community, the community health nurse imparts knowledge to clients and to colleagues. Client education can occur in informal one-to-one teaching and counseling sessions, and within the structure of planned *health-education programs.* Similarly, community health nurses teach their colleagues in one-to-one informal discussions.

Health education is a process; it contains intellectual, psychological, and social dimensions relating to activities that increase people's ability to make informed decisions on questions that affect their personal, family, and community well-being. Health education is based on scientific principles and facilitates learning and behavioral changes in both health personnel and consumers. Whether the nurse's education role is directed to the lay public or to colleagues, the teaching process is the same.

THE PROCESS OF HEALTH-EDUCATION PROGRAM DEVELOPMENT

The education process begins with planning the education program. In order to plan a client education or staff development program, you must answer the questions: *What? To whom? How? Why?* Health-education planning models serve as guides in the planning process. Recall from Chapter 5 that a model is a blueprint or a map that guides and gives direction to practice. It gives structure to our practice, thus insuring that all important components are considered.

Choosing a Health Education Model

The selection of a health-education model is the first step in the process of planning an education program. An education model starts the program on the right track and keeps it moving to a successful evaluation. Public health statistics such as morbidity and mortality rates, community and agency health goals, and the criteria for healthy community behavior can be placed into a planning model so as to answer the questions listed above.

It is important to study the intended purpose of a model before choosing one for use in health-education program development. Some health-education models are more concerned with a philosophy of how education occurs than how to plan an education program. For example, explaining behavioral change, specifically why a person does or does not change their health-affecting behaviors, is the focus of the Health Belief Model, the Fear Drive Model, the Dual Process Model, the Ajen–Fishbein Model, and the Health Promotion Model. In contrast, the Precede Model focuses on the planning process.

The behavioral change models, the Precede Model, and Nola Pender's Health Promotion Model are described in the following pages. You may choose to adapt various models to form your own.

Health Belief Model

The *Health Belief Model* appears in Figure 13-1. It focuses on the motivational determinants that direct health actions—in other words—what motivates people to comply with health-affecting behaviors. According to the model, the factors that determine (or motivate) health actions include

- Individual perception of *vulnerability* or *susceptibility* to a disease. (Affirmative responses to questions such as, "Are you likely to develop this disease?" or, "Do you worry about having this disease?" indicate high perceived vulnerability.)
- Individual perception of the *severity* of the disease. (A statement such as "Smallpox is not a health problem, people are not even vaccinated any

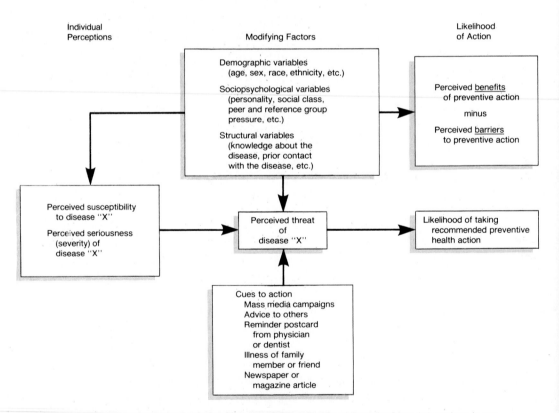

Figure 13-1. The Health Belief Model. (Becker MH: The Health Belief Model and Sick Role Behavior. In Becker MH (ed): The Health Belief Model and Personal Health Behavior, p 89. Thorofare, New Jersey, Charles B Slack, 1974)

more," indicates low perceived severity. In contrast, a statement such as "People die of cancer every day," indicates high perceived severity.)

- Individual perception of the *benefits* and feasibility of complying with the proposed health behaviors. (A statement such as, "I've changed my diet to decrease my risk of heart disease," indicates perceived benefits of compliance.)
- Individual perception of perceived *barriers* to health behavior. (A statement such as "A change of diet will be costly, I do not like the foods suggested and I do not have time for the extra preparation time," indicates that perceived barriers appear to outweigh benefits; compliance is unlikely.)

The Health Belief Model is based on the idea that people change (or do not change) behaviors, depending on their perception of a health threat. For example, the threat of cardiovascular disease to the middle-age overweight adults, the benefits of a risk-reduction behavior (diet modifications), and barriers to that behavior (inconveniences, cost, discomfort) are all weighed in a client's decision of whether or not to change a health-affecting behavior such as caloric intake. Demographic variables (*e.g.,* age, sex, and ethnicity) are modifying influences on the chances of an individual's making a change. The Health Belief Model focuses on disease prevention and the actions taken to avoid the consequences of illness and disease; therefore, it is considered a behavioral change model.

Fear Drive Model

The *Fear Drive Model,* shown in Figure 13-2, assumes that knowledge and understanding are insufficient to cause a health behavior change; the emotion of fear is necessary. Fear is the driving agent that motivates the change in habits or initiates health actions. A series of stages comprise the Fear Drive Model. First, the person receives a fear-inducing message, for example pain or impaired mobility; this is followed by an emotional response (usually fear). The person then experiences a subjective discomfort to the fear (usually worry); this motivates actions such as a change in lifestyle practices.

The Fear Drive Model proposes that fear can be used to produce behavioral changes. Indeed, levels of fear have been associated with behavior change, with high fear causing a greater change in health practices. However, there may be undesirable side effects such as producing negative health behavior. For example, the middle-age, overweight adult with a sedentary occupation stops an exercise program after reading about the death of a middle-age adult during aerobic exercise. The recipient of the fear message may develop

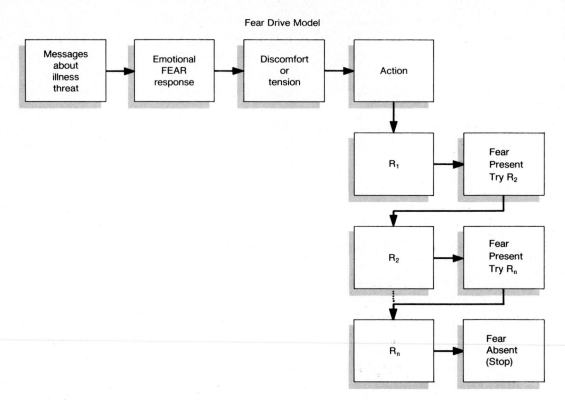

Figure 13-2.   The Fear Drive Model. (Leventhal H, Safer M, Panagis D: The impact of communications on the self-regulation of health beliefs, decisions, and behavior. Health Educ Q 10(1):7, 1983)

an attitude of hopelessness—a reaction that occurs more frequently in persons who have low self-esteem.

Dual Process Self-Regulatory Model

The *Dual Process Self-Regulatory Model* is shown in Figure 13-3. This model integrates fear and knowledge into a behavior plan. The processes of emotional arousal, cognitive awareness, and the planning of health actions are formulated subjectively from the participant's viewpoint. The processes proposed in the model are

- The *objective–cognitive process*—a health threat is generated and the individual plans a coping action. Both past experience and current information are used in the formulation of a plan.

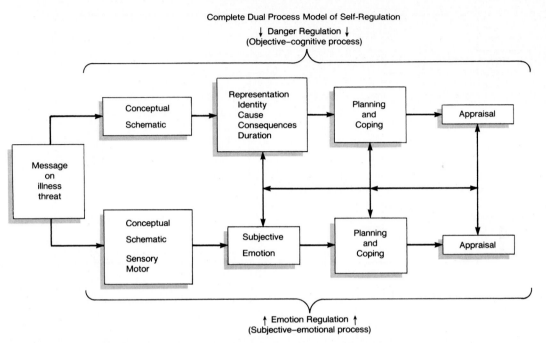
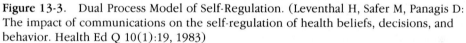

Figure 13-3. Dual Process Model of Self-Regulation. (Leventhal H, Safer M, Panagis D: The impact of communications on the self-regulation of health beliefs, decisions, and behavior. Health Ed Q 10(1):19, 1983)

- The *subjective–emotional process*—the health threat is communicated to the individual, resulting in an emotional reaction. The force of this reaction is dependent upon the type or strength of the health threat and if the individual perceives it as applying to himself or herself.
- *Interactions between cognitive* and *emotional processes* that result from health threats may be independent of each other. For example, people can have the knowledge that smoking is associated with lung cancer, but the emotional gratification from smoking is stronger than the fear of cancer—so they continue to smoke. Of course, other factors (*i.e.,* habit, nicotine addiction, etc.) that are involved in smoking continuation.

Ajen–Fishbein Model

The *Ajen–Fishbein Model,* shown in Figure 13-4, is based upon the premise that beliefs, attitudes, intentions, and behaviors are four different factors that are interrelated and that interact to determine behavior. To explain—a person's attitude is related to beliefs, but not always related to a certain belief (a

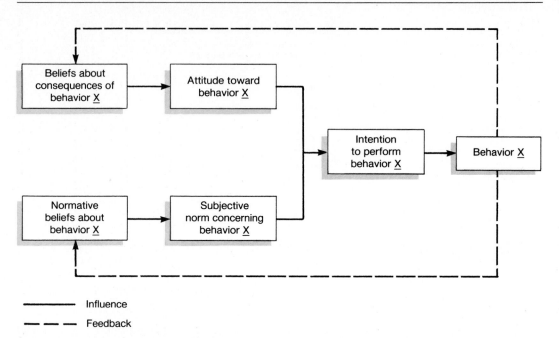

——————— Influence

— — — Feedback

Figure 13-4.   Ajen–Fishbein Model. (Fishbein M, Ajen I: Belief, Attitude, Intention and Behavior: An Introduction to Theory and Research, p 16. Reading, Massachusetts, Addison–Wesley Publishing Co, 1975)

person may feel that cancer is somehow related to health behavior, but not necessarily to smoking). Similarly, a person's attitude is related to his or her intentions but not necessarily to any one intention (a woman may feel that early prenatal care can insure a healthy pregnancy outcome, but she does not change her customary practice of not beginning prenatal care until the eighth month of pregnancy). Intentions can and do serve as predictors of behavior (a person who makes a written self-contract or goal of intentions is especially apt to change behavior). Although a person's attitude toward an object is related to overall behavior, it may not be related to a single act or repetitive behavior (a person may hold a generally positive attitude toward the importance of seatbelt use, but neglect to buckle up for every ride in a car).

To form new beliefs, it is necessary to perform a new behavior that is based upon new information. The Ajen–Fishbein Model assumes an arousal chain that links beliefs to attitudes to intentions to behavior. The performance of a new behavior then reacts with the belief component and the chain reaction is invoked again. A 24-year-old, physically fit male who smokes but also runs three miles a day, may believe that smoking is a health hazard; but he also may have the *attitude* that his health is excellent and therefore a health-affecting behavior change (*i.e.,* smoking cessation) is unnecessary.

The Health Belief, Fear Drive, Dual Process, and Ajen–Fishbein Models each focus on behavioral changes to avert illness or disease. The behavioral change, if adopted, protects the self from illness or disease. But what about health promotion—behaviors completed to promote and enhance health?

Health Promotion Model

Nola Pender's *Health Promotion Model,* shown in Figure 13-5, lists personal characteristics (*e.g.,* self-esteem and self-awareness) that facilitate or sustain health-promoting behaviors. Pender explains that behaviors that are initially begun to avoid a health risk, such as regular aerobic exercise to decrease the risk of cardiovascular problems, elicit internal positive feelings that motivate the person to continue regular exercise. What began as a disease-prevention behavior is transformed into a health-promotion behavior.

The Precede Model

Behavioral change models can be used in conjunction with program-planning models such as the Precede Model. The *Precede Model* is appropriate for planning both client-education and staff-development programs. The model, shown in Figure 13-6, consists of seven phases. Most phases begin with a diagnosis; the diagnosis acts to specify the health problem and gives direction to interventions. To demonstrate how the model works, a prenatal health-education program is presented in Figure 13-7 according to the phases of the model. (Notice that the model is used from right to left—we do not know why!)

Prior to the planning, an advisory committee to the project should be established that has both agency and community representatives. The Precede Model begins with Phase 1, which requires a social diagnosis. The social diagnosis identifies individual and community indicators of the quality of life (examples of social diagnoses include, high unemployment and substandard housing). Phase 2, the epidemiological diagnosis, identifies measures of health that affect individual and community quality of life (epidemiological diagnoses include, increased teenage-suicide mortality rate, and increased cardiovascular morbidity rate). For example, in the program outlined in Figure 13-7, the social diagnosis is teenage pregnancy; the epidemiological diagnosis is, high rate of low-birth-weight infants. A diagnosis may be derived from national, state, community, and agency health goals. (Recall from Chapter 9 and the objectives for the nation that a lowered infant-mortality rate was a major objective.) However, in planning a community-education or staff-development program, you must carefully study the agency goals and objectives and

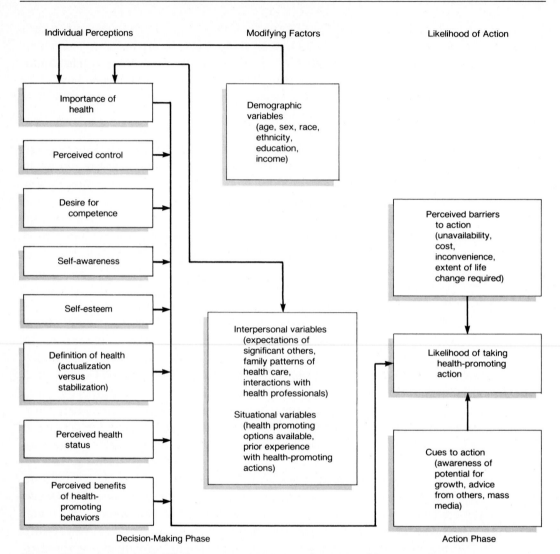

Figure 13-5. Pender's Health Promotion Model. (Pender, N: Health Promotion in Nursing Practice, p 66. East Norwalk, Connecticut, Appleton-Century-Crofts, 1982)

decide if they are applicable to your target groups and the assessed health needs of your community.

Phase 3, the behavioral diagnosis, considers the behavior of the health care provider and the community; both affect the health of the target population and therefore each area merits a diagnosis. For example, a behavioral diagnosis for the pregnant woman may be, lack of health maintenance practices (*i.e.,* balanced nutrition) or noncompliance with recommended medical care (*i.e.,* refusal to take daily iron supplementation). A behavioral diagnosis for the community health nurse would focus on nursing behaviors that would promote health maintenance and compliance behaviors of pregnant woman such as offering health-education classes or support groups. Notice the behavioral diagnoses in Figure 13-7 focus on the pregnant woman, as well as the nurse.

> STOP! Consider for a minute your assessed community. List one social diagnosis and one epidemiological diagnosis. What behavioral diagnoses follow? For the client? For the nurse?

Phase 4 lists *predisposing, enabling,* and *reinforcing factors* involved in health services. Predisposing factors consist of the *knowledge, attitudes, values,* and *perceptions* that are necessary for behavioral change. Figure 13-7 lists the knowledge to be included in prenatal education classes. Do you agree with the listing? Do you feel that additional topics should be included?

The *attitudes* of the prenatal patient and the nurse toward the pregnancy affect behaviors. Does the pregnant woman believe a healthy pregnancy is important? Does she believe her behaviors are important in the creation of a healthy baby? Assess the attitudes of both the patient and family and, in a similar fashion, assess the *perceptions* of patient, family, nurse, and health care team. Do the patient and family have a sense of control over the outcome of the pregnancy? Knowledge, attitudes, and perceptions are all interrelated in a person's *values.* Notice that the Precede Model lists the values of patient, family, and nurse, and those of their culture. What is important to one culture or ethnic group is not necessarily important to another. Prenatal care offered by health providers may be valued by one group of women, whereas another group may value family beliefs and traditional care recommendations more highly. Assess and record the values of each group to which you offer health education. Values, attitudes, and perceptions are predisposing factors that determine a person's receptiveness to health education.

The areas remaining under Phase 4 are *enabling factors* and *reinforcing factors.* Enabling factors include the feasibility of the staff and client complying with a proposed education plan. Can the prenatal patient afford to purchase the required servings of fruit per day? Is a program ethical? Should a community health nurse propose a program that is difficult or unsuitable for many clients? Is the staff receptive to teaching the proposed content? Is the staff qualified? Do sufficient resource materials exist? Learn to know your target group and what behaviors they can and cannot accomplish. Reinforcing

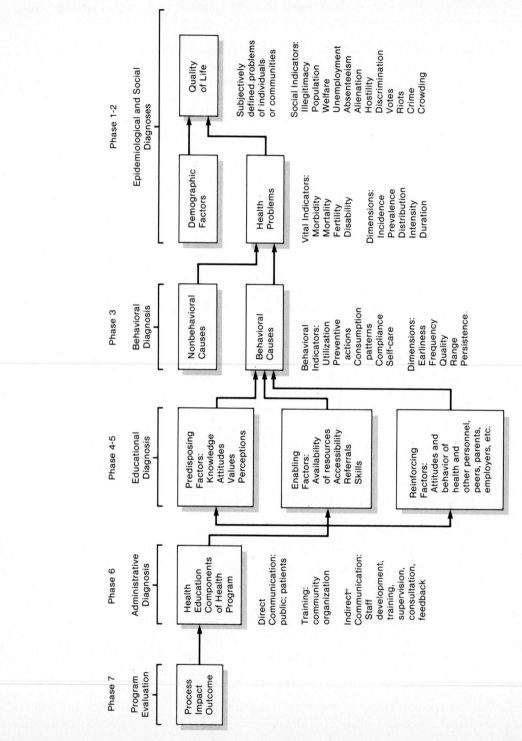

Figure 13-6. The Precede Model. (Green L et al: Health Education Planning, p 14. Palo Alto, California, Mayfield Publ, 1980)

Phase 1
Social Diagnosis

Quality of Life
Teenage pregnancy

Social Implications
Psychological and financial cost to family and community

Phase 2
Epidemiological Diagnosis

Demographic Variables
Mothers:
Age
Race
Education
Marital Status
Income

Health Problem
High rate of low birth weight infants

Phase 3
Behavioral Diagnosis

Nonbehavioral Causes
Health Care Delivery
Risk Factors

Behavioral Causes
Patient:
Noncompliance with nutritional recommendations and iron supplementation

Community Health Nurse:
Lack of prenatal classes for pregnant women

Phases 4–5
Educational Diagnosis

Predisposing Factors
A. Knowledge (for each trimester)
1. Physiological and psychological changes
2. Prenatal care, (i.e., hygiene, nutrition, exercise, rest)
3. Teratogens and other risks
4. Danger signs
5. Fetal growth and development
6. Preparation for childbirth
7. Sexuality
8. Labor, delivery, postpartum
B. Attitudes
1. Client and family
2. Nurses.
C. Values
1. Client and family
2. Culture
3. Nurse
D. Perceptions
1. Client
2. Family
3. Nurse
4. Health Care Team

Enabling Factors
Ability to comply with prenatal recommendations

Reinforcing Factors
Family, Peers, Health Care Team

Phases 5–6
Administrative Diagnosis

Lack of health education in the prenatal clinics

Health Education Components
A. Program objective
B. Client cognitive, affective, and behavioral objectives
C. Program content
D. Implementation

Phase 7
Program Evaluation

Process
Were all the necessary steps included throughout?

Impact
1. Program objective
2. Client objectives
   a. Knowledge
   b. Behavioral
3. Record keeping

Outcome
1. Health Goals
2. Social Goals

Figure 13-7. The Precede Model used in a prenatal education program.

403

factors refer to the use of handout materials, audio-visuals, practice sessions, and the assistance of client's family and peer group in maintaining behavioral changes.

Phase 5 is the ranking in order of priority of the predisposing, enabling, and reinforcing factors. This is completed simultaneously with Phase 4. It is usually during Phases 4 to 5 that additional assessment data are needed about client attitudes, resources, and health practices. During Phases 4 to 5 you will continually refer to your community assessment data for information on cultural practices, educational levels, and perceived values.

Phase 6 is the making of an administrative diagnosis. One administrative diagnosis for the prenatal education program was, lack of health education in the prenatal clinics. Additional components in Phase 6 include program objectives; client cognitive, affective, and behavioral objectives; specifics of program content; and implementation of the program. Each component of Phase 6 for the prenatal health-education program is presented in Figure 13-8.

Phase 7 of the Precede Model is program evaluation and consists of *process, impact,* and *outcome evaluation.* Process evaluation refers to the observation of all activities involved in the planning, development, implementation, and evaluation of a health-education program, whereas impact evaluation is concerned only with the effect of the health information upon the program participants (*i.e.,* as a result of the program were knowledge, behavior, or attitudes changed?). Outcome evaluation measures cost effectiveness or quality control.

> STOP! Before using Phase 7 of the Precede Model to plan an evaluation for a health-education program, review Chapter 10: *Evaluating a Community Health Program.*

Figure 13-9 is a copy of the Precede Model and can be used to plan your community health-educational program.

ASSESSING EDUCATIONAL NEEDS

When you assess educational needs, several categories should be considered. These are the education needs of the *target group,* the *agency,* and the *community* or *society* as a whole.

Target-Group Education Needs

To know about a *target group* information must be acquired on its demographic characteristics of age, sex, educational level, ethnicity, and income

Health-Education Component

A. Program Objectives
 1. Establish a prenatal education program that teaches
    a. The importance of early and consistent compliance with prenatal care
    b. The implications of nutrition, stress, exercise, and teratogens on fetal development
 2. Implement the program in one health center
 3. After 6 months
    Evaluate, revise, and offer the program at two additional health centers
 4. After one year
    Evaluate, revise, and offer the program in all eight health centers

B. Client Objectives
 Cognitive: Following a prenatal health education program, 90% of prenatal patients will demonstrate knowledge about importance of prenatal care and implications for fetal development
 Affective: Prenatal clients will share their attitudes, values, and perceptions regarding their current pregnancy
 Behavioral: Thirty percent will attend four prenatal classes
  Seventy percent will attend all scheduled prenatal appointments
  Fifty percent of prenatal patients will self-report eating prescribed diet, compliance with vitamin and iron supplementation, coping effectively with stress, and avoiding teratogens

C. Program Content
 1. Three slide–tape presentations (one presentation for each trimester), audio will be English and Spanish
 2. Three teaching manuals (one for each trimester). Manuals will include reinforcement materials, teaching strategies, and discussion questions
 3. Pretests and posttests for each slide–tape presentation that measure knowledge, attitudinal, and behavioral changes

D. Implementation
 1. Select health center for initial presentation
 2. Assign and orient nurse educator
 3. Secure audio-visual equipment and supplies
 4. Determine class size, dates, and time schedule
 5. Design and test slide–tape presentations
 6. Design and test teaching manuals
 7. Evaluation of slide–tape and manuals by staff and clients for
    a. Appropriateness
    b. Acceptability
    c. Clarity
    d. Accuracy of content
 8. Revise materials as needed

Figure 13-8. Phase 5 of the Precede Model—Health-Education Components for a Prenatal Education Program

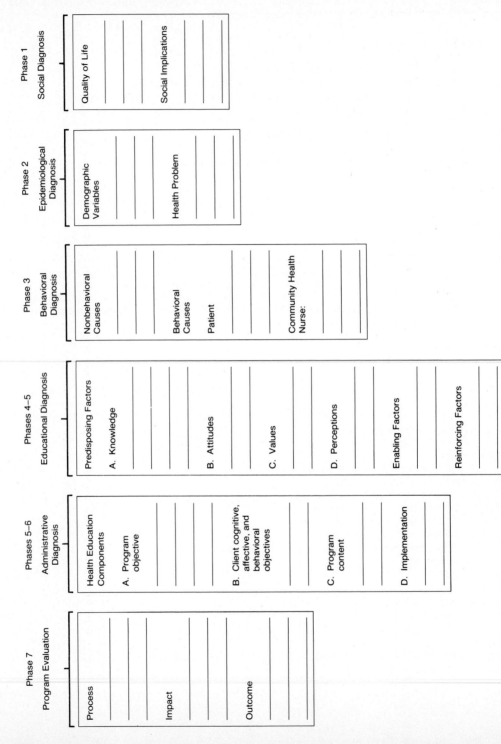

Figure 13-9. The Precede Model planning form.

406

levels. Other pertinent epidemiologic information may also need to be gathered such as morbidity, mortality, and fertility rates. It is necessary to assess what the members of the group already know, what they would like to know, and what they need to know. The target group's perception of what they need to learn can differ widely from the perception of an educational-program planner. *Always include at least one representative of the target population* in the planning and preparation of the education program.

Agency Health Education Needs

Assessment of an agency's policy, perception, and plans for handling client health problems is a strong prerequisite to program planning. If an agency has targeted health problems in specific groups (for example, prenatal education to pregnant women), a good part of the *who* and *what* questions are answered. Indeed, you may at this point proceed to the use of your chosen health-education planning model.

However, if this information is not available, you will need to complete an assessment of needs. You may choose to look at community morbidity and mortality rates associated with an agency's services. For example, an agency may offer a family health service (health maintenance and health promotion for infants, children, and women of childbearing ages) and also a communicable disease service (tuberculosis, Hansen's, immunizations, and sexually transmitted diseases (STD) surveillance and treatment). While studying the morbidity and mortality rates, you realize that the agency's service area has both a higher than average infant-mortality rate and also STD are at epidemic proportions. Client education might then consist of planning two programs: a client-education program that deals with STD and a program to lower infant-mortality rates.

Planning and preparing a program that is congruent with an agency's organizational and service goals affords certain benefits. Agency-administrative support and multidisciplinary-staff support are more likely to be present if the program matches agency goals. This is because the education component naturally enhances the quality of agency services.

Barriers to the planning and preparation of client-education programs can and do occur. A multidisciplinary committee to advise on program planning will assist in handling agency- and staff-imposed barriers. Members of such a multidisciplinary advisory committee might include a nutritionist, social worker, physician, and pharmacist. Representatives from agency administration also need to be on the advisory committee.

Community Health Education Needs

To thoroughly comprehend health-education needs of the *community,* it is necessary to assess its social, political, cultural, and economic structures. The planning process must consider optimal community health status, and determine what an education program can do to maintain and promote community health. Community nursing diagnoses profile the health problems of the community and are the building blocks for community health-education programs.

Community nursing diagnoses of potential and existing health problems, along with etiologies, are essential. It is crucial that the health problems have a possibility of an improved change. The chosen health problem should also be one for which agency support can be expected for change through use of educational strategies. You will also need to define exactly what population has the health problem. For example, if you have documented low-birth-weight infants as a health problem of your community, you must define the conditions of infants who are affected. What are the demographics of the mothers of the low-birth-weight infants? What is their age, race, and ethnicity? Do adolescent mothers give birth to a larger percentage of these infants? Are any lifestyle practices associated with these mothers? Is income or geographic location associated with the incidence of low-birth-weight infants? It is necessary to collect as much data as possible in an effort to know not only what the problem is, but also who has the problem; it is helpful when theories as to why the problem exists can be found in the area's literature. Developing a community nursing diagnosis affords a profile of the health problem and the population that is affected.

Another aspect of community understanding is to be cognizant of the *political ramifications* of health problems. Not only must you look to the agency for administrative support for health-education strategies, but also consider the viewpoint of other community agencies and institutions. Are community leaders concerned that an infant mortality rate of 17 per 1000 live births exists in low-income minority census tracts (CT) in your community?

Look also to the *economics* of the community that is affected by the health problem. If the health problem is completely or partially the result of low-income levels, how can an education program be of any value? Again, does the target community feel that the selected health problem is a priority? Survival needs may be the daily priority in a low-income, crime-ridden neighborhood. A pregnant teenager may be more concerned about her family's withdrawal of love and financial support than she is with following a recommended prenatal diet.

Cultural assessment must also be a part of education-program planning. Recommended lifestyle practices may not be compatible with the practices of a specific cultural group. When planning an educational program for a community group, it is essential to include throughout the program process input from persons of that culture. Dietary habits, language, values and beliefs, and family influence may all reflect cultural practices that the educator must take into account in education-program planning.

State, national, and *world health objectives* that focus upon specific diseases or health conditions are valuable guides in determining which health problems are considered of a priority nature. Generally, the health of women and children—world-wide, nationally, state-wide, and locally—are considered to be a first priority. "The future of a nation is dependent upon the health of its women and children" is a phrase from the World Health Organization (WHO) that is frequently quoted. However, certain situations such as the outbreak of a communicable disease or the discovery of a toxic chemical hazard could alter priorities.

Additional areas to assess include the resources of other agencies in the community and their perception of community health-education needs. Other agencies may provide needed education resources for your clients (*i.e.,* speakers, audio-visuals, and teaching materials). Assess the journals, books, and periodicals to learn what is perceived by others as current community health-education needs. This information can verify your community health-education program; a library search will provide articles and books of assistance.

Planning an education program for a specific target group considers *community health status,* as well as *target group* and *agency perceptions* of education program needs. A blending of these three factors in conjunction with an overview of the target group's quality of life furnish the background for education program development. After assessing and diagnosing the health and associated education needs of a target group, you are ready to move to the planning and program preparation stage.

Offering the Health-Education Program

To begin planning for a health-education program, you must first secure agency administrative support for the program. Secondly, you need to set up an advisory committee. This should consist of an interdisciplinary selection of health care providers from the agency and representatives from the target population. The purpose of this group is to comment on and evaluate program content and teaching strategies. They will also assist in the planning of implementation and evaluation methodology.

A written rationale for the proposed program is a third early-program-planning task—the rationale will answer the question of *why* the educational program is proposed. An example of a proposed program title along with the rationale follow.

Title: Health Promotion Information for Health Providers of the Elderly

Rationale

The increase in the number of older persons in the population has created an increased need for health-education programs that focus on maintaining and promoting the health of older persons. However, most health providers are unprepared to teach healthy lifestyle practices to the elderly. The term *health provider* means both professional (*e.g.*, registered nurse, social worker) and nonprofessional (*e.g.*, day-care worker, recreational department employee).

The next task is to set program activities, goals, and objectives. Examples of each for the *Health Promotion Information for Health Providers of the Elderly* program include the following elements.

Program Activities

To train a minimum of 70 health providers who currently work with the elderly to teach health promotion behaviors to the elderly.

Program Goal

Increased knowledge of health providers on how to increase health promotion practices among the elderly.

Objectives

Following eight one-hour classes, the health providers will be able to

- Identify risk factors specific to the elderly
- Describe at least five techniques for teaching health promotion behaviors to the elderly
- Teach to the elderly health promotion classes on stress reduction, exercise fitness, and healthy diet
- Refer the elderly to community resources that promote the health of the elderly (*e.g.,* nutrition, recreation, and housing programs)

Constraints of the program activities need to be identified, as well as possible remedies for these restrictions. In the program *Health Promotion Information for Health Providers of the Elderly,* it was necessary to cancel the last series of eight classes owing to budgetary constraints. Budgeting is a vital aspect of education-program planning. Time, staff, equipment, and supplies represent money. In most cases the nurse who is planning an educational program will be faced with budgetary constraints that dictate careful management of monies for staff, supplies, equipment, and printing.

When planning any program, the educational level of the target population must be considered. There are formulas available that, when applied to a program, determine its educational level (see Laubach and Koschnick, pp 12–15, 1977). One such formula is Gunning's Fog Index. To use the Fog Index, take a sample of 100 words from your teaching material and divide it by the total number of sentences to arrive at an average number of words per

READING LEVEL DETERMINED BY GUNNING'S FOG INDEX

Fog Index	*Reading Level*
17	College graduate
15	College junior
13	College freshman
11	High school junior
9	High school freshman
7	Seventh grade

PRINCIPLES OF TEACHING

Principles of Teaching

The teacher enhances the student's opportunity for self-fulfillment.

The teacher helps each student clarify individual aspirations for improved skills.

The teacher assists each learner to define the gap between aspiration and present level of performance.

The teacher helps the learner identify the life problems experienced because of gaps in knowledge or skills.

The teacher provides a climate conducive to learning (physical conditions) and an atmosphere of trust.

The teacher values each student.

The teacher encourages learner interactions.

The teacher exposes personal feelings in a spirit of mutual inquiry.

The teacher involves the student in a mutual process of objective formulation that considers the needs of learners, the agency, the teacher, the subject matter, and society.

The teacher shares ideas, provides options, and involves learners in the selection of learning materials and methods.

The teacher helps the students to organize themselves into project groups, learning teams, and to create independent study projects.

The teacher uses role-playing, discussions, and case studies in order to build on past experiences of learners.

The teacher adapts the presentation level to appropriate learner level.

The teacher helps the learner apply newly learned knowledge or skills by integrating them into life experiences.

The teacher and the learner are involved in the evaluation methodology.

The teacher helps the students to develop and use evaluation criteria.

---

sentence (*i.e.,* 8, 10, 12). Then add the average number of words per sentence to the number of words in the sample with three or more syllables (capitalized words, compound words, and syllables made by "es" or "ed" are not counted). The total sum is multiplied by 0.4. The Fog Index scores correlated to a reading level appear in the displayed material. Strive to provide materials that have a score of 10 or less.

Once the program is prepared, it is important to pilot test it on a group from the target group. Revisions are made according to the pilot-testing results.

PRINCIPLES OF LEARNING

Principles of Learning

Learning takes place when an individual is ready to learn.

Individual differences must be considered if learning is to occur.

Motivation either from without or within the person must be present.

What is learned in any situation is dependent upon the perception of the learner.

The learning process must be of relevance to the learner.

Learning is more effective if the message is of value to the learner.

Evaluation by the learner and the teacher is necessary to determine what learning has taken place.

(After: Leahy K, Cobb M, Jones M: Community Health Nursing, p 70. New York, McGraw-Hill, 1977)

Implementing the Health-Education Program

Implementation of the program can be a difficult and trying experience. Actually, implementation is the "fitting process." It is fitting the program into the existing service programs and service sites. It is a time of adjusting the program to the individual in each class, and of "polishing" and improving the curricula content and teaching methodology (educational methodology refers to teaching strategies and educational theories).

Teaching strategies refer to the materials and techniques that are used to transmit the information. Teaching materials consist of audio-visuals such as films, slides, tapes, video tapes, posters, charts, brochures, and pamphlets. Teaching techniques refer to the use of lectures, discussions, role-playing, self-programmed study, and simulations. Creative use of materials and techniques serve to stimulate student interest and to increase learning.

EDUCATIONAL THEORIES

Educational theories state how the teacher influences the student to learn and by what processes the student learns. Educational theories are multiple; specific theories may be applied to particular categories of learners or situations. In health-education programs, most participants are adults, therefore some assumptions from adult learning theories (presented below) may be helpful.

- Adults are motivated to learn if the message satisfies their interest and needs.
- Adult learning is life-centered rather than subject-centered.
- Adult education uses the rich resource of adult experience.
- Adults are self-directing so the teaching role becomes one of mutual inquiry.
- Adults are more individualistic, therefore the teaching process must be flexible.

Teaching and learning principles, shown in the displayed material, are presented to guide your educational program.

SUMMARY

Planning, preparing, and providing community health education is the teaching role of the community health nurse. This teaching role synthesizes the disciplines of nursing, public health, and education. To assess the need for health-education programs, consider community, agency, and target-group educational criteria. To develop a comprehensive health-education program, use a planning model. Finally, use the principles and theories of teaching and learning to implement a health-education program that is adaptable to specific community groups.

REFERENCE

Laubach RS, Koschnick K: Using readability: Formulas for easy adult materials. Syracuse, New York, New Readers Press, 1977

SUGGESTED READINGS

Planning Models

Becker M (ed): The Health Belief Model and Personal Health Behavior. Thorofare, New Jersey, Charles B Slack, 1974
Fishbein M, Ajen I: Belief, Attitude, Intention and Behavior: An Introduction to Theory and Research. Reading, Massachusetts, Addison-Wesley, 1975
Green LW, Kreuter MW, Deeds SG, Partridge KB: Health Education Planning: A Diagnostic Approach. Palo Alto, California, Mayfield, 1980

Pender NJ: Health Promotion in Nursing Practice. East Norwalk, Appleton-Century-Croft, 1982

Planning Community Health Education Programs

American Nurses' Association: Standards for Continuing Education in Nursing. Cabinet on Nursing Education, Council on Continuing Education Task Force on Revision of Standards for Continuing Education. Kansas City, American Nurses' Association, 1984

Breckton D: Community Health Education. Rockville, Maryland, Aspen Publishers, 1985

Bigge ML: Learning Theories for Teachers. New York, Harper and Row, 1982

Knowles MS: The Adult Learner: A Neglected Species. Houston, Gulf Publishing, 1973

Knowles MS: Self-Directed Learning. Chicago, Follett Publishing, 1975

Knox AB: Adult Development and Learning. San Francisco, Jossey–Bass, 1977

Knox AB: Assessing the Impact of Continuing Education. San Francisco, Jossey–Bass, 1979

O'Doyle K: Evaluating Teaching. Lexington, Massachusetts, Lexington Books, 1984

14

The Management Role in Community Health Nursing

OBJECTIVES

This chapter focuses on the role of the nurse manager within the practice of community health nursing. As a student, you may question whether or not you will have a true management role. That is, are there management responsibilities attached to the role of a beginning practitioner, or are those responsibilities more appropriately assumed by senior staff members who hold the more formal titles of supervisor, clinic manager, coordinator of health services, or director? This is an important question, which must be answered if you as a beginning practitioner are to understand and carry out the functions and responsibilities of a community health nurse. After studying this chapter you will be able to

- Use the management process to implement community health nursing interventions
- Perform skills of the management role, including
     Effective communication
     Delegation of tasks
     Completion of employee performance evaluation
     Allocation of resources
     Preparation of a budget
     Marketing of a community health program

INTRODUCTION

To learn about the functions and responsibilities that are associated with management within community health nursing, it is critical to have a definition of the terminology. *Management* means "to direct," "to take charge," or "to control." Management is an ongoing process; it is never static. The process is multifaceted because it uses and blends a variety of skills and activities to achieve specified results. It can be viewed as a linking of individuals, or the organizing of people around issues or problems. It is a dynamic process that revolves around the interaction between people and an organization. To achieve desired outcomes, management depends on the abilities that are possessed by individuals, material resources, and technology. The nurse manager uses both interpersonal and technical skills as took to achieve desired outcomes.

THE MANAGEMENT PROCESS

The *management process* has "inputs" of people, money, equipment, materials, and energy that are used or transformed to achieve the organization's objectives. The results of this transformation are known as "outputs" and can take many forms, which may include, but are not limited to, services rendered, products produced, and problems resolved.

In examining the role of management within any organization, it is important to recognize that the activities of management are essential to the maintainence of the functions of the organization. When management is not fully integrated at every level into the structure of an organization, the survival of the organization is threatened. The management process can be thought of as five steps, including

1. Decision making or planning
2. Arrangement of people and their functions into cohesive units
3. Implementation of the planned changes
4. Communication of changes to all affected
5. Evaluation of outcomes

These five steps form the structure or framework for maintaining an organization. Management can also be considered a process of *linking* decisions to people who, in turn, carry out the decisions in order to accomplish goals and objectives for promoting and maintaining health.

Management functions form a managerial system that, when applied, assists users at any level in the organization to become more effective managers. A beginning-level community health nurse can take these functions and apply them in an endless variety of practical ways. The nurse who is able to effectively apply a managerial system will be able to plan more effectively to achieve goals and objectives in such areas as type and quality of services provided, health behaviors expected, community actions effected, and personal nursing growth.

Application of the management process can and should occur at all levels within the organization. Keep in mind that the management process is applicable in all settings that use human and physical resources. The application below demonstrates the use of the five parts of this process on a community health nursing issue that you can expect to encounter.

Application

As a beginning community health nurse you are employed in a community health center that is located in a large city. The center is in an area where health services and resources are limited and those that are available are not readily accessible owing to problems with transportation and hours of service. The population groups using the services of the center have changed dramatically. An analysis of the previous year's demographics reveals an increasing service demand by women and children, and a significant demand by the elderly and teenagers. At present the majority of services are directed at women, infants, and preschoolers. The issues facing the center are

- How should the composition of services be reorganized to meet the changing demographics and corresponding health needs of the service population?
- In what ways can the center respond to the demand for a change in services?
- What constraints and obstacles will the center encounter in redesigning services (*e.g.,* lack of prepared staff, inadequate resources)?

All staff are expected to assist the agency director to determine how potential changes in service delivery will impact on the center. As manager of the family planning services team, you will be expected to contribute to each step of the management process, beginning with the *decision making or planning step.* Your contributions to the planning step might include: evaluating the role of nursing in providing family planning services (*i.e.,* what are nurses presently doing in the clinic and what skills are within the educational preparation of the nurses?); assisting in the determination of non-nursing functions and the selection of the staff member who is best prepared to complete these tasks; suggesting methods to determine the cost of proposed services and the expected health benefits; and proposing staff composition, range of services to be provided, and methods that could be used to provide services.

The second step of the management process, *arrangement of people and their functions in cohesive units,* involves organizing resources to meet the goals of the center. This activity requires the cooperation of all staff. Your functions may include the following: discussing change theory with the staff and everyone's natural resistance to change (refer to Chapter 8 for a discussion of change theory); assisting the team to identify anticipated problems and solutions as the structure and service priorities of the center are changed; maintaining continuity of care and service delivery for present clients; and informing clients of the plan to change services and exactly what events to expect and when.

The third step, *implementation of the planned changes,* must involve all staff. The management role includes the following: implementing the policy changes, initiating the new services, modifying old procedures to facilitate the new services, and rewriting objectives to reflect the new services.

The step of *communicating changes to all affected individuals* is vital to ensure success of the new services. As the manager you will need to interact with the staff at the center, as well as related departments in the same building or even several hundred miles away. Decide which departments need information about the change in services and communicate with them. Ask yourself which departments are important in facilitating the offering of new services. For example, if family planning services are to be extended to teenagers in the evening and on Saturday, then corresponding changes in hours of operation for the pharmacy are important. The pharmacy department must be given information about the expansion of the family planning services and ample time to change their own services.

Lastly, *evaluation of outcomes* is completed to establish if goals were accomplished. As with any plan, evaluation is necessary in order to determine if the plan is being implemented as designed and to initiate alternative plans if needed. Management roles during evaluation include the following: establishing outcome criteria for evaluating services, determining cost of offering the new services, and establishing client satisfaction with the new services.

A discussion of the process of management, with particular application to the beginning community health nurse, has been presented. The text below presents an indepth discussion of two important areas of the management role: interpersonal and technical skills.

INTERPERSONAL SKILLS
OF THE MANAGEMENT ROLE

The interpersonal skills necessary in the management role encompass several areas, including communication, delegation, and employee evaluation.

Communication

Effective management depends upon clear *communication.* Communication between people can be written, verbal, or nonverbal and is influenced by a multitude of variables, especially culture, beliefs, and values. We each have an established pattern for communicating with family, friends, colleagues, and clients. The willingness to continually analyze, change, and refine methods of communication so that we remain sensitive to what others are saying, as well as objective and non-judgmental, is a major skill and is characteristic of the effective manager in community health nursing.

Communication is the only way to exchange information. Whether we are giving an order to a waiter, introducing ourselves and describing our role to a client, explaining the dangers of crossing the street alone to a toddler, or disagreeing with a co-worker, we are communicating both directly and indirectly. Sometimes we communicate effectively, and sometimes ineffectively. If we can recognize why we are successful in one encounter and fail in another, we can learn about ourselves and our communication abilities. Evaluating oneself is very difficult. Begin by asking, "What do I want to communicate?," "Why is the message important?," and "What is the response that I expect?" Frequently, we are very effective in communicating information, but because the expected response is not received, we may mistakenly evaluate the communication as ineffective or as a failure. Always begin by clarifying the *what, why,* and *who* of the communication. Once the purpose is firmly justified in your mind, choose a vehicle for delivering the communication. Sometimes several methods of communication may be appropriate. For example, if a new policy is to be implemented, everyone who will be affected (including, most importantly, clients) needs to have the policy in writing; this should be followed by open-discussion periods, during which questions and concerns can be communicated. In contrast, information affecting one or two people is perhaps best presented during a one-to-one encounter or one-to-two encounter.

Several management decisions are required before any information is exchanged. These decisions may include the following: how to state the information (which words to use), the setting and time of the information exchange, the expected response, follow-up activities to allow for reaction and questions, and evaluation measures to determine the effectiveness of the communication. It is helpful to list communication strategies by considering the benefits and deficits of each. Always assess the recipient(s) and their preferred method of communication. Some people demand written communication and attach a high value to all communication that is transmitted in writing; others are insulted and angered by written information, feeling that it implies an absence of trust. One aspect of communication is delegation, which is one of the interpersonal skills of the management role.

Delegation

Delegation is the act of assigning a task or tasks to a person or group. This may seem easy enough. But what tasks are best delegated? To whom? When? For what purpose? Employee job descriptions, staff educational preparation, agency policies, and agency operating procedures all are useful in making delegation decisions. Like communication, delegation is a process that begins with decision making and ends with evaluation. Once the decisions are made as to what tasks to delegate and to whom, it is important to provide supervision and guidance.

Delegation, in and of itself, may appear at first to be a simple process. Further assessment reveals, however, that delegation is a management function. In organizing services, the nurse manager must delegate tasks and other assignments to health care personnel on a daily basis. *Delegation,* the act of delegating, assigns one person to act for another, but with the final responsibility remaining with the person who made the assignment. Delegating, therefore, is defined as a management tool that provides for the extension of the manager through other workers. The ultimate responsibility, however, remains with the manager.

Delegation begins with the *decision making or planning step.* The nurse manager assesses the nature of the tasks to be delegated and the complexity of the tasks, as well as the time that will be needed to complete them. In a clinic setting, for example, the community health nurse manager will want to decide which tasks should be completed by a nurse, and which tasks can be delegated to non-nursing personnel.

In deciding on staffing patterns, the community health nurse manager will need to decide who can assume the tasks of scheduling appointments, answering the telephone, staffing reception areas, conducting intake interviews, taking health histories, completing physical assessments, collecting samples for the laboratory, counseling and educating clients, scheduling reappointments, and maintaining the quality of the clinic rooms.

It is obvious the community health nurse manager cannot and should not complete all of these tasks. Appropriate delegation at all levels will perform the next step of the management process, which is *arranging people and their functions into cohesive units.* For example, to use the professional nursing staff to schedule appointments, to answer the telephone, and to staff the intake area would be a costly misuse of nursing expertise and time. These functions would be more appropriately delegated to clerks, intake interviewers, or volunteers.

The third step, *implementation of the delegation plan,* must involve the entire staff. Deciding on the final plan, reordering and matching positions and tasks, and deciding on the methods to be used to institute the delegation of tasks all reside with the nurse manager. The methods used to *communicate the delegation of tasks* to the persons affected is the fourth step in the process. This determines to a great extent the outcome of the delegation. Individuals need to know not only what tasks have been added to their area of responsibility, but also what tasks have been eliminated and, when possible, a simple, realistic explanation should be provided. The community health nurse manager becomes responsible for not only coordinating the delegation of tasks with all appropriate staff but also for communicating with those persons who are directly or indirectly affected.

Evaluation of outcomes is the final step, the examination of how the delegated changes have affected delivery of services, how staff have responded to the changes, and how those who have been served evaluated the services. Are there differences evident? Are the costs and benefits consistent with changes? How were services improved? Can staff see the relationship between their delegated tasks, their position, and their level of responsibility in relationship to the outcomes of the services provided? If the answers are positive, the delegation plan and methods selected were appropriate to the situation.

Employee Evaluation

A major part of the community health nurse manager's role is performing employee evaluations. The function of employee evaluation is sometimes perceived as a dreaded task by both manager and employee. Frequently, managers have not been formally trained in the process and are just told to do it. Consequently, the experience may be negative for both the manager and the employee despite an employee rating of outstanding. Prior to performing an employee evaluation, read the agency's personnel manual or the agency's policy and procedures documents. (It is important for both manager and employees to read official agency documents and for sessions to be provided to discuss the documents.) Then review job descriptions and make yourself familiar with the performance level expected for each employee.

The purpose of an employee evaluation is to measure and communicate to the employee a picture of his or her accomplishments toward the goals and objectives of the organization. Employee job descriptions should reflect the goals and objectives of the organization, as well as standards of role performance. (Chapter 16 discusses standards of practice [expected performance levels] for community health nurses according to educational preparation.) It is helpful to compare the nursing job descriptions of a health agency to the practice standards.

The process of employee evaluation should be standardized and objective; an evaluation can be considered as a scheduled feedback session for an employee. It should be in writing and should include sections for employee self-evaluation, as well as for evaluation by the nurse manager. The evaluation should be reviewed during a one-to-one session with time allowed for discussion. An evaluation can encourage an employee to achieve individual potentials and can challenge further growth. A performance evaluation should identify the employee's strengths and weaknesses in role performance and thus provide the information necessary for planning educational and professional development goals.

Unfortunately, performance evaluations tend to be annual and to be the *only* instance of evaluation. The employee may be totally surprised by the evaluation and unable to account for reasons for either positive or negative performance. Meaningful feedback must be given during the entire year. It is important for the manager to make notes and keep records of specific occasions or incidents, both positive and negative, that are critical to job performance. Incidents provide documentation for the annual performance evaluation. The most valuable asset of an organization are its employees. Employee evaluation time should be an event that both the manager and employee anticipate positively.

The interpersonal skills of the management role have been reviewed. These skills include, but are not limited to, communication, delegation, and employee evaluation. Of equal importance, however, are other skills of the management role that may be categorized as technical skills.

TECHNICAL SKILLS
OF THE MANAGEMENT ROLE

The community health nurse in the management role must have expertise in many areas of technical skills. One very important category of technical skill is resource allocation. Without appropriate resource allocation many worthwhile programs may be inadequate or unsuccessful.

Resource Allocation

The allocation of both human and material resources is a crucial skill of the management role in community health nursing. To understand how resources are allocated, a discussion of some basic principles of systems is useful. Recall that a system is a whole that functions because of the interdependence of its parts. The parts of a system are usually termed *subsystems.* An organization can be considered a system composed of subsystems. Examples of subsystems within an organization might include the nursing staff, the clerical personnel, nursing services, and laboratory functions. Each subsystem of the organization is a resource. Additionally, a community is a system composed of subsystems, and it functions because of the interdependence of its subsystems. In the Rosemont sample case, when the community subsystems were assessed, the data were analyzed to determine health needs.

> STOP! Consider the assessed health needs of your community (*e.g.,* inadequate primary care services for the elderly, inaccessible dental services, lack of hospice care, no recreational program for youngsters). Form a mental picture of those services that are needed, or list them on a piece of paper. Now consider the services that are available from any organization in the community (*e.g.,* the health department) and form a second mental picture of those available services, and list them. Superimpose one system on the other, looking for matches between needs and services, and you have begun the process of resource allocation.

Resource allocation is the process of *matching* the assessed needs of a community to the available resources in the organization. To allocate resources, an assessment and analysis of the organization must be first completed. How can an organization be assessed? You've completed an assessment and analysis of a community, can that same process be applied to an organization?

Our familiar Community Assessment Wheel can also be used as an organizational assessment model (see Fig. 6-1). People are still the core of the model. In an organization, the people are the agency personnel—the nursing personnel, clerical staff, and laboratory technicians. Beginning with the physical environment subsystem, what should be assessed? Perhaps you want to assess the size and condition of the building or buildings, the number and size of rooms inside the building, and the condition and function of each room. How much space is allocated to group education, private counseling, and client physical examination? Equally important, how do staff feel the space should be used? For example, do staff want additional space for group education, or for a lounge and eating area for themselves? (Or both?) What are the priorities of administration for the space? Have policies been mandated that new services be provided (*e.g.,* blood-pressure screening) that will in turn require space?

Once an assessment of each subsystem in the community is completed, before resources can be allocated or matched, we must identify the community's need for that resource. For example, what are the ages of the clients who use the agency's physical resource of space? All children need to play. If children are served by the agency, is there an area for play? If the predominant populations served are generally aged, frail, or handicapped, are there access ramps and railed stairs? In addition, because most health facilities provide care to both healthy and ill individuals, is the space so divided that ill individuals are not in contact with healthy persons? Once each subsystem has been assessed and the needs of the community have been considered, the process of allocating each resource begins—the act of matching resources to health needs. The process of resource allocation is the same for each subsystem of the organization.

Conflict during resource allocation is inevitable. Community health needs always exceed available resources. It must be decided which programs will receive allocated resources and which programs must be postponed. How are allocation-of-resources decisions made? Established goals and objectives based on the community nursing diagnosis and agency directives can help in making difficult decisions. For example, in official public health agencies, such as state, county, and city health departments, legislative action results in laws that must be enacted. It is law in all states that immunizations be provided, as well as screening tests and treatment for sexually transmitted diseases (STD) and tuberculosis.

Creative use of nursing time can meet both required services and assessed health service needs. For example, all states require immunization services and most persons who require immunizations are children. Children must be accompanied to immunization appointments by a parent or guardian. (We now have access to both a parent and a child, both of whom usually are healthy and receptive to health information.) During immunization administration, a major nursing responsibility is to inform the parent (and child, if old enough) about the purpose and importance of an immunization, as well as how to assess for adverse reactions (*i.e.,* fever, lethargy) and to perform the correct home treatments (*i.e.,* type, dosage, and administration of antipyretics). Therefore, as the "required service" of immunizations are completed, health information can be offered.

> SOMETHING TO CONSIDER: It is a known fact that when parents learn information and thus increase their confidence in their ability to care for their children, feelings of parental worth and self-esteem are elevated. With experience, parents can feel competent to assess their child physically for illness and to initiate care. As a result, the anxiety and stress surrounding common childhood illnesses are reduced for all family members. In turn, the child's health is improved as parents offer early assessment and prompt intervention. What began as a "required service" can be combined with creative nursing to have major health promotion implications. (As always, it is important to assess what information parents and children desire to have. To establish educational needs, a survey or questionnaire can be helpful. Refer to Chapter 8 for a discussion on how to design, distribute, and analyze a survey instrument.)

Goals and objectives

Resource allocation should produce the best possible mix of health services to meet assessed community health needs, fulfill legal mandates, and be consistent with established agency policy. *Goals and objectives* can facilitate resource allocation. As with community health program planning and the essential partnership relationship that must exist between a community health nurse and the community, organizational goals and objectives require the active involvement of staff and personnel. If they have been agreed upon mutually, the staff will feel a sense of ownership, and responsibility for the completion of the goals and objectives. Usually staff have the best appraisal of whether or not a goal is realistic, timely, and measurable. Goals and objectives can be used to direct services and allocate resources, but equally important, goals can generate budgets, and design job descriptions and employee performance evaluations.

When beginning the process of goal setting, consider these five questions.

What are the primary elements to consider? (*i.e.,* space, personnel, budget, time)

Who needs to be involved? (*i.e.,* laboratory staff, clerical personnel)

What are the obstacles? (*i.e.,* inadequate physical space, lack of prepared staff, insufficient time)

What is the role of the nurse manager? (*i.e.,* supervisor, evaluator, teacher)

What is the role of each person involved? (*i.e.,* home-care nurse specialist, referral nurse)

Once these questions have been answered, you are ready to specify the goals and objectives. (Refer to Chapter 8 for a discussion of the process of writing goals and objectives, and for sources in the Suggested Reading list.)

During the writing of goals and objectives, it is most effective for the community health nurse manager to first *expect* staff participation in the process (by arranging formal blocks of time for this purpose away from service delivery) and then to *facilitate* that process (with instruction and examples). After nursing diagnoses and health problems have been identified, each staff member should individually answer the above five questions. For example, if the assessed community need is for improved access of teenagers to health information and primary care, and the goal is to establish a health clinic for teenagers that will be located at the public high school, then each of the what and who questions must be answered with regard to the clinic for teens. Mutual goal setting requires consensus, or the agreement, of the group. One method of achieving consensus is to use either the nominal group or Delphi techniques.

Nominal group technique

Recall from Chapter 10 that the nominal group uses a structured group meeting, during which all individuals are given a judgment task such as to list the obstacles that block the implementation of a teen clinic at the high school. Each staff member is asked to write down their ideas and to not discuss them with others. At the end of 5 to 10 minutes, all members present their ideas and each is recorded so all members can see the list, but the ideas are not discussed as they are being recorded. Once all obstacles have been presented, a discussion follows, during which time ideas are clarified and evaluated. (Frequently, additional information will resolve an apparent obstacle.) Following the discussion, there is a vote on the priority ranking of the obstacles that the group wants to address. The nominal group technique allows for all individuals to present their ideas before the entire group. Involving the entire group decreases the problem of selective perception and promotes individual participation because each individual was involved in the decision-making process.

Delphi technique

A modification of the Delphi technique is helpful if staff are separated by distance and cannot convene for regularly scheduled meetings. The Delphi technique involves a series of questionnaires and feedback reports to all staff. For example, a list of potential obstacles to the teen clinic could be distributed to all staff members by mail, accompanied with questions about the validity of these obstacles. Staff can independently generate their responses and return the questionnaire. Based on the responses of the group, a feedback report and questions are sent again to the staff. Using the feedback information, the respondents evaluate their first responses and complete the questionnaire again. The process continues for a predetermined number of feedback rounds, or until consensus is reached.

Summary

Obviously, resource allocation is an important skill of the nurse manager in community health nursing. To effectively allocate resources, begin by assessing the resources of the organization, match the resources to the assessed health needs of the community, and then use goals and objectives to establish the best possible service delivery plan. This is an exciting and challenging role. However, equally exciting and challenging to the nurse manager is the technical skill of marketing, for to ensure success, all programs must be marketed.

Marketing

Marketing is the act of buying and selling, and is a basic function of any society. However, only in recent years have seminars, books, and media attention been directed to the process of selling health. Community health nurses have always taught and stressed the importance of health promoting practices (such as balanced nutrition and adequate rest) and the environmental health requirements of clean air and safe food. However, as was discussed in Chapter 1, the health care system changed dramatically in the 1980s—deregulation of the system by the government initiated fierce competition between health agencies that subsequently produced advertising directed at potential consumers. Alternative delivery systems (ADS) proliferated alongside new reimbursement arrangements such as diagnostic related groups (DRG). Services such as screening and immunizations, once offered exclusively by official nonprofit agencies (*e.g.,* the health department) to targeted populations (*e.g.,* the indigent), were now offered to the same clients by private for-profit agencies. What does all this mean for the manager in community health nursing?

The public, regardless of age, ethnicity, or geographic location, wants convenient and affordable health care that meets perceived needs and is delivered in a professional, caring manner. Community health nurses are in the best position to offer acceptable and affordable health care because of their unique partnership with the community. Marketing parallels the nursing process. To market community health nursing services, first assess what needs exist and identify who or what is the target of the nursing product. For example, the homeless population may have a high incidence of STD, or the young unmarried persons in a community may feel isolated and experience stress-induced illnesses of depression and anxiety. Once needs have been assessed (following community assessment and analysis), the planning of needed services begins. As always, it is important to include consumers in the planning process in order to establish what types of services and service providers are acceptable.

Once a plan is completed, then resources (*e.g.,* space, personnel, supplies) must be allocated to the service. The board of the agency or chief executive officer will probably need to be convinced of the need for the program (and the associated reallocation of the budget). Present the plan to the board along with clearly identified goals, objectives, a time schedule for implementation, and expected outcomes that can be measured in terms of improved health. Presentation to administration is a vital part of the marketing process.

Once the plan is approved, then market to the target population in the community. Media releases such as public service announcements, flyers, and notices in community-gathering places, as well as notices in local newspapers, will inform the community about the specifics of the program. Allow sufficient time to adequately inform the community about the service and then be prepared with adequate staff and supplies to provide the service that has been marketed.

The final step in the marketing process is the evaluation of the program. Use the goals and objectives for measurement. Ask the consumers about satisfaction. Query staff about their perceptions of the adequacy of service delivery and associated cost. Finally, measure whether or not the program has improved health. Is there a lower rate of STD among the homeless after a screening, diagnosis, treatment, and education program? Do young unmarried persons report less perceived isolation and fewer stress-induced illnesses after implementation of support groups, a crisis hotline, and stress-reduction classes?

Budgeting

Frequently budgets are thought of as time-consuming, necessary evils. However, with appropriate skills, constructing a budget can become a time-efficient skill, which in turn will greatly aid the community health nurse manager.

Budgeting is actually the translation of organizational goals and objectives into dollars and cents. A budget is a tool that the nurse manager can use to estimate future needs and resources. The purpose of a budget is also to apportion systematically the expenditures of resources that will occur during a given period of time.

In determining the content of a nursing budget, there are three categories of activities that most agencies use to group costs. These categories are *manpower costs, operational costs,* and *capital expenses.* Probably the largest expense in the nursing budget will be the manpower costs of the salaries and employee benefits of nurses and other support staff. The operational costs most often are charges for utilities, rent, cost of supplies, travel expenses, janitorial services, and so forth. Capital expenses include such items as major pieces of equipment, the cost of bulk buying of supplies, or the construction or renovation of a building. Capital expenses are long-range in nature versus the short-range scope of operational expenses. The nurse manager must be familiar with the agency's formal budget policies, procedures, forms, calendar, and process for gaining final approval of the budget.

When the nurse manager is beginning the budget process for the purpose of planning a new program, there are several considerations that need to be examined. First, the manager must be clear on the goals and objectives for the new service. Statistical data regarding the population to be served—how many clients, average number of visits, and so forth—are needed to plan the budget. Specifying the time period that the budget will cover is also important. Many budgets use a fiscal year, and many are subdivided into monthly, quarterly, or semiannual periods. Once these areas have been covered, the manager begins to identify and justify all expenditures in the categories of manpower, operational, and capital expense.

The manpower category must take into consideration the skills of the nursing staff that will be needed to deliver the service, and if this staff will work full-time or part-time on delivering the service. The number and type of staff needed must be converted to the agency pay scale and allocated based on the amount of time spent delivering particular services. Other personnel expenses should be charged to the new service when they can be identified as adding expenses to the program. Examples might be a clerk assigned on a part-time (50%) basis or additional laboratory personnel needed one-quarter time (25%) to support the new service. If personnel services are provided to the agency at no cost, (*e.g.,* a nurse consultant from the state health department) then that cost should not be charged to the service. Computation of fringe benefits such as retirement, insurance, and so forth should follow agency policy. Frequently, 33% of salary equals fringe benefits.

In the operational expenditure category, the major items of expense are rent, staff travel, supplies, utilities, and other miscellaneous costs. If rent is paid, the amount may be based on a flat fee that has been negotiated with the landlord to cover a specified period of time. That fee may or may not include certain utilities or housekeeping expenses. Often the service may be held in a building that is shared by other agencies or with other programs within the nurse manager's agency. One way of determining the amount that the new program should be charged is to base the rent on the percentage of square footage that it occupies in the building. Utilities and supplies may be computed in somewhat the same manner. The cost of supplies and equipment should be based on the kind of program and standard of care to be delivered. An example would be if every child served in the Child Health Program, either at 6 months of age or at admittance, were to have a hematocrit performed; the nurse manager should be able to estimate how many capillary tubes would be needed.

Travel expenses are based on the agency's rates of reimbursement for mileage and per diem. When possible the nurse manager may want to look at historical data of already-established programs and estimate travel expenses based on that data. Again, the manager may find that the best way to estimate travel is to base it on standards of care (average number of home visits for a high-risk infant and average distance that will be driven). Other considerations are staff meetings that require travel and continuing-education needs of staff and the incurred expenses.

In the category of capital expenses, the nurse manager will have to determine the major items such as furniture and office equipment that are needed. The expenditure with these items will be based either on actual costs, or on estimates obtained from retail companies or the agency's purchasing agent. If

Time period of budget: _____

Budget title

Category description	Source of funds	Budgeted amount	Expenditures	Balance
Salaries: Employee benefits:				
Operational costs:				
Capitol outlay:				
Budget total				

Figure 14-1.   Budget Format

a comparable amount of equipment is to be replaced every year, a standard cost can be used. When a major expenditure is necessary, agencies usually adjust the cost over several years by some method of depreciation. Depreciation simply spreads the cost over the expected lifespan of the item.

Another part of the budget that the nurse manager needs to estimate is income generated by the program. This will depend on the kind of agency in which the manager is employed. In most official agencies, income is generated through third-party reimbursement (*e.g.,* private insurance or Medicare), or through fees that are charged for services to individual clients or groups of clients. It is important to know if the income generated by a program remains with the program or returns to the total budget of the agency. How closely the nurse manager must balance program expenditure with program income will be determined by agency policy, philosophy, and funding source.

To evaluate your understanding about budgets, use Figure 14-1 and the following information to draft an annual and monthly budget for a new child health program.

Data Input

The State Health Department will provide one salary for a public health nurse at $28,000 with no employee benefits. They will also provide $5000 to be used for physician fees. The city government will budget $50,000/year and the program has received a grant of $17,000/year from a private foundation. The total monies committed to the new child health program is $100,000.

A facility shared by two other agencies is available. The total rent for the facility is $2000/month. The new program will need at least one-third of the total space. Utilities have averaged $250/month for each of the other two agencies. Most of the clinic equipment will be donated by a local civic group, but supplies, office equipment, desks, chairs, and waiting room furniture must be purchased by the child health program.

SUMMARY

The management role in community health nursing includes the use of the management process to link resources and accomplish goals and objectives. Management is a dynamic process that requires decision making, interpersonal skills, and the technical expertise of resource allocation, budgeting, and marketing. It is the manager who must be aware of community health needs and proceed to match those needs to services and resources of the health agency. Management requires ongoing assessment of the organization, and the ordering in priority of services, and the evaluation of outcomes. Regardless of your position and job description in community health nursing, management skills will be important to optimally perform your role as a community health nurse.

SUGGESTED READINGS

The Management Process

Clark CC, Shea CA: Management in Nursing: A Vital Link in the Health Care System. New York, McGraw-Hill Co, 1979

del Bueno DJ, Sheridan DR: Developing prospective managers, Part 3. J Nurs Adm 14(6):23–27, 1984

del Bueno DJ, Walker DD: Developing prospective managers, Part 1. J Nurs Adm 14(4):7–10, 1984

Jackson–Webb ML: Team building: Key to executive success. J Nurs Adm 15(2):16–20, 1985

Kraegel JM: Planning Strategies for Nurse Managers. Rockville, Maryland, Aspen Publications, 1983

McClure ML: Managing the professional nurse, Part I. J Nurs Adm 14(2):15–21, 1984

McClure ML: Managing the professional nurse, Part II. J Nurs Adm 14(4):7–10, 1984

Peterson ME, Allen DG: Shared governance: A strategy transforming organizations, Part 1. J Nurs Adm 16(1):9–12, 1986

Sheridan DR, DiJulio JE, Vivenzo K: Developing prospective managers, Part II. J Nurs Adm 14(5):23–28, 1984

Communication

Kraegel JM: Planning Strategies for Nurse Managers. Rockville, Maryland, Aspen Publications, 1983

Marriner A: Guide to Nursing Management, pp 154–163. St. Louis, CV Mosby, 1980

Munn HE Jr, Metzger N: Effective Communication in Health Care: A Supervisor's Handbook. Rockville, Maryland, Aspen Publications, 1981

Roberts KH, O'Reilly CA III: Failures in upward communication in organizations: Three possible culprits. Academy of Management Journal 17(2):205–213, 1974

Spradley BW: Community Health Nursing Concepts and Practice. Boston, Little, Brown & Co, 1981

Budget

Hanlon JJ, Pickett GE: Public Health Administration and Practice. St. Louis, Times Mirror/Mosby Publication, 1984

Kraegel JM: Planning Strategies for Nurse Managers. Rockville, Maryland, Aspen Publication, 1983

Marriner A: Guide to Nursing Management, pp 32–37. St. Louis, CV Mosby, 1980

Employee Evaluation

Burchett SR, DeMeuse KP: Performance appraisal and the how. Personnel 62(9):29–37, 1985

Kaye BL: Performance appraisal and career development: A shotgun marriage. Personnel 61(2):57–66, 1984

Metzger N: Personnel Administration in the Health Services Industry. New York, SP Medical and Scientific Books/Division of Spectrum Publications, Inc, 1979

Moravec M: How performance appraisal can tie communication to productivity. Personnel Administrator Jan:51, 1981

Meyer AL: A framework for assessing performance problems. J Nurs Adm 14(5):40–43, 1984

Resource Allocation

Kirkpatrick SL: Nurses: Leaders in wellness. Occup Health Nurs 33(9):450–452, 1985

Sheahan SL, Aaron PR: Community assessment: An essential component of practice. Health Values: Achieving High Level Wellness 7(5):12–15, 1983

Marketing

Dugan DB: Expanding nursing's practice terrain: Imperatives for future viability. Pub Health Nurs 2(1):23–32, 1985

Skinner P: Community Health Services: Marketing Community Health Services. New York, National League for Nursing, 1979

15

The Research Role in Community Health Nursing

OBJECTIVES

In Chapter 2, the steps of the research process were carefully delineated and the development of a research study was described. In this chapter, emphasis has been placed on the need for research and the means for integrating research into the staff-nurse role. After studying this chapter, you will be able to

- Describe the importance of research for the profession and for the practice of the community health nurse
- Briefly describe the history of research in community health nursing and the needs that have been identified for the present and future in community health nursing
- Analyze the causes and solutions for problems in the dissemination and use of research findings
- Use research findings
- Conduct research

INTRODUCTION

In Chapter 2 research was defined as "a structured process used to acquire new knowledge or verify existing information" accomplished "through verifiable examination of data and empirical testing of hypotheses." The activities suggested by this definition may not fit your picture of the everyday activities of a beginning community health nurse, but take time to consider the importance of research for the discipline of nursing and for the field of community health nursing.

In tracing the history of nursing research, Notter (1974) indicated that it was not until the middle to late 1950s that research became a goal for the nursing profession. The 1960s brought the beginnings of the focusing of nursing research on clinical practice. Prior to that time, the majority of the studies were of nurses and were conducted by non-nurses (Notter, 1974). It was not until the 1970s that clinical practice was dealt with in a significant portion of the nursing research.

Community health nursing has its own history of research. History buffs will enjoy reading "Abstracts in Public Health Nursing (1924–1957)" by Hilbert (1959). This compilation includes brief descriptions of all published research related to public health nursing during the specified time period. Reviews of more recent research related to community health nursing have been completed by Highriter (1977, 1984) and cover the periods from 1972 to 1976, and 1977 to 1981. In her most recent review, Highriter (1984) recommended that community health nursing develop a theoretical framework for practice, use that framework as a basis for research, and focus on major practice problems. She further recommended increased use of experimental and quasi-experimental designs, and of replications of previous studies. She clearly believes that community health nursing has made progress but, like in other specialties, a great deal more needs to be done.

Although our history indicates that nursing is a relative newcomer to research, the field's leaders have identified its essential place. Schlotfeldt (1960) stated the need to develop nursing theory as a guide to practice and in order to yield a body of scientific knowledge for the profession. The position of the American Nurses' Association (ANA) (1981b) is

> *Accountability to the public for the human use of knowledge in providing effective and high quality services is the hallmark of a profession. Thus, the preeminent goal of scientific inquiry by nurses is the ongoing development of knowledge for use in the practice of nursing.*

Development of nursing theory and of a body of scientific knowledge cannot be accomplished by academicians working in isolation. Practitioners at all levels must be involved to achieve real progress.

The needs of the profession as a whole may not be uppermost in the mind of the beginning community health nurse. But on a daily basis, she needs to be knowledgeable with regard to research findings, and then apply them to clinical practice with clients. This role as a consumer of research, and the nurse's role in using, sharing, and conducting research will be described in this chapter.

The ANA Commission on Nursing Research (1981a) has delineated the research activities that are appropriate to nurses prepared at various educational levels. For nurses prepared at the baccalaureate level in nursing, appropriate activities are

1. Reads, interprets, and evaluates research for applicability to nursing practice
2. Identifies nursing problems that need to be investigated and participates in the implementation of scientific studies
3. Uses nursing practice as a means of gathering data for refining and extending practice
4. Applies established findings of nursing and other health-related research to nursing practice
5. Shares research findings with colleagues

Basically, the research role of the community health nurse has two levels: consumer, or conductor. All nurses must be responsible consumers of research if they are to provide quality care to clients. In addition, some nurses will also be involved in conducting research.

THE CONSUMER ROLE

Everyone understands what *consumer* means: one that consumes (uses), or one that purchases. But in research, what does the consumer role mean to the community health nurse? It means using existing research, but—is the existing research valid and reliable, and how frequently has use been documented?

Research Utilization

Using research findings may appear to be an easy task. Nursing students are often instructed that their practice must be research-based, therefore they believe that it is! This idea has become an accepted tenet, one so widely written and spoken that if the author of this chapter had a nickel for each time a nurse said her practice was research-based she could happily retire to a Caribbean island! But can you identify a research base for all of your practice? For both the process and the content of your interventions? And then relate them to client outcomes? No one can do this.

So much of nursing practice has been based upon tradition and intuition. Over 15 years ago, the report of the National Commission for the Student of Nursing and Nursing Education (Lysaught, 1970) stated

> *In the past, nursing has not conducted sufficient research into its own practice. . . . Of necessity, nursing practice today consists of stereo-typed techniques sprinkled liberally with personal idiosyncrasy. . . . Since we have not developed valid means for assessing the effects of varied interventions, it is almost impossible to define optimum nursing care.*

Some progress has been made in terms of increasing the number and significance of nursing research studies. There are relevant research findings in existence; and nursing is slowly building its necessary research base, but the research findings are not readily implemented into practice. However, if you are going to provide quality care to clients, it is necessary to know the relevant research findings and use them in practice. A number of nurse leaders have addressed research-utilization issues and their articles are recommended in order to develop a more complete understanding of the issues (Fawcett, 1982; Horsley *et al,* 1978; Krueger, 1978, 1979; Loomis, 1985; Stetler, 1985; in the Suggested Readings list). The primary problems that interfere with the utilization of research findings by practitioners and staff nurses are

1. There is no systematic process to move results of research studies from the researchers to the practitioners.
2. When research findings are published, in numerous and diverse publications, they are usually written in a form suitable for communication with other researchers, not with practitioners.
3. Because of the form in which the reports are written, it may be difficult for practitioners to understand the report and evaluate the quality of the study.
4. It usually is inappropriate to attempt to use research findings unless certain criteria regarding quality, generalizability, and replication have been met.
5. The staff nurse does not have the time, nor usually the inclination or access to the publications, to search out a number of studies on a similar topic, evaluate their quality, synthesize their results, and develop a plan for implementing the findings.

To solve these problems, the federally funded Conduct and Utilization of Research in Nursing (CURN) project (under the Division of Nursing from

1977 to 1982) developed a model for facilitating the use of research findings. Project staff reviewed all extant nursing research, identified similar studies, and assessed their quality and the similarity of findings. Where an area of research met all the criteria and was determined to be ready to be implemented into practice, a protocol was developed. It is indicative of the state of research in nursing that there were only ten areas where protocols could be developed (CURN Project, 1982).

- Pain: Deliberative nursing interventions
- Structured preoperative teaching
- Reducing diarrhea in tube-fed patients
- Preoperative sensory preparation to promote recovery
- Preventing decubitus ulcers
- Intravenous cannula change
- Closed urinary-drainage systems
- Distress reduction through sensory preparation
- Mutual goal setting in patient care
- Clean intermittent catheterization

Each protocol is a "written document that transforms the individual studies in a research base into a synthesized whole, translates research jargon into clinical jargon, and addresses issues surrounding the use of the new knowledge in practice" (CURN Project, 1983). In addition, the CURN Project published the text *Using Research to Improve Nursing Practice: A Guide,* which offers useful, detailed guidelines for implementing research (CURN Project, 1983).

Research on Research Utilization

Identifying and testing methods to promote the use of research findings has become an area of research in and of itself. Major findings from studies on research use or dissemination are

1. Nurses' awareness of research that questions restrictions on myocardial infarction patients was significantly correlated with the number of journals and the hours per week spent reading (Kirchoff, 1982).
2. Nurses' knowledge of the Centers of Disease Control's (CDC) guidelines for the prevention of catheter-associated urinary-tract infections was positively associated with participation, external resources, and professional continuing learning. Participation was defined as the level of nurse participation in nursing department activities, the nursing department's level of

participation within the hospital, and the means of communication between staff nurses and nurse administrators. External resources were defined as the number of outside speakers presenting at the hospital per year (paid for by the nursing department). Professional continuing learning was measured by a scale, which included items regarding amount of reading, participation in professional associations, and enrollment in courses and workshops (Butler, 1986).

3. Nurses were not knowledgeable regarding proper temperature-taking techniques even though research findings in reference to these techniques had been in the literature for more than five years (Ketefian, 1975).

4. Nurses in community agencies reported that their practice was based upon research findings (who would say otherwise?) and that the majority of their agencies were supportive of implementing research findings. However, only about one-fourth had access to research journals in their agency libraries (Krueger, 1982).

While these studies have not been sufficiently replicated to generalize to all settings, the findings do suggest that the individual nurse must assume responsibility for being up-to-date in her practice.

To summarize, nurses' activities related to being knowledgeable were: subscribing to professional journals, reading professional journals, enrolling in workshops and educational courses, and participating in professional committees in the worksetting. Other activities such as the nursing department's participation within the rest of the agency, the means of communication between nursing administrators and staff nurses, and the agency's financial support of external speakers are not under the control of the staff nurse. But staff nurses can encourage, promote, or bargain for organizational and administrative mechanisms to enhance their continued learning.

In addition to considering the approaches suggested by the research studies, an additional option is a "Journal Club" in the workplace. As a group, the club selects an article of interest each month, each member reads it, and the group meets to discuss, evaluate, and analyze its implications for practice. After they have reviewed a number of research reports regarding similar studies, Journal Club members may be able over time to develop a protocol for research to be implemented into practice.

As long as you acknowledge that the responsibility for being an informed practitioner is yours, you will be able to develop creative ways to keep up to date. Unsurprisingly, being knowledgeable about research findings is essential to conducting research.

THE CONDUCTOR ROLE

As a conductor of research, your role will include setting priorities for research. Also included in this role is recognition that to obtain the most useful results, research should be based upon a solid framework. However, one of the most important aspects of the role as conductor of research is the first step—initiation of research—or getting started.

Priorities for Research

As was stated in Chapter 2, you are not yet expected to conduct research that will solve the nation's health problems. The carefully described epidemiological study of the validity of Spanish-surname infant-mortality rates (Chapter 2) might be difficult for a staff level nurse to conduct independently, especially when the competing needs for services are considered. However, research is rarely a solo activity. The nurse may identify a need through her observations of her practice and then recruit others to be involved in the study or even to conduct most of it. More importantly, this type of epidemiological study may have already been conducted through the state department of public health; thus, it is crucial to review available data prior to beginning a study.

In addition to being very clear that the study you want to do has not already been done and sufficiently replicated, give some thought to what the priorities for the research are in terms of both your practice and the needs of the profession. The ANA has determined priorities for research, (1981a) stating that priority should be given to the nursing research projects that would generate knowledge to guide practice in

1. Promoting health, well-being, and competency for personal care among all age groups
2. Preventing health problems throughout the life-span that have the potential to reduce productivity and personal satisfaction
3. Decreasing the negative impact of health problems on coping abilities, productivity, and life satisfaction of individuals and families
4. Ensuring that the care needs of particularly vulnerable groups are met through appropriate strategies
5. Designing and developing health care systems that are cost-effective in meeting the nursing needs of the population
6. Promoting health, well-being, and competency for personal health in all age groups

Lindeman (1975) surveyed priorities for clinical nursing research. The majority of the 15 most important areas that needed research related to quality of nursing care and evaluation of patient outcomes. Bloch (1975) emphasized the importance of evaluating nursing care in terms of both process and outcomes. Community health nursing practice was considered by Barkauskas (1982) from the perspective of an educator. She identified the need to describe and document practice, and to obtain data regarding the effectiveness of preventive services.

As an example of describing and documenting practice, a number of researchers have demonstrated the effects of home visits upon maternal–infant clients (Carpenter *et al*, 1983; Hall, 1980; Kelly, 1983; Olds *et al*, 1986; Stanwick *et al*, 1982; in the Suggested Readings list). However, none of the authors has reported explicitly what occurred during these home visits. While the intent of these studies may have been to describe and document nursing practice, insufficient attention was given to the process. Without specific descriptions of the process and content of the home visits, it is not possible to effectively replicate the studies, nor to use the findings.

In reference to obtaining data regarding effectiveness of preventive services, Fagin (1982) stated there is data to substantiate nurses' effectiveness in health care delivery; however, "the plethora of data about nursing contributions is unknown to the public and barely known to nurses themselves."

In these studies, researchers did demonstrate effectiveness in health care delivery in terms of outcomes of services. However, the effectiveness of delivery was not directly linked to nursing interventions. This was also true for nurses in Santa Clara County, California, who, to avoid an 87% budget cut, were forced to identify their contributions and describe them to community leaders, decision makers, and clients (Couser *et al*, 1986). The nurses labeled their effort as an "effective marketing campaign," but the information they so efficiently disseminated provided data regarding cost-effectiveness of nursing services; and their campaign could not have been successful without these data.

Chapter 10 described the need to evaluate health programs and offered guidance in regard to nonexperimental and experimental designs for evaluation. Although there may be a gray area between where program evaluation ends and research begins, the experimental approaches to program evaluation are certainly research. It is often difficult to document the prevention of an illness or injury, but community health nursing must have such records in order to ensure the practice's survival; this is especially true during periods of concern over cost containment. There is a universal recognition of the need for nursing to test alternative interventions and to document their effectiveness, but it must also be understood that epidemiologic or descriptive re-search may be required in order to identify a problem so that such testing can be possible.

The general, formal definition of research appeared at the beginning of this chapter, but within this definition are varying levels of formality in project design. Some in the field refer to two different kinds of research—*R*esearch and *r*esearch. Research with *R* refers to formal studies, developed step-by-step, that follow the guidelines in Chapter 2. Research with *r* refers to the less formal studies. These may include analysis of a diary of your work with certain types of clients, a conscious attempt to use two different interventions with two similar groups and compare the results, or a summary of your observations of the characteristics of attendees at a specific clinic. Research spelled with *r* is part of your everyday practice; it is incorporated into data collection and analysis, in addition to its use in the intervention and evaluation components of the nursing process.

Framework for Research

Whether it is through research with *R* or *r*, there is general agreement on the need to evaluate community health nursing practice. Using a framework to guide the research will yield more useful results. A relevant conceptual frame-work, based upon a systems approach, was developed by Flynn (1977) to evaluate community health nursing practice. Assumptions within the design of this framework are: (1) community health nurses view the community as their clients, (2) the impact of community health nursing services will need to be measured in relation to services to individuals/families in population groups, and (3) community health nurses work in collaboration with interdisciplinary health care providers. Flynn identified four dimensions in the framework:

The *environment* surrounds structure, process, and outcome. The environment is viewed through several levels of analyses (such as city, county, state, and nation). A wide range of variables are incorporated in the environment: population characteristics, including demography, lifestyle, and health levels; level of health technology; health legislation; and geographic characteristics, including climate and transportation.

Structure is the particular community health nursing organization that is under study. It may be a health program, a one-nurse agency, an interdisciplinary community health center, a state health department, or any unit or organization providing community health nursing services. Structure variables include: organization size, policies, finances, staffing patterns, and so forth.

Process incorporates the interface between community health nursing organization or program, and the client. Examples of process variables are: nursing-client encounter (*e.g.,* home visit, clinic visit, telephone), the client's health problems, the nursing services provided, and the utilization of the services by the client.

Outcome is the result of the community health nursing practice on clients' health knowledge, behaviors, and attitudes. Outcome variables include: morbidity, health knowledge, immunization levels, consumer prices, satisfactions, and so forth.

This framework indicates that structure, process, and outcome interact with the environment of which they are a part. Structure, process, and outcome directly influence each other. Change in any one part of the system creates change in other dimensions of the system.

Flynn presented tabular examples of variables within each component of the framework. Process variables and their indicators, with outcome indicators for each variable, are illustrated in Table 15-1. These process variables and indicators are subdivided according to the three levels of prevention (primary, secondary, and tertiary). A review of Table 15-1 will provide helpful examples for the development of research studies to measure process and outcome of nursing interventions.

Use of Flynn's research framework for the evaluation of community health nursing practice suggests a quantitative approach to research; this approach was described in Chapter 2. The term *quantitative* refers to data being measured in numerical terms. However, *qualitative* research uses some of the research steps outlined in Chapter 2, but collects the data, analyzes and reports it through narrative descriptions, rather than with numerical values. Qualitative research can contribute a great deal to increasing the quality of care provided by nurses. Owing to the type of priorities and needs that have been identified for community health nursing, this book has been focused on the quantitative approach. Qualitative approaches could offer an excellent possibility for research you might conduct in the field. Two relevant articles in the Suggested Readings list, Oiler (1982) and Swanson *et al* (1982) will help you identify how you might use the qualitative approach in research.

Guide for Getting Started

To initiate a study requires careful planning. Chapter 2 gave specific examples of activities related to the steps of the research process. Guidance is provided below on the all-important first two steps.

TABLE 15-1.   INDICATORS OF COMMUNITY HEALTH NURSING SERVICES AND OUTCOMES OF THESE SERVICES

Process Variables and Indicators	Outcome Indicators
Primary prevention (health promotion and specific protection)	
Assistance in identifying growth and development behavior appropriate for family members	Knowledge of growth and development; expectations of children's behavior appropriate to age and sex
Assistance in social and psychological adjustment to changing lifestyles	Social and psychological satisfaction and functioning
Assistance in identifying strengths and weaknesses of communication patterns	Knowledge of family communication patterns
Assistance with planning normal diet within a fixed budget	Adequate family nutrition habits
Assistance in obtaining immunizations and boosters	Increased immunization level in the population and decreased reporting of immunizable disease
Secondary prevention (early diagnosis and prompt treatment)	
Consumer advocate in health planning for health-screening program	Identification of early disease states
Educate to participate in health-screening programs	Increased participation in screening clinics; identification of early disease states
Referrals to other health team members to meet specialized needs	Appropriate utilization of community health resources
Assistance in adjusting treatment regimen to family lifestyle	Compliance with treatment regimen, reduction of disability limitation
Tertiary prevention (rehabilitation)	
Disease control counseling including medications and special diets	Compliance with medication and special diets; reduction in further complications
Provision of home nursing care to the sick including medication administration, bathing, assistance with exercises	Family maintained as a group without institutionalization of sick member; reduction in discomfort of sick member; maintenance of activities of daily living
Assistance in identifying alternatives in order to cope with illness and management of health care	Family selfhelp established; appropriate utilization of community health resources

(Flynn BC: Research framework for evaluating community health nursing practice. In Miller MH, Flynn BC (eds): Current Perspectives in Nursing: Social Issues and Trends, p 41. St Louis, CV Mosby, 1977)

Step 1. Identify an area of interest

You are eminently qualified to identify problems in practice because your practice places you on the "front line," where you are the expert concerning problems in the process or outcome of services to clients. Even if you are not going to personally conduct the proposed research, your input is vital to those who will. Also, do not rule out conducting small studies by yourself or with the help of colleagues. Even for a small study, a consultant may be very helpful.

Step 2. Review the literature to formulate a problem statement based on theory and research

To identify relevant literature for review, computerized bibliographic searches are great time-savers. Contact a local professional library for assistance, and request printouts that provide an abstract for each article. The librarian will be able to assist in identifying the "key words" to use for your computer search. Read each abstract and select those that appear to be relevant to the problem under study. Obtain those articles (and I like to have my own photocopies of each), and read them to determine which ones are relevant. Now you are ready to conduct your analytic review of the literature. It is useful to have a set of criteria for evaluating each of the published research studies and to prepare a summary of the evaluations. Criteria for evaluating research are shown in Table 15-2. A form to use in summarizing studies (that includes an example of its use) is provided in Table 15-3. Even if you never progress to the next steps in the research process, this step will give you valuable information for practice purposes.

Here are two thoughts that may provide some reassurance as you begin your work.

1. Don't forget that your background as a practitioner enables you to contrast the research designs, findings, and implications against your knowledge of the practice setting—the real world—and that is a very valuable evaluation.
2. If statistical formulas and techniques seem like Greek to you (pun intended), focus attention on design, method, and interpretation of results. If it becomes crucial to your project, you can seek others' evaluation of the statistics used.

After completing most of the information in Tables 15-2 and 15-3, you may want to consult an experienced researcher to validate your conclusions and to make plans for steps 3 through 12 of the research process, which were outlined in Chapter 2. How do you obtain such a consultant? If your agency does not employ a nurse researcher, the faculty of the local school of nursing is the best resource. From informal networks, you can obtain information about the research interests of doctorally prepared faculty. Call and talk with those who have interests relevant to your topic and explore their availability to assist you. You might be wondering why they would want to help you, if you do not have money to hire them. The reward system for faculty places highest priority on conducting research and publishing results (Young-Graham, 1986). Faculty researchers need access to clinical settings and to the perspective offered by staff nurses. Therefore, you do have something to offer. If you are willing to work out an agreement to collaborate, it can be a "win–win" situation for each of you.

From the beginning, be sure to clearly specify your plan for collaboration. Clearly spell out in writing, in advance, who will own the data, the plan for publishing the results, and the roles that you and your collaborator will fill in the project. As you develop the project, will outside funding be necessary? If so, then agree on the way that each of you will contribute to the preparation of the grant proposal, the operation of the project, and the authority for expenditure of funds. (It is possible to have one principal investigator with one or more co-investigators, or to be co-principal investigators.)

The remainder of the research steps (3 through 12) are described and applied in Chapter 2. It is useful to consult with a researcher as needed throughout all of the steps. The extent of involvement between you and the consultant will be determined by the size and scope of the study, the confidence you feel with regard to your ability to perform the steps, and the resources available—both your personal time and the access to consultants.

TIME OUT: Some questions to ask before accepting a community health nursing position

- Are research findings considered to be of value?
- Is there support for implementing research findings into practice?
- Is assistance provided to help the nurse to keep up to date?
- What are the expectations about conducting research?
- Is research built into the workload?
- Is consultation available?
- Is financial support available?

If you decide that this is not the time for you to initiate your own project, there are other ways you can contribute to the conduct of nursing research.

TABLE 15-2.   CRITERIA FOR EVALUATION
OF RESEARCH REPORTS

Criteria	Questions to ask in evaluating research reports
The problem	Is it clearly stated, significant, relevant? Is the research question one that can be answered through an empirical study?
Review of literature	Does the literature directly relate to the problem? Are the references current? Are the previous studies critically analyzed? Are the implications for this study clearly stated?
Conceptual framework	If a theoretical or conceptual framework is used, does it fit the problem?
Hypotheses, or research questions	Are these clearly stated, logical? Are they congruent with the framework used and with the review of the literature? Are they measurable?
Subjects	Are the population and/or sample clearly identified and described? Are the means of obtaining the subjects clearly stated? Are the population and/or sample appropriate in terms of size and characteristics? Is the response rate adequate?
Data collection	Are the data collection methods appropriate to the purpose of the study? Are the instruments clearly described, including their source, reliability and validity? (If you are interested in comprehensively evaluating questionnaires, review Babbie (1973) and Selltiz, Wrightsman, and Cook (1976) for guidelines for constructing questionnaires.)
Research design	Is the design appropriate to the purposes of the study? (Review Chapters 2 and 10 regarding potential designs.) Is the design appropriately executed?
Data analysis	Is the process adequately described? Is the type of analysis appropriate for the types of data collected? Are results of both descriptive and inferential statistics appropriately presented? Are results clearly presented and related to the study's research questions?
Interpretation of the findings	Is each result discussed in terms of study's hypotheses/research questions and the literature review? Are alternative explanations for the findings discussed?

(continued)

TABLE 15-2. (Continued)

Criteria	Questions to ask in evaluating research reports
	Are limitations of the study clearly described? Is the discussion sufficiently tentative and unbiased? Is the distinction made between practical and statistical significance?
Implications	Are the implications discussed in terms of the research questions, the conceptual framework, and their relevance for practice? Are the implications appropriate with consideration of the study's limitations and generalizability?
Recommendations	Are recommendations made for improving the study and for future studies? Are recommendations for nursing actions congruent with the study's findings?

(Adapted from Polit DF, Hungler BP: Nursing Research: Principles and Methods, pp 581–592. Philadelphia, JB Lippincott, 1983)

One way is through providing morale and "go-for" support for projects in your agency. Another way is to take advantage of opportunities to serve as a data collector. You will be trained for your task and will learn more about research through your exposure to the entire project. Acting as a data coder for a project can also provide good experiential learning. Thus, there are a number of options for the nurse who values research and wants to contribute to the conduct of research in the field.

SUMMARY

There is a very great need for nursing research to ensure the success, recognition, and perhaps even the survival of the profession. Community health nursing, because of its reliance on public funds, may have an even greater need to document its effectiveness than do other nursing specialties whose costs are hidden in room charges. Providing quality care to our client, the community, requires a research base. Some of that research base presently exists, but is not being used. The problems involved in disseminating and utilizing research findings can be at least partially ameliorated by staff nurses who are committed to continued learning. Much of the research base for community health nursing practice is still to be developed. If we are to provide quality care:

TABLE 15-3. FORM FOR SUMMARIZING RESEARCH STUDIES

Summary of Research Findings
Topic: Home Visits to Maternal-Infants

Study (citation)	Subjects (*n*, sampling)	Aims, hypotheses or questions	Interventions	Measures	Results	Comments
Hall, Nursing Research 29(5): 317–321, 1980	*n* = 30 normal deliveries from community hospital. Random assignment to: Experi = 15 Control = 15 Age 18–30, Married Primip Uncomplicated vaginal delivery	Does structured informative at-home nursing intervention concerning infant behavior affect primiparas' perceptions of their newborns?	*Experi:* Structured informative nursing intervention. A standard teaching plan with specific goals through home visit 2–4 days post discharge *Control:* Testing only	Broussard's Neonatal Perception Inventories I and II Time 1: 1–2 days P.P. hospital Time 2: 1 mo after delivery	1) NPI scores higher for Expe. group at Time 2 than at Time 1 and higher than Con. group's 2) Expe. group had lower expectations of baby and higher perceptions of baby and higher perceptions of own 3) At 1 mo visit, comments similar by both Expe. and Con. groups 4) Other nonquantifiable observations shared—Expe. —"seemed more assured."	1 person was both investi. and intervener. Not blind study. No control for investi. bias. Relatively small sample. Would have been better to formalize collection of "subjective observations" to attempt to make more objective

1. Staff nurses will need to be more knowledgeable regarding research findings relevant to their practice.
2. Staff nurses will need to be more involved in generating knowledge through participation in research projects.

Your involvement is essential as community health nursing moves to document the effectiveness of its services and to provide a research base for its practice.

REFERENCES

American Nurses' Association Commission on Nursing Research: Guidelines for the Investigative Function of Nurses, p 2. Kansas City, Missouri, American Nurses' Association, 1981(a)

American Nurses' Association Commission on Nursing Research: Research Priorities for the 1980's: Generating a Scientific Basis for Nursing Practice. Kansas City, Missouri, American Nurses' Association, 1981(b)

Babbie ER: Survey research methods. Belmont, CA: Wadsworth Publishing Co., 1973

Barkauskas VH: Public health nursing practice: An educator's view. Nursing Out 30:384–389, 1982

Bloch D: Evaluation of nursing care in terms of process and outcome: Issues in research and quality assurance. Nurs Res 24:256–263, 1975

Butler PWM: Hospital embedding—diffusion mechanisms and nurses' knowledge of an innovation. Dissertation Abstracts International (University Microfilms No. 86-21256) 47(6):2368B, 1986

Couser S, Daly G, Grisham J, Rieder B: Health in the balance. Nurs Out 34:25–27, 1986

CURN Project: Mutual Goal Setting in Patient Care. New York, Grune & Stratton, 1982

CURN Project: Using Research to Improve Nursing Practice: A Guide, p 2. New York, Grune & Stratton, 1983

Fagin CM: Nursing's pivotal role in American health care. In Aiken LH (ed): Nursing in the 1980's: Crises, Opportunities, Challenges, pp 459–473. Philadelphia, American Academy of Nursing/JB Lippincott Co, 1982

Flynn BC: Research framework for evaluating community health nursing practice. In Miller MH, Flynn BC (eds): Current Perspectives in Nursing: Social Issues and Trends, pp 35–45. St. Louis, CV Mosby, 1977

Highriter ME: The status of community health nursing research. Nurs Res 29(3):183–192, 1977

Highriter ME: Public health nursing evaluation, education, and professional issues: 1977–1981. Ann Rev Nurs Res 2:165–189, 1984

Hilbert H: Abstracts of studies in public health nursing (1924–1957). Nurs Res 8(2):42–115, 1959

Ketefian S: A diffusion survey of coronary precautions. Nurs Res 31:196–201, 1975

Kirchoff KT: A diffusion survey of coronary precautions. Nurs Res 31:196–201, 1982

Krueger JC: Using research in practice: A survey of research utilization in community health nursing. West J Nurs Res 4(2):244–248, 1982

Lindeman CA: Priorities in clinical nursing research. Nurs Out 23(11):693–698, 1975

Lysaught JP (ed): An Abstract for Action, p 84. New York, National Commission for the Study of Nursing and Nursing Education/McGraw-Hill, 1970

Notter LE: Essentials of Nursing Research. New York, Springer, 1974

Polit DF, Hungler BP: Nursing Research: Principles and Methods, 2nd ed. Philadelphia, JB Lippincott Co, 1983

Schlotfeldt RM: Reflections on nursing research. Amer J Nurs 60:492–494, 1960

Selltiz C, Wrightsman LS, Cook SW: Research methods in social relations (3rd ed.). New York, Holt, Rinehart and Winston, 1976

Young-Graham K: Narrowing the reward gap between research and practice. Public Health Nurs 3(4):213–214, 1986

SUGGESTED READINGS

Carpenter RG, Gardner A, Jepson M, et al: Prevention of unexpected infant death. Lancet 1(8327):723–727, 1983

Fawcett J: Utilization of nursing research findings. Image: The Journal of Nursing Scholarship 14(2):57–59, 1982

Hall LA: Effect of teaching on primiparous' perception of their newborn. Nurs Res 29(5):317–321, 1980

Haller KB, Reynolds MA, Horsley JA: Developing research based innovation protocols: Process, criteria, and issues. Res Nurs and Health 2:45–51, 1979

Horsley JA, Crane J, Bingle JD: Research utilization as an organizational process. J Nurs Admin 8(7):4–6, 1978

Kelly M: Will mothers breast feed longer if health visitors given them more support? Health Visitor 56:407–409, 1983

Krueger JC: Utilization of nursing research: The planning process. J Nurs Admin 7:6–9, 1978

Krueger JC: Research utilization: What is it? Real or superficial dissemination. West J Nurs Res 1(1):72–75, 1979

Krueger JC: Using research in practice: A survey of research utilization in community health nursing. West J Nurs Res 4(2):244–248, 1982

Loomis ME: Knowledge utilization and research utilization in nursing. Image: The Journal of Nursing Scholarship 17(2):35–39, 1985

Oiler C: The phenomenological approach in nursing research. Nurs Res 31:178–181, 1982

Olds DL, Henderson CR Jr, Tatelbaum R, Chamberlin R: Improving the delivery of prenatal care and outcomes of pregnancy: A randomized trial of nurse home visitation. Pediatrics 77(1):16–28, 1986

Stanwick RS, Moffat MEK, Robitaille Y et al: An evaluation of the routine postnatal public health nurse home visit. Canadian J Public Health 73:200–205, 1982

Stetler CB: Research utilization: Defining the concept. Image: The Journal of Nursing Scholarship 17(2):40–44, 1983

Swanson JM, Chenitz WC: Why qualitative research in nursing? Nurs Outlook 30:241–245, 1982

Treece EW, Treece JW: Elements of Research in Nursing. St. Louis, CV Mosby, 1982

16

Issues and Opportunities for Practice

OBJECTIVES

The focus of this chapter is on the current trends in health care and the major issues that affect community health nursing. The ways in which the profession is responding to these issues and what you as an individual nurse can do will also be addressed. After studying this chapter, you should be able to

- Describe major trends and issues that affect health care
- Describe the community health nursing's involvement in issues that affect health care
- Determine relevant sources of information about these issues
- Begin active participation in professional organizations in order to address issues of concern to community health nursing

INTRODUCTION

Almost 100 years ago Lillian Wald introduced the term *public health nursing* to emphasize that "the nurse's peculiar introduction to the patient and her organic relationship with the neighborhood should constitute the starting point for a universal service to the region" (Wald, 1941). Wald's development of the historic Henry Street Settlement was in response to needs that she saw on the lower East Side of New York City.

This book has provided you with tools and examples to use when applying the nursing process in a community-as-client situation. These are the essentials of your practice in the community, but looking at the field in general, in what direction is health care moving? Where will the community health nurse fit in? How can you keep abreast of changes and influence their direction in a positive way as Wald did when she recognized that work for social betterment is an appropriate role for nursing?

TRENDS AND ISSUES

The United States is in the midst of a revolution in health care; in its financing, in the way it is delivered, and in who assumes "responsibility" for the country's health. The major issues confronting us as a concomitant to this revolution were summed up by Joseph A. Califano, former Secretary of Health, Education and Welfare.

> *Science serves up biomedical breakthroughs that hold the promise of miraculous cures and the threat of unacceptable costs. The aging of the population—in the first quarter of the next century 60 million Americans will be over 65—signals the dawn of a four-generation society, in which it will be common to have two generations of the same family in retirement, on Medicare, receiving Social Security and nursing care (Califano, 1986).*

Aging Population

The *graying of America* is one of the major population trends that is affecting health care, and it will continue to have an effect well into the next century. By the year 2030, it has been predicted that the proportion of older people in the population will have reached 20%. As this group grows, so will the need for long-term care and also there will be increasing need for innovative health promotion programs that are aimed at the over-65-year-old. Concern will continue on issues such as how to plan for retirement and how not to lose the experience and wisdom of the older population.

At the same time that the population ages, there will be a decrease in the group between the ages of 18 and 25. Therefore, there will be increasing needs in the field of health care and a decreasing pool of young workers to address those needs. There is an increasing shortage of nurses in critical areas, and projected needs for community health nurses are for many times the number of professionals who are available. There is a chronic shortage of nurses prepared in the care of the elderly, whether they are in institutions or in the community.

Consider, too, that the nursing population, as a "sample" of the general population, is aging also. Most of us will work longer than have former generations, and with this "graying of nursing" the benefits of our deeper, richer experience will become available to consumers.

New High-risk Groups

Traditional high-risk groups with which public health professionals have been concerned (pregnant teens, and persons with hypertension for example) are being joined by other diverse, at-risk aggregates. Examples of high-risk groups with unique health care needs are the Southeast Asian refugees, the homeless, runaway youngsters, and the growing population of chronically underfed people. *Can you think of others in the community who might be identified as having special needs?* Recall examples of community health practice from Chapter 12 that described the practice role. The challenge of providing adequate, accessible, and acceptable health care to these groups is one that community health nurses welcome. It may be a major way for us to demonstrate our strengths and capabilities.

Cost Containment

Another area of interest and concern for community health nurses revolves around the cost of care: who will pay for it, and how to deliver services that are cost efficient and effective. Currently, reimbursement mechanisms are controling the types of services that are being made available in the health care industry. Prospective payment systems are forcing shorter hospital stays (they pay a set amount for each diagnostic category) so that patients are sent home "quicker and sicker." Home health care has become a "boom" field and has expanded to include highly technical care that was previously only available on an inpatient basis.

At the same time that funding sources (insurers, Medicare) are being focused on cost containment, the number of persons without any form of insurance is rising. When workers become unemployed, they lose their job benefits, as well as income. Often this affects a whole family if there is one wage earner and the other family members were covered under that person's insurance.

Nursing's philosophy that health care is a right rather than a privilege and that care should be continuous and comprehensive must be scrutinized in light of concerns about cost. One nursing leader warns that nursing's "belief in comprehensive care may be a real threat to the survival of nursing in its present form" (Stevens, 1985).

The challenge to all of nursing is clear: demonstrate that nursing not only makes a difference in the health of clients, but also that it does this in a cost-effective way. This has been well demonstrated in the use of nurse practitioners to deliver primary health care, but much more research is needed.

Self-care and Prevention

Technology of the past ten years (and more) has developed at such an accelerated rate that premature infants weighing less than a pound can not only be kept alive, but can grow and develop to become healthy people. Human transplant programs routinely extend people's lives for months and years. However, a concomitant development of ethical guidelines or processes to assist people in making decisions about the use of the technology has *not* occurred.

At the same time that the complex, life-saving technology was being developed, it was also discovered that the vast majority of health problems could be appreciably diminished or prevented altogether by *self-care,* guided by the assumption of a sense of *self-responsibility* for personal behavior. Joseph Califano put it succinctly when he reported that "smoking has killed and maimed more Americans than all our wars and automobile accidents combined" (Califano, 1986). (Recall the chapter on the role of the community health nurse educator and the models that can be used to affect health behavior.)

The concepts of self-care and health promotion have been part of nursing since the days of Florence Nightingale. Indeed, a focus on the client doing for himself and concomitant emphasis on health versus disease are two of the unique features of community health nursing—of all of nursing, some would say.

Nursing has a grand opportunity to demonstrate its concern for self-care and to contribute to health promotion through the National Center for Nursing Research (NCNR) in the National Institutes of Health (NIH). Authorized after a two-year struggle, the NCNR will move nursing research into the mainstream of scientific research and should add a focus on health to what now might be more correctly referred to as the "National Institutes of Disease."

Expectations for the NCNR were summarized by the National League for Nursing (NLN) (1986)

As the focal point of the nation's nursing research activities, the center will encourage high quality nursing research, provide leadership to expand the pool of experienced nurse researchers, and serve as a base for interaction with other areas of health care research.

Findings from research conducted at the center should help nurses add to the scientific basis for nursing interventions. The center will also play a pivotal role in conveying the importance of nursing research to the consumer. Nursing's contributions to treating chronic illness and to the psychosocial dimensions of health care, as well as the proven cost-effectiveness of nursing practice, can be publicly demonstrated and promoted through the visible new center.

Scope of Practice and Education

The scope of public health nursing continues to expand and diversify. Practice in the community encompasses virtually all of nursing practice. Significant changes include the expanded roles (*e.g.,* nurse practitioners), and the rapid expansion of home health services. Previously described measures for cost containment and concerns for the aging population have created new challenges and opportunities for community-based nursing practice.

EXAMPLE: Consider the trends and issues that have been discussed and how practice reflects these changes. For instance, nurses who work with Southeast Asian refugees must learn about a culture that is new and different to them and they must be open and willing to change their usual way to approach problems.

In 1980 two publications set the stage for defining the scope of practice in the community: The Public Health Nursing Section of the American Public Health Association (APHA, 1980) and the American Nurses' Association (ANA, 1980). Each organization independently published a document that described the role of the public health/community health nurse. (The two documents are summarized in Chapter 5, Nursing Models). A third document, *Nursing: A Social Policy Statement* (ANA, 1980), delineated the nature and scope of all of nursing practice. It was in the social policy statement that nursing was succinctly defined as "the diagnosis and treatment of human responses to actual or potential health problems." Nursing was described as a segment of the health care system with four defining characteristics: boundary, intersections,

COMMUNITY-FOCUSED FUNCTIONS

ASSESSMENT

1. Identifies pertinent information about community.
2. Gathers descriptive data about the community.
3. Assesses health-related learning needs of populations.
4. Participates in identifying community health states and health behaviors, including the knowledge, attitudes, and perceptions of groups regarding health and illness.
5. Collects pertinent information about community in a systematic way.
6. Aids in community health surveys.
7. Includes members of the community as partners in the assessment process.
8. Uses basic statistics and demographic methods to collect health data.
9. Collaborates with other health care providers to assess the community.
10. Consults with community leaders to describe the community.

ANALYSIS

11. Identifies common and recurrent health problems that have potential for illness consequences.
12. Identifies health needs of help-seeking and nonseeking populations.
13. Describes health capability of community based on assessment.
14. Applies selected epidemiologic concepts in analyzing assessment data (population-at-risk, incidence, prevalence, for instance).
15. Describes present community health problems in the perspective of time (recognizes trends).

16. Describes and analyzes resources available including patterns of utilization.
17. Analyzes data for relationships and clues to the community's health.
18. Aids/participates in analysis of community health data base.
19. Forms ideas and hypotheses concerning data gathered in community assessment to derive inferences for nursing programs.
20. Includes members of the community in analyzing assessment data.

PLANNING

21. Assists in developing plans to meet needs arising from gaps or deficiencies identified.
22. Develops service priorities and plans for intervention based on analysis, community expectations and accepted practice standards.
23. Participates in planning community health programs.
24. Determines priorities for community health care based on information gathered during assessment.
25. Participates with community leaders in planning to meet identified health needs.
26. Participates with others in developing health plans applicable to the community at large.
27. Develops service objectives of identified community problems.
28. Uses knowledge of change process in planning community programs.
29. Plans for communitywide or age-specific screening programs.
30. Includes members of the community as partners in planning community health programs.

(continued)

COMMUNITY-FOCUSED FUNCTIONS (Continued)

IMPLEMENTATION

31. Mobilizes the community's collective resources to help achieve higher community health goals.

32. Functions as a health advocate for the community.

33. Serves as vital link in the communication network between all kinds of community agencies and clients.

34. Seeks opportunities to participate with other disciplines in projects to bring about changes in the availability, accessibility, and accountability of health care and related systems.

35. Sets up immunization campaigns with community leaders and public health officials.

36. Initiates and monitors disease prevention programs in the community.

37. Educates the community through media regarding health issues.

38. Organizes community groups to work on alleviating community health problems.

39. Acts as a catalyst/potentiator for community change.

40. Sets up ongoing community health educa-

tion programs with community leaders and public health officials.

EVALUATION

41. Monitors health services for desired quality.

42. Continually validates appropriateness of public health programs (discusses with residents, collects more data, for example).

43. Contributes information for use in evaluation of nursing programs.

44. Evaluates community response to nursing intervention.

45. Ensures necessary community health program evaluation data are collected accurately and systematically.

46. Analyzes results of service in relation to proportion of population served.

47. Promotes systematic evaluation of community resources.

48. Evaluates the impact of nursing activities on the health of the community as a whole.

49. Includes members of the community as partners in evaluating health programs.

50. Analyzes results of service in relation to whether community program objectives were reached.

© 1981, E. Anderson

(Anderson ET: Community focus in public health nursing: Whose responsibility? Nurs Out 31:46, 1983)

dimensions, and core. (Consider how these characteristics parallel aspects of the Community-as-Client Model).

Having three documents that addressed the role and scope of practice— two specifically for the community health nurse—and each with a slightly different focus—created further confusion rather than clarification. In addition, the nurses who responded to one survey of community health nurses indicated that while some agreement existed on functions of the nurse (Anderson, 1983), there was no clear statement of educational preparation needed or how various levels of practitioner were defined. (See the displayed material for a list of the generally recognized functions.)

An invitational conference, "Essentials of Public Health Nursing Practice and Education" (Anderson *et al*, 1985) was held to address the critical issues summarized above. Representatives from the American Nurses' Association (ANA), NLN, the Association of State and Territorial Directors of Nursing (ASTDN), the Association of Graduate Faculty in Community Health/Public Health Nursing (AGFCH/PHN) and the Public Health Nursing Section of the American Public Health Association (APHA) together with staff of the Division of Nursing, Department of Health and Human Services, were included in this division-funded, APHA-sponsored conference. The representatives from these groups included educators, practicing public health nurses, and administrators from the practice and education arenas, and from both rural and urban areas.

Along with identification of critical issues, the outcome of the "consensus conference" was a general agreement on educational preparation: to practice as a *generalist* in public health nursing, a baccalaureate degree is needed; and to practice as a *specialist,* a master's degree is necessary. Consensus was also reached on specific definitions and areas of content for each of the levels of practice. These are summarized in the displayed material, *Areas of Consensus in PHN Practice.*

A consensus was reached on the definitions of the terms public health nurse and community health nurse. The public health nurse is a nurse "who has received specific educational preparation in public health nursing . . . [and has a baccalaureate degree] so that she has the initial qualifications to practice in an official public health agency" (Anderson 1985). The community health nurse was defined as a nurse who works in the community, so that the practice is defined by the setting, a limited "definition."

Recommendations of the consensus conference have been widely disseminated and surveys of nursing directors in public health (ASTDN members), graduate educators (AGFCH/PHN members), and undergraduate educators (attendees at the Tenth Annual Public Health Nursing Conference sponsored by the School of Public Health at the University of North Carolina at Chapel Hill) indicate general agreement with the levels and content. In addition, the creation of the guideline, *Standards of Community Health Nursing Practice* (see the displayed material), provide tangible affirmation of agreement.

The *Standards* use the terms public health nursing and community health

AREAS OF CONSENSUS IN PUBLIC HEALTH NURSING PRACTICE

	Generalist	*Specialist*
Education	Baccalaureate degree	Master's degree
Focus	Individuals/families/groups in the community who are in need of nursing care or at-risk of a health problem	Aggregates/population groups
Function	Service to individuals/families/groups Gather data to identify aggregates-at-risk	Assess and intervene at the aggregate level (apply the nursing process)
Preparation needed	Defined block of time to practice applying public health theory in the community Clinical experiences in community-based agencies serving a broad range of clients	Socialization through experiential learning in master's program Faculty with doctoral preparation that includes both public health and nursing

Content	(Assumes prior content and experience in maternal–child health, including prenatal care; assessment and gerontology with accompanying experiences outside the hospital)
	  Transcultural nursing
	  Emphasis on prevention
	  Introduction to epidemiology and biostatistics
	  Research
	  High-risk groups
	  Health care system and regulation
	  Politics
		Epidemiology
		  Biostatistics
		  Community assessment
		  Nursing theory
		  Program planning and evaluation
		  Management
		  Economics
		  Politics
		  Interventions at aggregate level
		  Social and community change
		  History of public health
		  Issues

(Anderson ET, Meyer AT: Consensus conference on the essentials of public health nursing practice and education. Report of the Conference, September 5–7, 1984, Maryland, Division of Nursing, US Department of Health and Human Services, 1985)

STANDARDS OF COMMUNITY HEALTH NURSING PRACTICE

Standard I. *Theory*
   The nurse applies theoretical concepts as a basis for decisions in practice.
Standard II. *Data Collection*
   The nurse systematically collects data that are comprehensive and accurate.
Standard III. *Diagnosis*
   The nurse analyzes data collected about the community, family, and individual to determine diagnoses.
Standard IV. *Planning*
   At each level of prevention, the nurse develops plans that specify nursing actions unique to client needs.
Standard V. *Intervention*
   The nurse, guided by the plan, intervenes to promote, maintain, or restore health; to prevent illness; and to effect rehabilitation.
Standard VI. *Evaluation*
   The nurse evaluates responses of the community, family, and individual to interventions in order to determine progress toward goal achievement and to revise the data base, diagnoses, and plan.
Standard VII. *Quality Assurance and Professional Development*
   The nurse participates in peer review and other means of evaluation to assure quality of nursing practice. The nurse assumes responsibility for professional development and contributes to the professional growth of others.
Standard VIII. *Interdisciplinary Collaboration*
   The nurse collaborates with other health care providers, professionals, and community representatives in assessing, planning, implementing, and evaluating programs for community health.
Standard IX. *Research*
   The nurse contributes to theory and practice in community health nursing through research.

(American Nurses' Association: Standards of Community Health Nursing Practice. Kansas City, Missouri, American Nurses' Association, 1986)

nursing synonymously, but agree with the generalist–specialist levels. A preliminary diagram of community health nursing roles is presented in Figure 16-1 and is an attempt to illustrate the relationship of the various definitions. Note that community health nurse is used as an ''umbrella'' term and that it encompasses all of those below it. Perhaps there are others that belong under community health nursing. Can you think of any?

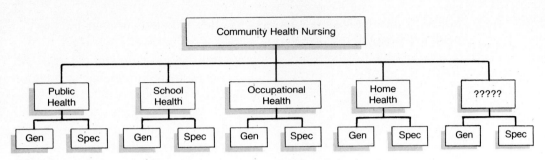

Figure 16-1. The "umbrella" of Community Health Nursing.

THE FUTURE

The consensus conference acted as both a catalyst and as a synthesizer. As a catalyst the findings sparked lively discussion of the issues and recommendations. As a synthesizer it brought together persons with diverse backgrounds and views and facilitated the achievement of some agreement on the issues, definitions, and the directions in which the field is headed. The agenda for the future that was proposed by the consensus conference group forms a base from which to propose strategies for the future. You may use them to guide your career planning. Note how these strategies address the major issues identified earlier in the chapter.

Demonstrate Accountability

Adapt marketing techniques to gain support for nursing services needed in the community. Use facts and figures to back up your demands. Understand the importance of cost containment and include cost-benefit information in any proposal that you promote. Take the initiative in showing how nursing services are cost effective. Participate in research that will document the cost effectiveness of care.

Strengthen Education for Practice

There is a shortage of baccalaureate-prepared nurses to fill staff-level positions in public health agencies. Efforts to facilitate the new graduate moving into these positions will need to be accelerated. The truism that a year of "med-surg" will prepare nurses to work in public health is being seriously questioned by nursing leaders. Innovative models in both education and practice need to be explored.

Certification of both the generalist and the specialist through the ANA should be supported. As you accrue the necessary requirements (in addition to the degree requirement, a certain amount of practice is mandatory), plan to acquire certification. The National Council Licensing Exam ("state boards") measures minimum competency levels to practice safe nursing care—certification is additional documentation that you are knowledgeable and proficient in a special area. Beyond initial certification is advanced certification at the master's level. The advanced certification examination for the community health nurse specialist is expected to be completed in 1989.

Meet Increased Demand for Community Nursing Services

The aging population and other high-risk groups, such as persons with Acquired Immune Deficiency Syndrome (AIDS), will place increasing demands for community nursing services. Planning for effective use of scarce nursing resources will test the skills of nursing administrators, who will need to be adept at dealing with rapid change. These administrators will need to develop skills in dealing not only with a changing population of clients, but in supervising older workers. It will be an opportunity to use their expertise, and to learn from the experience that older workers bring to the job.

Being computer literate is already a prerequisite for most health care positions. Nurses will be called upon increasingly to assist in decisions that have ethical and legal ramifications. With much of sickness care moving into the community, community health nurses will be expected to advise consumers about such diverse topics as living wills and decisions about death with dignity.

Become knowledgeable about the legal and ethical concerns of practice. Attend mock trials and professional conferences sponsored by the district nurses' association or your local Sigma Theta Tau chapter. If possible, attend hearings of your State Board of Nurse Examiners. Keep abreast of current legal and ethical issues by reading professional journals, attend ethics "rounds" if available, and read outside of the nursing literature as well, so that you broaden the base of information from which you must make decisions.

Support Health Promotion

As a national priority health promotion and disease prevention is more talk than substance. To increase support for these activities, decision makers at all levels need to become oriented to the importance of health promotion and disease prevention. Community health nurses as "health promoters" are in an excellent position to affect policy decisions. Many of the strategies that have already been covered need to be used to promote health. In particular, being informed and informing others (consumers, legislators) are keys to affecting policy decisions.

Nurses have played an important role in many health promotion decisions. They have testified at local, state, and national hearings on the importance of prenatal care; they have influenced legislation on smoking in the workplace and on mandating use of child restraints in automobiles. And through innumerable calls, letters and other forms of contact nurses are affecting policy decisions daily.

Become an active health promoter through local organizations such as the American Lung Association and by personally epitomizing what you "preach." Strive to be a role model for health. If you need help, such as weight reduction or smoking control, don't be afraid to ask—there is a nurse who can assist you.

Strengthen Practice

Promote community health nursing. Educate consumers, lawmakers, and the media about the value of community health nursing. Take advantage of every opportunity to speak to groups, whether they be church groups or neighborhood committees, about health issues and nursing's concern. (It is all right to think of this as speaking for *one* nurse—*you*—so that you won't be intimidated by the idea of being an official spokesperson for nursing.) Initiate discussion of current events and issues with colleagues, business acquaintances, and others. Be articulate and conversant about the health and health care (especially nursing) implications of these events.

Become actively involved as a "consumer" in your own community. Begin by volunteering for a committee in an organization you support (or would like to know more about) such as the Parent Teacher's Organization (PTO), the American Lung Association, the March of Dimes, or Chamber of Commerce. Show that you can do more than attend meetings by volunteering for a specific task and then follow through with it.

Join your professional organization. Be an active, contributing member of your local district nurses' association. Serving on the governmental affairs or legislative committee is an excellent way to learn what is happening in your community and also contribute in a positive manner to promote the profession.

Be a good citizen. This may sound like advice from a ninth grade civics class, but it is probably one of the major methods through which community health nursing can be strengthened and promoted. Vote, write letters, voice an informed opinion, be politically aware and active at all levels, and advocate for the health of your community. It is only through individual commitment to the tenet, "Health for all," that collectively we can reach this goal.

REFERENCES

American Nurses' Association: A Conceptual Model of Community Health Nursing, p 9. Kansas City, Missouri, American Nurses' Association, 1980

American Nurses' Association: Nursing: A Social Policy Statement. Kansas City, Missouri, American Nurses' Association, 1980

American Nurses' Association: Guide to Community-based Nursing Services. Kansas City, Missouri, American Nurses' Association, 1985

American Nurses' Association: Standards of Community Health Nursing Practice. Kansas City, Missouri, American Nurses' Association, 1986

American Public Health Association: The Definition and Role of Public Health Nursing in the Delivery of Health Care. Washington, DC, American Public Health Association, 1980

Anderson ET: Community focus in public health nursing: Whose responsibility? Nurs Out 31:44–48, 1983

Anderson ET, Meyer AT: Consensus conference on the essentials of public health nursing practice and education. Report of the Conference, September 5–7, 1984. Maryland, Division of Nursing, U.S. Department of Health and Human Services, 1985

Califano JA: A revolution looms in American health. New York Times, March 25, 1986

National League for Nursing: The League's 1986 legislative agenda. Public Policy Bulletin 4(4):1–4, 1986

Stevens BJ: Tackling a changing society head on. Nurs & Health Care 6(1):27–30, 1985

Wald L: Foreword. In Wales M (ed): The Public Health Nurse in Action. New York, Macmillan, 1941

Index

Page numbers in *italics* indicate illustrations; those followed by t indicate tables.

during immediate post-
war years, 354–357
patterns of change in,
368–370
during World War II,
352–354
Public health services. *See also*
Community health
program; Health care
services
in community assessment,
187–189, 193t
analysis of, 249–251, 252–
253t
Public policy, 102
Public transportation, in community assessment,
221

Qualitative research, 446
Quantitative research, 446
Quasi-experimental research,
56, *59*
Questionnaire
survey, 321
for validation of nursing diagnosis, 281–285,
285–287t

Radiation, as pollutant, 129
Rail service, in community assessment, 222
Randomization, 55
Rate(s)
adjusted, 24–25
calculation of, 21, 23t
calendar year, limitations
of, 22–24
commonly used, 22, 23t
in community health assessment, 21–22
crude, 24

defined, 20–21
vs. proportion, 22
specific, 24
Ratio level of measurement, 54
Recreation, in community assessment, 232–234,
233t
analysis of, 266
Refreezing, 104, 279–280, 279t
Reinkemeyer's stages of
planned change, 278–
279, 279t
Relative risk, 25–26
of homicide, 26
and odds ratio, 27–29, 29t
Reliability, 66–68
coefficients of, 68
as correlation coefficient, 66
defined, 44, 66
and equivalence, 67
and internal consistency, 68
inter-observer, 44
inter-rater, 67
and internal consistency, 68
intra-observer, 44
intra-rater, 67
measurement of, methods
of, 66–68, 70–71, 72t
parallel forms, 67
as percentage of agreement,
66
sample specificity of, 66
of screening tests, 44–45
and stability, 67–68
test-retest, 67
Religion, in community assessment, 175–176
Research
defined, 16, 437–438
epidemiologic approaches
to, 35–42
ethical issues in, 55–56
experimental, 55–56, *59*
framework for, 445–446

history of, in community
health nursing, 438–
439
nonexperimental, 56–60, *59*
priorities for, 443–445
prospective, 20, 57–60
purposes of, 47–48, 48t
qualitative, 446
quantitative, 446
quasi-experimental, 56, *59*
and research/Research di-
chotomy, 445
retrospective, 20, 57, 58–60
subjects of, protection of,
64, 84
utilization of, 439–442
Research design, selection of,
55–60, *59*
Research process, 16, 47–88
communication of results of,
85–88
community health nurse's
role in, 380–382
conductor role in, 443–451
consumer role in, 439–442
focus of, 48
formulation of problem
statement in, 50–52,
448–449
formulation of research
questions or hypoth-
esis in, 52–53
identification of area of interest in, 49–50, 448
implementation of method-
ology in, 85–88
initiation of, 446–451
interpretation of results of,
85–88
limitations of, 81–84
literature review in, 50–52,
448–449
evaluation criteria for,
450–451t
summarization form for,
452t